Series in BioEngineering

The Series in Bioengineering serves as an information source for a professional audience in science and technology as well as for advanced students. It covers all applications of the physical sciences and technology to medicine and the life sciences. Its scope ranges from bioengineering, biomedical and clinical engineering to biophysics, biomechanics, biomaterials, and bioinformatics.

More information about this series at http://www.springer.com/series/10358

Regina Padmanabhan · Nader Meskin ·
Ala-Eddin Al Moustafa

Mathematical Models of Cancer and Different Therapies

Unified Framework

Springer

Regina Padmanabhan
Electrical Engineering Department,
College of Engineering
Qatar University
Doha, Qatar

Nader Meskin
Electrical Engineering Department,
College of Engineering
Qatar University
Doha, Qatar

Ala-Eddin Al Moustafa
Medical Basic Science Department,
College of Medicine
Qatar University
Doha, Qatar

ISSN 2196-8861 ISSN 2196-887X (electronic)
Series in BioEngineering
ISBN 978-981-15-8642-2 ISBN 978-981-15-8640-8 (eBook)
https://doi.org/10.1007/978-981-15-8640-8

This Springer imprint is published by the registered company Springer Nature Singapore Pte Ltd.
The registered company address is: 152 Beach Road, #21-01/04 Gateway East, Singapore 189721, Singapore

"Much is known but unfortunately in different heads"

—(Werner Kollath, A German scientist, 1892–1970).

Preface

Accurate and reliable model representations of cancer dynamics are milestones in the field of cancer research. Mathematical modeling approaches are abundantly used in cancer research as these quantitative approaches can contribute to validate various hypotheses related to cancer dynamics and thus to elucidate complexly involved interlaced mechanisms. This book presents a comprehensive review of various mathematical models as well as control strategies currently available to analyze cancer dynamics under various therapeutic interventions. The knowledge gaps that restrict the development of effective mathematical models pertaining to cancer are also highlighted. It is envisaged that further exploring these areas can contribute to the pursuit to gain deeper understanding of the underlying mechanisms involved in cancer dynamics towards tailoring appropriate control strategies for the eradication of cancer.

Why is this book needed? Technologies in the area of health sciences and engineering are developing at a very fast pace and the scientists dwell so deep that each of these streams is narrowing down to more specific areas of research that itself comprises of vast knowledge. Consequently, even though conceptual and technical information is building up at an exponential rate, the application of this knowledge and realization of useful healthcare devices is happening at a comparatively slower pace. In order to combat this inefficacy and bridge the gap, more interdisciplinary research works, and course curriculum need to be introduced in academic, industrial, and clinical organizations.

Even though a compendium of information on the topic of cancer dynamics, therapy methods, and related mathematical models are there in literature, there exists no work which discusses the inter-relation and knowledge gaps in the mathematical models of all the existing therapy methods together. This book aims to provide basic guidelines to follow while developing mathematical models of cancer dynamics. First, a general mathematical model is provided and all important mechanisms that should be addressed while modeling this disease are listed. Then, existing mathematical models of cancer dynamics that present the effect of various therapeutic interventions are rigorously reviewed. As explained in the forthcoming chapters, most of the existing mathematical models are a special case of the general model as many of them explore the cancer dynamics from a certain perspective and ignore the effect of other mechanisms. Moreover, many recent literature surveys highlight the need for improved mathematical models that address many clinically observed mechanisms that are yet to be incorporated into models.

Given that there exist wide scopes for mathematical modeling in this area, it is imperative to have a handbook that provides guidelines for the model development. Hence, the exposition of this book is kept as simple as possible by defining a set of common parameters for all therapy modes and following the same throughout the book. This allows the reader to compare and contrast all the therapy-based models developed to date under one heading. This book is expected to bridge the gap between biologists and engineers and hence, in-depth analysis of the complex biological aspects of the disease is not presented. Rather many simplified illustrative diagrams of the biological phenomena are provided for the engineers to easily comprehend and build mathematical models or design control strategies for the optimal and patient-specific drug dosing and prediction of treatment outcomes. The presentation of this book is in such a manner that any new information in this area fits the general model and thus can be easily translated to a mathematical model for cancer.

Organization of the book: This book includes 11 Chapters. Chapter 1 is a general overview of the mechanisms involved in the tumor growth and interaction with its environment, types of therapeutic strategies used for management of the disease, and a general model of the tumor dynamics.

Chapter 2 details various methods commonly used for data collection, interpretation of the data, and model building. This chapter deals with the process of transforming raw time-series data into a mathematical model.

Chapters 3–9 involve a review of various mathematical models in literature categorized based on the mode of therapy. In these chapters, the evolution of models from one cell population to many are not discussed for brevity. Instead, the most evolved models in terms of the considered number of cell populations and biochemical factors are presented and the assumptions involved and mechanisms addressed are listed with respect to the general model discussed in Chap. 1.

In Chap. 10, a survey on various control strategies used for cancer therapy is presented and the relevant research works are categorized based on control solutions such as optimal, adaptive, or patient-specific solutions. Finally, in Chap. 11, many clinically observed phenomena which are not explained through existing mathematical models are discussed followed by recommendations for future work.

Doha, Qatar

Regina Padmanabhan
Nader Meskin
Ala-Eddin Al Moustafa

Acknowledgement Authors acknowledge funding from the internal grant No. QUUG–CENG–19/20–3 from Qatar University. The findings reported herein are the sole responsibility of the authors.

Contents

Abbreviations

2D	Two-dimensional
3D CRT	Three-dimensional conformal radiation therapy
3D	Three-dimensional
6TGN	6 Thioguanine nucleotide
ACI	Adoptive cellular immunotherapy
ACT	Adoptive cell transfer
ACTH	Adrenocorticotropic hormone
AD	Androgen-dependent
ADCC	Antibody-dependent cellular toxicity
ADT	Androgen deprivation therapy
a-FGF	Acidic fibroblast growth factor
AI cell	Androgen-independent cell
AI	Artificial intelligence
AIC	Akaike information criterion
ALL	Acute lymphocytic leukemia
AML	Acute myeloid leukemia
ANN	Artificial neural network
ANOVA	Analysis of variance
APC	Androgen presenting cell
AR	Androgen receptor
AR+	Androgen receptor-positive
ART	Adaptive radiation therapy
BCG	Bacillus Calmette-Guerin
BCGF-1	B-cell growth factor-1
BED	Biologically effective dose
b-FGF	Basic fibroblast growth factor
BM	Bone marrow
CAR	Chimeric antigen receptor
CAS	Continuous androgen suppression
CCC	Concordance correlation coefficient

CCR	C-C chemokine receptor
CD	Cluster of differentiation
CHL	Classical Hodgkin lymphoma
CML	Chronic myelogenous leukemia
CR	Complete response
CSC	Cancer stem cell
CSF	Colony-stimulating factor
CTL	Cytotoxic T lymphocytes
CTLA-4	Cytotoxic T-lymphocyte-associated protein 4
CV	Coefficient of variation
CXCL	Chemokine receptor ligand
CXCR	Chemokine receptor
CXCR	C-X-C chemokine receptor
DAPT	Dual-antiplatelet therapy
DC	Dendritic cell
DCV	Dendritic cell vaccine
DEC	Distributed evolutionary computing
DFS	Disease-free-survival
DHT	Dihydrotestosterone
DNA	Deoxyribonucleic acid
DRAM	Delayed-rejection adaptive metropolis
EA	Evolutionary algorithm
ECM	Extracellular matrix
EKF	Extended Kalman filter
EMT	Epithelial to mesenchymal transition
ER	Estrogen receptor
ERD	Extrapolated response dose
FDA	Food and drug administration
Fib	Fibrinogen
FIM	Fisher-information matrix
FLC	Fuzzy logic controller
FOXP3	Forkhead box P3 is a protein
FSH	Follicle-stimulating hormone
G phase	Growth phase
GA	Genetic algorithm
GFF	Goodness of fit
GLMNET	Generalized linear model via elastic net
GM-CSF	Granulocyte-macrophage colony-stimulating factor
GnRH	Gonadotrophin-releasing hormone
HDL	High-density lipoprotein
HER2	human epidermal growth factor receptor 2
HIF	Hypoxia-inducible factor
HPV	Human papillomavirus
HSA	Human serum albumin
HSC	Hematopoietic stem cell

HTM	Hydroxytamoxifen
IAS	Intermittent androgen suppression
IFN	Interferon
IgG	Immunoglobulin G
IGRT	Image-guided radiation therapy
IL	Interleukin
IMRT	Intensity-modulated therapy
IP	Interior-point
iPSCs	Induced pluripotency of stem cells
ITIM	Immunoreceptor tyrosine-based inhibitory motif
IWRES	Individual weighted residuals
KP model	Kirschner–Panetta model
LAK	Lymphokine-activated killer
LH	Luteinizing hormone
LM	Levenberg-Marquardt
LMA	Levenberg-Marquardt algorithm
LQR	Linear quadratic regulator
LSC	Leukemia stem cell
M phase	Mitotic phase
Mab	Monoclonal antibody
MCMC	Markov-chain Monte-Carlo
MCV	Mean corpuscular volume
MDR	Multiple drug-resistant
MEK	mitogen-activated protein kinase
MHC	Major histocompatibility complex
MIMO	Multi-input multi-output
MPC	Model predictive control
MRAC	Model reference adaptive control
mRNA	messenger RNA
MSE	Mean squared error
MTD	Maximum tolerated dose
NK	Natural killer
NLME	nonlinear mixed-effects
NLS	Nonlinear least squares
NMA	Nelder-Mead algorithm
NMPC	Nonlinear MPC
NMSE	Normalized mean squared error
NN	Neural network
NSCLC	Non-small cell lung cancer
NSE	Normalized standard error
ODE	Ordinary differential equation
ONYX-15	Oncolytic virus
OOC	Organ-on-chip
OV	Oncolytic virotherapy
PB	Peripheral blood

PD	Pharmacodynamics
PD-1	Programmed death receptor-1
PDE	Partial differential equation
PDF	Probability density function
PD-L1	Programmed death-ligand 1
PID	Proportional-integral-derivative
PK	Pharmacokinetics
PRCC	Partial rank correlation coefficient
PSA	Prostate-specific antigen
RBC	Red blood cell
RFPT	Robust fixed-point transformation
RISC	RNA-induced gene silencing complex
RL	Reinforcement learning
RMSE	The root mean squared error
RNA	Ribonucleic acid
S phase	Synthetic phase
SAEM	Stochastic approximation expectation maximization
SAH	Staphylococcus aureus ®-hemolysin
SBC	Schwarz Bayesian criterion
SDRE	State-dependent Riccati equation
SERM	Selective estrogen receptor modulator
siRNA	Short interfering RNA
SMC	Sliding mode controller
SQP	Sequential quadratic programming
SRT	Stereotactic radiation therapy
SSE	Sum of squared errors
TAA	Tumor-associated antigens
TAF	Tumor angiogenic factors
TCR	T cell receptors
TGF	Transforming growth factor
TIL	Tumor-infiltrating leukocyte/lymphocyte
TM	Tamoxifen
TNF	Tumor necrosis factor
TNP-470	Trinitrophenol-470
TSC	Tumor static concentration
TSE	Tumor static exposure
TST	Testosterone
TVDT	Tumer volume-doubling time
VEGF	Vascular endothelial factor
VMAT	Volumetric modulated arc therapy
WBC	White blood cell

Chapter 1
Background

1.1 Introduction

The 17 million new cases of cancers reported in 2018 and a predicted yearly number of 23.6 million new cases by 2030 substantiate that there will be a staggering increase in the rate of incidence of the cancer disease [1, 2]. Moreover, surveys suggest that by 2030, over 20 million people will die annually due to cancer. These statistics call for tireless collaborative efforts from multiple disciplines of science and technology to foster healthcare-related to this disease. Cancers include a large family of diseases that involve repeated and uncontrolled division and spreading of cancer cells. Tumors can be either solid ones, formed of masses of tissue, or can be cancer of blood like leukemia. Tumors can be classified as comparatively harmless and non-spreading benign tumors or maliciously spreading malignant ones. The process of the advancement of tumors from the primary site to different sites is known as metastasis.

Currently, oncologists use several therapeutic measures to restrict the tumor growth and to eventually eradicate cancer. However, the survival rate of the patients heavily depends on the type and stage of cancer when diagnosed, the age of the patient, and on the type of the treatment strategies adopted. For instance, pancreatic and prostate cancer report the least (6%) and the most (99.2%) survival rates, respectively [3]. The usual treatments for cancer management include surgery, chemotherapy, radiation therapy, targeted therapy, immunotherapy, hormone therapy, and stem cell transplantation. In many cases, in order to eradicate cancer completely and to avoid the chance of cancer relapse, it is important to use multiple treatment modes together or intermittently which is referred to as a combination therapy [4–7].

Combination therapies are often attempted to reap the advantages of synergistic cancer treatments while keeping the side effects due to treatments to the minimum. For instance, some chemotherapeutic drugs can be used to enhance the susceptibility of tumors to radiotherapy. Thus, an orderly combination of chemotherapy and then radiation therapy shows an improvement in patient outcomes. Another case is the combination of chemotherapy or radiotherapy with the stem cell therapy [8]. High

R. Padmanabhan et al., *Mathematical Models of Cancer and Different Therapies*,
Series in BioEngineering, https://doi.org/10.1007/978-981-15-8640-8_1

doses of chemotherapy and radiation therapy can destroy hematopoietic stem cells (HSC) that generate all kinds of blood cells. Therefore, stem cell transplantation procedures are used after such treatments for the restoration of blood-forming stem cells.

In general, the development of associated mathematical models has fostered the evolution of many assistive devices in the area of healthcare [9–11]. Typically, mathematical models can aid associated experimental and clinical studies by providing mechanistic insights about the disease and effects of the current drug administration regimes to subsequently revamp current treatment methods. Similar to many other areas of healthcare, cancer research also makes use of quantitative mathematical models to accelerate its quest for the betterment of patient care. Cancer dynamics involves many complex mechanisms and is influenced by several inter-related biological factors. Analysis of such complex and interlaced phenomenon with multiple interlaced parameter influence can be significantly simplified using appropriate mathematical models. For instance, mathematical models enable one to predict the behavior of the system in a future time scale and to analyze the effect of each and every variable or parameter on the overall cancer dynamics. These parameters can be related to the patient physiology, disease type, and treatment modality. Such predictions and analyses are often difficult to make, maybe risky, or costly to implement using an in vivo/vitro experimental setup or a clinical trial.

In this book, the term *cancer dynamics* is used to refer to the overall mechanisms involved in the initiation, progression, and regression of cancer. Figure 1.1 depicts an illustration of the progression and regression trajectory of cancer dynamics. Cancer dynamics involves linear or nonlinear, continuous or discontinuous growth and decay of many cell populations and cell signaling biochemicals. Cancer cells, normal cells, immune cells, and endothelial cells are a few examples of cell populations at the site of cancer. Hormones, enzymes, antigens, cytokines, growth factors, and externally applied therapeutic agents (drugs) are a few examples of biochemicals whose concentration can significantly influence the progression or regression trajectory of cancer dynamics. These influences of the cell populations or biochemicals can be viewed and analyzed concerning their effects at the cellular level to the overall system (organism) level using a mathematical model.

Factors such as the proliferation rate, mutations involved, and metabolic changes that alter the dynamics of cancer cell populations vary considerably according to the stage of cancer. Irrespective of the type of cancer, one of the important factors that specify the type of treatment to be followed is the grade and stage of disease at the time of its diagnosis. As shown in Fig. 1.1, the development of blood vessels in a tumor plays an important role in the tumor growth progression as well as in its regression with the help of therapy. For instance, the vasculature of the tumor is initially poor and so it adversely affects the supply of nutrients and oxygen that facilitates the tumor growth. Similarly, with poor vasculature, it is difficult to effectively transport and distribute intravenous chemotherapeutic agents to the site of the tumor. Efficacy of the radiation therapy treatment is also hindered due to the insufficient oxygen supply from the immature vasculature of the tumor [12]. Interestingly, research on

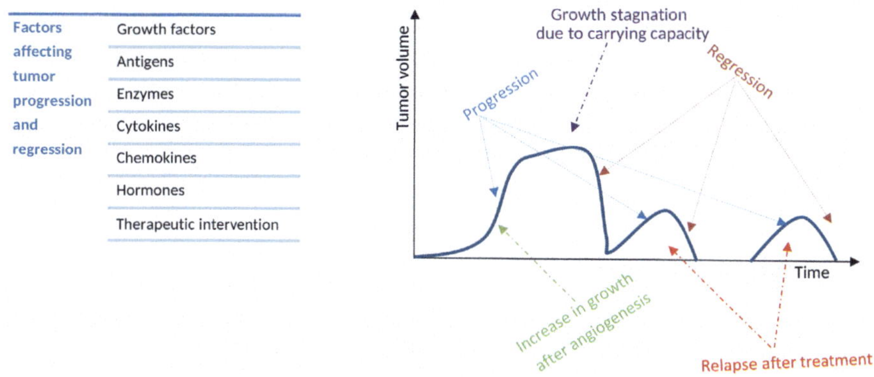

Fig. 1.1 Factors affecting cancer dynamics and an illustrative diagram showing the progression and regression trajectory of cancer dynamics. Angiogenesis in a tumor can result in an exponential increase in cancer growth. The progression of cancer growth is restricted by the carrying capacity of the tumor micro-environment. Therapeutic interventions can facilitate the tumor regression

pro-angiogenesis is also gaining attention for its ability to target more amount of drugs to the site of cancer and thus to facilitate an effective therapy [13].

Some specific areas of cancer research that is being benefited currently and can be improved further with the help of mathematical models are the investigation on tumor initiation, tumor growth, the reaction of the immune system to tumor growth, development of the vascular network in the tumor (angiogenesis), response to various treatment modes, metastases of the tumor, intra-tumor heterogeneity, drug toxicity, and drug resistance, to name some. Characteristics such as incidence-probability of developing cancer with respect to age, lifestyle, and dynamics of mutation acquisition that leads to cancer are more useful in building mathematical models that can be used to predict the incidence of cancer [14].

In general, partial differential equations (PDE) and ordinary differential equations (ODE) are used to model the progression and regression of cancer. The PDEs are used to model the cancer dynamics when more than one independent variable comes into the picture, for instance, oxygen diffusion with respect to time and space [14, 15]. Moreover, partial differential equation-based models can account for shapes of various solid tumors and assist in spatio-temporal analysis. However, ordinary differential equation-based models are more suitable for depicting the time-dependent progression and regression of cancer which allow comparatively easier dynamical analysis with respect to the inherent mechanisms involved. The focus of this book is to provide guidelines for the development of ODE-based mathematical models to represent the mechanisms that affect the progression of cancer and its regression due to various therapeutic interventions. Towards this end, a general mathematical model of cancer dynamics is developed and then a detailed review of the existing mathematical models based on the type of therapy is presented.

The main aim of this book is to identify knowledge gaps that restrict the development of effective mathematical models pertaining to the disease towards tailoring appropriate control strategies for the eradication of cancer. Toward this goal, this book is mainly focused on the mechanisms that affect the progression of cancer and its regression due to various therapeutic interventions.

1.2 Tumor Dynamics

1.2.1 Basic Mechanisms Involved in Tumor Growth

When it comes to the development of mathematical models to represent cancer dynamics and associated therapies, it is essential to understand the fundamental mechanisms of cancer dynamics. This subsection presents some of the basic mechanisms and in vivo factors that promote tumor growth. Irrespective of the type of the therapy used, the basic mechanisms involved remain more or less the same. It should be noted that a tumor that successfully thrives in an organism is a bunch of surviving abnormal/mutated cells with the ability to outrival the inherent tumor inhibiting mechanisms (e.g. tumor suppressor genes, immune response) in the body of that organism to a certain extent. Towards developing mathematical models that can account for the realistic mechanisms involved in the tumor growth, it is important to analyze the factors that promote and inhibit the tumor growth in an organism.

Even though, the exact mechanism that triggers the onset of cancer is still unknown, radiation, gene mutation, lifestyle, chemicals, etc. are identified as possible contributing factors. There is an enormous number of physiological, cellular, and molecular mechanisms and complex signaling pathways involved in the growth and regression of tumor dynamics. Many of which are still unknown to us. Throughout this book, known mechanisms are presented to illustrate how mathematicians or engineers look at such biological phenomena to derive the associated mathematical model. Looking from a cellular and macroscopic level, the progression of various types of cancer involves the following main steps [16]:

- At the cellular level

1. Anomalous cells undergo fast proliferation and cell-cycle deregulation without control.
2. The encounter of an immune cell with anomalous cell results either in destruction, inhibition, or survival of the anomalous cell. These actions by the immune cells are regulated through the cytokine signals.
3. Surviving cancer cells often proliferate aggressively.
4. Tumor cells, host cells, and immune cells share available resources such as nutrients and oxygen and fight for existence.

- At the macroscopic level

1. As the tumor grows, it moves farther away from the existing blood vessels which in turn restricts the growth of the tumor.
2. Angiogenesis is initiated to extend the existing blood vessels in the host tissues towards the tumor environment and thus the tumor grows further.
3. Once the tumor growth is restricted by the carrying capacity of the tumor environment, often tumor cells get into the extended vascular network in the tumor environment and advance to other areas of the body through the circulatory system and metastasize.
4. Mechanisms classified under macroscopic level also include the diffusion of oxygen, nutrients, chemical agents, etc.

1.2.2 Various Cell Populations in a Tumor Micro-environment

Typically, the tumor micro-environment includes both living and dead cells (necrotic cells). Living cells, which are in an actively multiplying stage are called as proliferating cells and in a dormant stage are called as quiescent cancer cells. The natural death of cells is often referred to as apoptosis. The dead cells are removed or ingested by the macrophages and the process is referred to as phagocytosis. Figure 1.2 shows the types of cells in a tumor. Depending upon the availability of nutrients and oxygen in the environment, the cells in the dormant stage can transition to proliferating cells or necrotic cells. A three-layer structure is generally identified for tumors which includes: (1) the proliferating cells that form the outer boundary layer, (2) the dead cells that form a necrotic core, and (3) the quiescent cells that lie in the middle between the necrotic core and outer proliferating layer [16, 17].

When it comes to the mathematical modeling of cancer dynamics, along with the growth and death pattern of various cell populations, it is important to account for the interaction between these cell populations in terms of their competition and survival [18]. The *carrying capacity* of the tumor micro-environment depends on resource (nutrients and oxygen) availability in the tumor micro-environment. Note that blood is the carrier that supplies resources. Blood tissue mainly includes platelets that help in blood clotting, red blood cells (RBCs) which carry oxygen and nutrients, and white blood cells (WBCs) which are the immune cells. Figure 1.3 shows various cell populations in the human blood. All of these cells are derived from the hematopoietic stem cells (HSC) by cell differentiation which means that the cell lineage (i.e. the developmental history) of all these cells tracks back to the hematopoietic stem cells. These cells serve various functions involved in immunosurveillance and immune response mechanisms to facilitate immunity. Another important cell type that comes into picture while investigating the cancer dynamics is the endothelial cells that line the blood and lymph vessels.

Tumor-immune interaction is a complex mechanism, which involves numerous cell types and protein-protein interactions. The immune system includes different types of cells such as natural killer cells, macrophages, cytotoxic T cells, helper T cells, regulatory T cells, memory T cells, dendritic cells, etc. [19]. It can be seen from Fig. 1.3 that all these cells are derived from myeloid progenitors and lymphoid progenitors by cell differentiation. These cell populations play a very significant role in mediating the immune response that restricts the tumor growth.

Apart from the quiescent and proliferating stages mentioned earlier, the cell types shown in Fig. 1.3 can be in cell differentiating stage after which the cells mature to a hunting stage (active or attacking). Such cell differentiation is prevalent in blood cells involved in immune actions. The cell types listed in Figs. 1.2 and 1.3 are used repeatedly to explain the cancer dynamics using various models in Chaps. 3–9. Another category of cell populations that are significant in the perspective of mathematical modeling of cancer dynamics is those that are segregated with respect to the response to therapy such as the cells that are sensitive to therapy and resistive to therapy. This category includes the drug-sensitive cell, drug-resistive, hormone-dependent cells, and hormone-independent cells.

1.2.3 Tumor-Immune Interaction

Tumor-immune interaction is a common mechanism that needs to be discussed in association with all mathematical models irrespective of the therapy used. However, in the case of immunotherapy, the tumor-immune interaction is boosted for its potential benefits. The response of the immune system against tumor progression can be broadly classified under two headings: innate immune action and adaptive

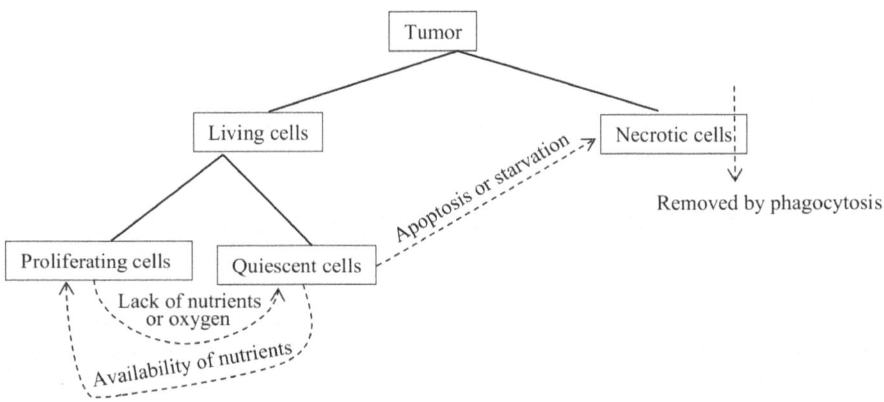

Fig. 1.2 A tumor can have both living and dead (necrotized) cells. Dead cells are removed by the process called phagocytosis. Living cells remain as proliferating cells or become quiescent cells when there is a lack of nutrients or oxygen. Quiescent cells can transition to proliferating type when resources for growth are available

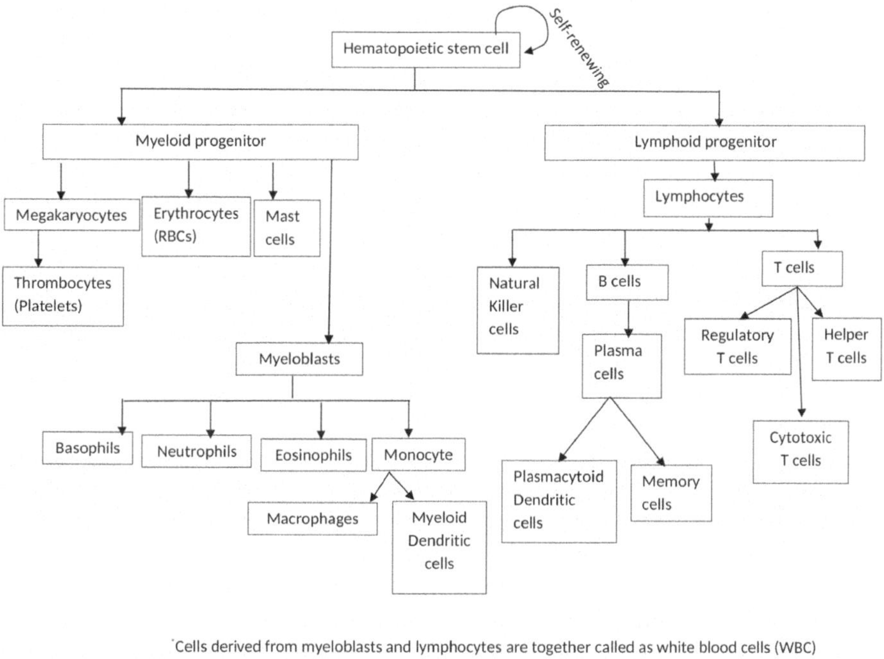

Fig. 1.3 Cell types in blood and bone marrow derived from hematopoietic stem cells. Hematopoietic stem cells are capable of self-renewal

immune action. Innate immune action involves rapid response called as phagocytosis mediated by macrophages, natural killer cells, and neutrophils to remove pathogens and unwanted cells. Adaptive immune action is a relatively slow immune response which involves identification of the pathogen or abnormal cells, preparing and activating specific immune cells to facilitate immune actions, and also memorizing the pathogen-specific counter activity so as to annihilate the same pathogen quickly at the next encounter. These activities involve many types of cell signaling pathways to ensure that only harmful invaders are attacked and the host's normal cells are not harmed (autoimmunity) [19–21].

Typically, substances that initiate an immune action and production of antibodies in the body are called antigens. The immune system is capable of identifying and marking (labeling) the antigens that are present on most of the pathogens. These antigens are basically proteins that are unique for each pathogen. Some of the immune cells such as dendritic cells and macrophages use their receptors to identify the antigens present on the surface of the pathogens and abnormal cells (cancer cells). There are many immune response pathways that are in place to combat tumor progression [20, 21]. Such pathways basically facilitate the immune response by increasing the number of helper immune cells and activating the proliferation of killer immune cells. These mechanisms can result in a constant influx of tumor-infiltrating leukocytes

(TILs) into the tumor micro-environment or a nonlinear increase in the proliferation and activation of immune cells.

The cell signaling proteins such as cytokines are capable of regulating growth, mutation, suppression, and activation of various immune cell populations. For instance, these proteins are involved in the activation and proliferation of naive T cells (cytotoxic T cells before activation), macrophages, etc. [20]. Apart from mediating the immune response, some cytokines are identified to exhibit pro-tumor and anti-tumor properties such as involvement in tumor inhibition, invasion, and metastasis (e.g. TGF-β, IL-23) [22]. These proteins can also enhance and suppress the tumor growth [21]. The anti-tumor action of the immune system is a cumulative effect of several interlaced mechanisms and involves several cell types and cell signaling proteins. However, for simplicity, the active cells of the immune system which are mainly involved in inducing these activities are sometimes, in general, referred to as "immune cells" or "effector cells" [23].

It should be noted that, even though the presence of cancer invokes an immune response in the patient, the level of immunogenicity is patient-specific and it also varies according to the type of cancer [24]. All these activities of the immune system may eventually lead to the destruction of most of the cancer cells, however, oftentimes the cancer cells evade from the immune system and grow uncontrollably. Such a situation necessitates the use of external adjuvants either to boost the immune system and to overcome the immunosuppressive mechanisms produced by malignant tumors or to directly facilitate tumor lysis [21].

1.3 Cancer Therapies

Oncologists use several therapeutic measures to restrict the tumor growth and eventually eradicate cancer. In many cases, in order to eradicate cancer completely and to avoid the chance of relapse, it is important to use multiple treatment modes together or intermittently which is referred to as a combination therapy. In this book, mathematical models are categorized according to the type of therapy (monotherapy) or therapies (combination therapy) used. Various modes of therapies discussed are as follows:

1. *Chemotherapy*: which involves the use of one or more therapeutic drugs to manage cancer disease.
2. *Immunotherapy*: which involves the use of one or more therapeutic agents to boost the immune system to facilitate effective cancer cure.
3. *Anti-angiogenic therapy*: which involves the use of one or more anti-angiogenic agents to limit blood vessel development in tumors and thereby to facilitate cancer cure.
4. *Radiotherapy*: which involves the use of radiation as a therapeutic agent to facilitate cancer cure.

5. *Hormone therapy*: involves the use of hormones or other agents that regulate hormone production in the body to kill cancer cells.
6. *Miscellaneous therapies*: such as stem cell therapy, nanomedicine mediated therapy, gene therapy, and radiovirotherapy which involve the administration of one or more therapeutic agents to facilitate cancer cure.
7. *Combination therapy*: which involves the use of multiple agents from different treatment modalities mentioned in (1)–(6) to facilitate more effective cancer cure than that can be accomplished by using monotherapy.

Most of the therapy modes mentioned above involve many complex mechanisms and multiple cell types and hence it is difficult to portray the overall involved cancer dynamics using single-cell and two cell-based models. Moreover, many of the existing reviews point out that oversimplified mathematical models such as the ones with single-cell and two cell dynamics are too generic and hence not suitable for illustrating the effect of therapy on cancer dynamics [15]. Hence, in later parts of this book, instead of going in a retrospective manner, the available mathematical models in literature are analyzed which involve two or more cell populations to depict the cancer dynamics under various treatment modes.

1.4 A General Model of Tumor Dynamics and Effect of Therapy

In this section, a general mathematical model of cancer dynamics is discussed. An essential starting step towards developing mathematical models of cancer dynamics with adequate complexity is to identify the most important cell populations that are involved in the process.

Figure 1.4 shows a simplified illustration of a general cell dynamics in the tumor micro-environment where inward and outward arrows denote mechanisms that contribute to the increase and decrease of cell numbers, respectively. Typically, the dynamics of each cell population is an aggregate of several basic mechanisms which involves parameters such as growth rate, death rate, competition rate, survival rate, carrying capacity, etc. Consequently, a general form that brings together all the essential mechanisms involved in cancer dynamics gives a more intuitive idea regarding the pros and cons of the available mathematical models. More specifically, by comparing the available models in various therapy modes with the general model, it will be easy to see the simplifying assumptions used in model building. As shown in Fig. 1.4, each of the ith cell population may undergo proliferation (growth), apoptosis (death), and cell transition. Cells of the same cell population and different cell populations compete for nutrients. A predator-prey type of competition occurs between certain cell populations.

As mentioned earlier, the mathematical models discussed in the available literature focus mainly on specific cell population and the associated cell dynamics. Hence, a general model for a given cell population can be written as:

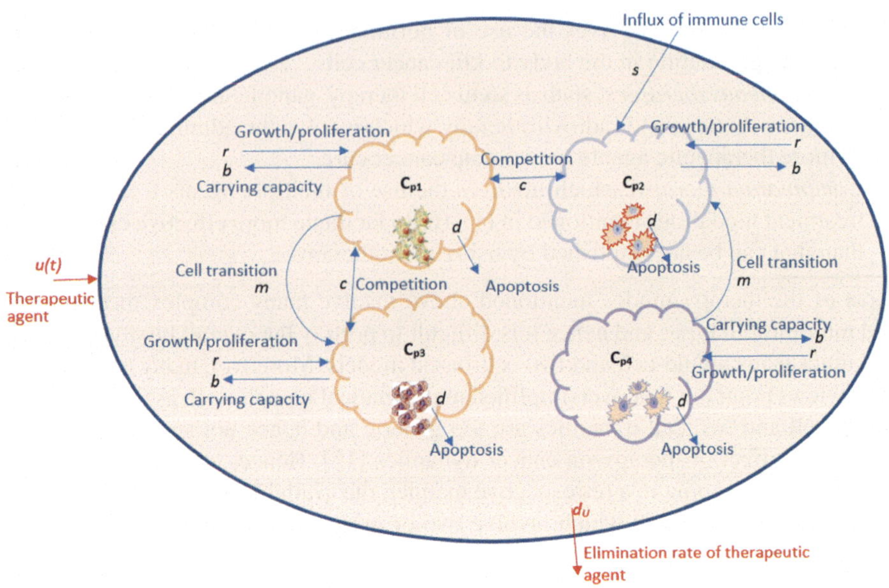

Fig. 1.4 Illustration of cell dynamics in a tumor micro-environment

$$\begin{aligned}\frac{\mathrm{d}C_{\mathrm{p1}}(t)}{\mathrm{d}t} &= \overbrace{\mathscr{G}\left(r(t), C_{\mathrm{p1}}(t-\tau), C_{\mathrm{p2}}(t)\right)}^{growth} - \overbrace{\mathscr{A}\left(d(t), C_{\mathrm{p1}}(t)\right)}^{apoptosis} - \overbrace{\mathscr{K}\left(b(t), C_{\mathrm{p1}}(t)\right)}^{carrying\ capacity} \\ &\quad \pm \overbrace{\mathscr{C}\left(c(t), C_{\mathrm{p1}}(t), C_{\mathrm{p2}}(t-\tau)\right)}^{competition} \pm \overbrace{\mathscr{M}\left(m(t), C_{\mathrm{p1}}(t-\tau), C_{\mathrm{p2}}(t)\right)}^{cell\ transition} \\ &\quad \pm \overbrace{\mathscr{D}\left(a(t), C_{\mathrm{p1}}(t-\tau), U(t-\tau)\right)}^{effect\ of\ therapy}, \quad C_{\mathrm{p1}}(0) = C_{\mathrm{p10}}, \end{aligned} \tag{1.1}$$

$$\frac{\mathrm{d}U(t)}{\mathrm{d}t} = \mathscr{D}_{\mathrm{c}}\left(d_{\mathrm{U}}(t), U(t-\tau), u(t)\right), \quad U(0) = U_0, \tag{1.2}$$

where $r(t)$ and $d(t)$ are the growth and death rates, $b(t)$ and $c(t)$ are the reciprocal carrying capacity and competition rate, $m(t)$ and $a(t)$ are the mutation (cell transition) rate and drug induced cell-kill rate, $d_{\mathrm{U}}(t)$ and τ are the drug decay rate and time-delay, respectively. Note that (1.1) represents the general dynamics of one cell population ($C_{\mathrm{p1}}(t)$) and its interactions with another cell population ($C_{\mathrm{p2}}(t)$) in the tumor micro-environment. It should be noted that $C_{\mathrm{p1}}(t-\tau)$, $C_{\mathrm{p2}}(t-\tau)$, and $U(t-\tau)$ denote the time-delay version of the variables $C_{\mathrm{p1}}(t)$, $C_{\mathrm{p2}}(t)$ and $U(t)$, respectively. The time-delay τ is considered in the general model (1.1)–(1.2) to represent the delayed interactions between different cell populations involved in the cancer dynamics. As it will be seen in the next chapters, most of the presented models in the literature do not consider the time-delay and consequently, $\tau = 0$.

Table 1.1 Parameter notations used in this chapter

Parameter	Description
$a(t)$	Fractional cell-kill rate due to therapy
$b(t)$	Reciprocal carrying capacity
$c(t)$	Competition rate between cell populations
$d(t)$	Death rate or depletion rate
$r(t)$	Growth rate
$m(t)$	Mutation (cell transition) rate
$d_{\mathrm{U}}(t)$	Depletion (elimination) rate of therapeutic agent from tumor site

In (1.1)–(1.2), the function $\mathscr{G}\left(r(t), C_{\mathrm{p1}}(t-\tau), C_{\mathrm{p2}}(t)\right)$ defines the growth of $C_{\mathrm{p1}}(t)$ with respect to the growth rate $r(t)$ and the influence of another cell population $C_{\mathrm{p2}}(t)$, $\mathscr{A}\left(d(t), C_{\mathrm{p1}}(t)\right)$ accounts for the natural death (apoptosis) of the cell population $C_{\mathrm{p1}}(t)$ in terms of the death rate $d(t)$, $\mathscr{K}\left(b(t), C_{\mathrm{p1}}(t)\right)$ quantifies the effect of resource availability in the environment in terms of the reciprocal carrying capacity $b(t)$, $\mathscr{C}\left(c(t), C_{\mathrm{p1}}(t), C_{\mathrm{p2}}(t-\tau)\right)$ quantifies the interaction between the two cell populations $C_{\mathrm{p1}}(t)$ and $C_{\mathrm{p2}}(t-\tau)$ in terms of the competition rate or interaction rate $c(t)$, $\mathscr{M}\left(m(t), C_{\mathrm{p1}}(t-\tau), C_{\mathrm{p2}}(t)\right)$ denotes the mutation of one cell population to other in terms of the mutation rate $m(t)$, $\mathscr{D}\left(a(t), C_{\mathrm{p1}}(t-\tau), U(t-\tau)\right)$ accounts for the effect of therapy on the cell population in terms of the intensity or concentration of the therapeutic intervention $U(t-\tau)$ and the cell-kill rate due to the therapeutic intervention $a(t)$, and finally $\mathscr{D}_{\mathrm{c}}(d_{\mathrm{U}}(t), U(t-\tau), u(t))$ describes the rate of change of drug concentration in the site of the tumor with respect to the drug depletion rate $d_{\mathrm{U}}(t)$ and the drug input $u(t)$.

Note that, the number of various cell types can increase or decrease in response to therapy. For instance, the number of cancer cells will decrease in response to chemotherapy or immunotherapy, however, in response to immune-boosting therapy, the number of immune cells will increase. Hence, the term $\pm\mathscr{D}\left(a(t), C_{\mathrm{p1}}(t-\tau), U(t)\right)$ is used to denote the effect of therapy on a general cell population.

The parameter τ in (1.1) and (1.2) is used to account for the possible time-delays that can affect tumor dynamics. Unavailability of resources can contribute delay in growth function, delay in the immune response can affect the time of the predator-prey type of competition between cells, the delay involved in cell transition of a resting cell to hunting cell, drug mixing delay, and delay due to the time taken by the therapeutic agent to show a certain result, etc. are possible examples of having time-delay in a cell population dynamics. Table 1.1 summarizes the list of parameters that are defined in (1.1)–(1.2).

The parameters $r(t)$, $d(t)$, $b(t)$, $c(t)$, $m(t)$, $a(t)$, and $d_{\mathrm{U}}(t)$ can be time-varying or constants according to the underlying mechanism under study and the simplifying assumptions involved. In most cases, constant parameters are used. According to the characteristic behavior of the significant cell populations involved in the cancer dynamics, the functions defined in (1.1) and (1.2) are modeled using logistic, exponential, Gompertz, Von Bertalanffy, Michaelis–Menten, and power laws. All these growth models are elaborated in Chap. 2 of this book. Typically, as shown in Fig. 1.4, the growth function $\mathscr{G}\left(r(t), C_{\mathrm{p1}}(t-\tau), C_{\mathrm{p2}}(t)\right)$ may include the effect of one or more of the mechanism such as mitosis or proliferation, the influx of cell population as in the case of immune cells, increase in the cell population due to transition of one population to other, etc. Note that, when the transition (mutation) of cells from one cell type to another cell occurs, the number (volume) of cells of the former decreases while that of later increases. Hence, in (1.1), since a general cell population $C_{\mathrm{p1}}(t)$ is considered, the term $\pm\mathscr{M}\left(m(t), C_{\mathrm{p1}}(t-\tau), C_{\mathrm{p2}}(t)\right)$ is used to denote the transition pattern of cells, where $m(t)$ is the associated cell transition (mutation) rate.

1.5 Summary

In this chapter, an overview of the mechanisms involved in the tumor growth, tumor interactions with the environment, types of therapeutic strategies used for management of the disease, and a general model of tumor dynamics are presented. Chapter 2 provides various methods commonly used for data collection, model building, and model validation. Next, in Chaps. 3–9, various mathematical models in literature categorized based on the mode of therapy are presented. As explained in the forthcoming chapters, most of the existing mathematical models are a special case of the general model (1.1) and (1.2) discussed in this chapter. Most of the models explore the cancer dynamics from a certain perspective and ignore the effect of other mechanisms. Thus, the main aim is to first detail the important biological aspects of each therapy mode and then compare each model in Chaps. 3–9 with the general model (1.1) and (1.2) to clarify the mechanisms addressed in each model and main assumptions involved in the model development. Various control methods that have been used with each treatment methods discussed in Chaps. 3–9 are reviewed in Chap. 10. Finally, the research gaps identified in the area of each therapy mode are listed at the end of the upcoming chapters and in Chap. 11.

References

1. Worldwide cancer statistics, Technical report, Cancer Research, UK, https://www.cancerresearchuk.org/health-professional/cancer-statistics/worldwide-cancer
2. Cancer statistics, Technical report, National Cancer Institute, https://www.cancer.gov/about-cancer/understanding/statistics
3. Cancer survival rate statistics by type of cancer. Statistics from the period between 2003 and 2009, www.cancer.gov/statistics. Accessed 31 Aug 2019
4. R. Bayat Mokhtari, T.S. Homayouni, N. Baluch, E. Morgatskaya, S. Kumar, B. Das, H. Yeger, Combination therapy in combating cancer. Oncotarget **8**, 38022–38043 (2017)
5. K. Khan, R. Kerbel, Improving immunotherapy outcomes with anti-angiogenic treatments and vice versa. Nat. Rev. Clin. Oncol. **15**, 310 (2018)

6. F.F. Teles, J.M. Lemos, Cancer therapy optimization based on multiple model adaptive control. Biomed. Signal Process. Control **48**, 255–264 (2019)
7. N. Babaei, M.U. Salamci, Mixed therapy in cancer treatment for personalized drug administration using model reference adaptive control. Eur. J. Control **50**, 117–137 (2019)
8. J.A. Child, G.J. Morgan, F.E. Davies, R.G. Owen, S.E. Bell, K. Hawkins, J. Brown, M.T. Drayson, P.J. Selby, High-dose chemotherapy with hematopoietic stem-cell rescue for multiple myeloma. N. Engl. J. Med. **348**(19), 1875–1883 (2003)
9. B. Verma, S. Ray, R. Srivastava, Mathematical models and their applications in medicine and health. Health Popul. Perspect. Issues **4**(1), 42–58 (1981)
10. D. Bertsimas, J. Silberholz, T. Trikalinos, Optimal healthcare decision making under multiple mathematical models: application in prostate cancer screening. Health Care Manag. Sci. **21**, 105–118 (2018)
11. J. Chase, J.C. Preiser, J. Knopp, A. Pironet, Y.S. Chiew, C.G. Pretty, G. Shaw, B. Benyó, K. Moeller, S. Safaei, M. Tawhai, P. Hunter, T. Desaive, Next-generation, personalised, model-based critical care medicine: a state-of-the art review of in silico virtual patient models, methods, and cohorts, and how to validation them. Biomed. Eng. Online **17** (2018)
12. D. Klein, The tumor vascular endothelium as decision maker in cancer therapy. Front. Oncol. **8**(367) (2018)
13. G. Lupo, N. Caporarello, M. Olivieri, M. Cristaldi, C. Motta, V. Bramanti, R. Avola, M. Salmeri, F. Nicoletti, C.D. Anfuso, Anti-angiogenic therapy in cancer: downsides and new pivots for precision medicine. Front. Pharmacol. **7**(519) (2017)
14. P.M. Altrock, L.L. Liu, The mathematics of cancer: integrating quantitative models. Nat. Rev. Cancer **15**, 730–745 (2015)
15. R. Eftimie, J.L. Bramson, D.J.D. Earn, Interactions between the immune system and cancer: a brief review of non-spatial mathematical models. Bull. Math. Biol. **73**(1), 2–32 (2011)
16. N. Bellomo, L. Preziosi, Modelling and mathematical problems related to tumor evolution and its interaction with the immune system. Math. Comput. Model. **32**(3), 413–452 (2000)
17. A. Friedman, A hierarchy of cancer models and their mathematical challenges. Discret. Contin. Dyn. Syst. Ser.-B **4**(1), 147–159 (2004)
18. L.G.D. Pillis, A. Radunskaya, A mathematical tumor model with immune resistance and drug therapy: an optimal control approach. Comput. Math. Methods Med. **3**(2), 79–100 (2001)
19. M. Robertson Tessi, A. El Kareh, A. Goriely, A mathematical model of tumor-immune interactions. J. Theor. Biol. **294**, 56–73 (2012)
20. J. Maher, E. Davies, Targeting cytotoxic T lymphocytes for cancer immunotherapy. Br. J. Cancer **91**(5), 817 (2004)
21. F.D. Barber, Recent developments in oncology immunotherapy, adverse effects part 2. J. Nurse Pract. **14**(4), 259–266 (2018)
22. S. Lee, K. Margolin, Cytokines in cancer immunotherapy. Cancers **3**(4), 3856–3893 (2011)
23. D. Kirschner, J.C. Panetta, Modeling immunotherapy of the tumor-immune interaction. J. Math. Biol. **37**(3), 235–252 (1998)
24. T. Blankenstein, P. Coulie, E. Gilboa, E. Jaffee, The determinants of tumour immunogenicity. Nat. Rev. Cancer **12**(4), 307–313 (2012)

Chapter 2
Time Series Data to Mathematical Model

In this chapter, various steps involved in building and validating mathematical models using the data of tumor dynamics observed experimentally are discussed. Initial attempts to model the tumor growth were based on the assumption of having a constant tumor volume-doubling time (TVDT). However, later on, it became apparent that the TVDT does not remain the same throughout the growth period. Subsequently, many mathematical models evolved. For instance, the logistic model, Gompertz model, and Von Bertalanffy model which were originally coined in the early 1800s for describing human population growth, human mortality rate, and length-age dependence of fish growth, respectively, have been later on adapted to represent tumor dynamics [1–3]. Many such ecological and biological models are currently extensively used to analyze tumor growth dynamics [3–5].

As it will be seen in later chapters of this book, several mathematical models have been developed to derive more insight into cancer dynamics and its treatment. However, our understanding of the biological and theoretical aspects of the initiation and progression of this highly complex disease is quite incomplete. Hence, several theoretical and experimental studies are ongoing worldwide to dissect the biological pathways that favor cancer progression so as to come up with improved treatment options for the eradication of this disease. Theoretical analysis is primarily conducted by using appropriate mathematical models that are developed based on the experimental evidence of cancer dynamics [6, 7]. In this chapter, first in Sects. 2.1 and 2.2, experimental designs and data collection for developing mathematical models of cancer are presented, followed by model fitting and validation in Sects. 2.3 and 2.4. Equilibrium point analysis and non-dimensionalization are discussed in Sect. 2.5 and a chapter summary is presented in Sect. 2.6. Tables 2.1 and 2.2 summarize the notations used in this chapter.

R. Padmanabhan et al., *Mathematical Models of Cancer and Different Therapies*, Series in BioEngineering, https://doi.org/10.1007/978-981-15-8640-8_2

Table 2.1 Parameter notations used in this chapter

Param.	Description	Param.	Description
a	Effect of therapy	b	Reciprocal carrying capacity
k	Carrying capacity	c	Competition rate
d	Growth-suppressive factor	r	Growth rate
m	Mutation (cell transition) rate	s	Immune cell influx rate
α	Immune threshold rate	p	Exponent quantifying relative growth rate
β	Decrease in proliferation rate	I_{max}	Maximum drug effect
n	Hill coefficient	g	Half-saturation concentration
N	Maximum number of data	i	Number of data
θ	Parameter set	θ_{k}	Normalization constant
θ^*	Dimensionless variable	θ_{r}	Reference variable
θ_{s}	Scaling parameter	Γ	Number of parameters in θ
y_{N}	Normalised data	y_{min}	Minimum value of observed data
y_{max}	Maximum value of observed data	μ	Mean of observed data
σ	Standard deviation of observed		

Table 2.2 Different types of cells and biochemicals in this chapter

Variable	Variable description
$k(t)$	Dynamic carrying capacity
$N(t)$	Amount of normal cells
$A(t)$	Amount of cancer cells
$E(t)$	Amount of immune cells
$U(t)$	Drug concentration
$C_{\text{p}}(t)$	General cell population
$C_{\text{p}_\text{s}}(t)$	Drug sensitive cells
$C_{\text{p}_\text{d}}(t)$	Damaged cells

2.1 Experimental Design

As mentioned in Chap. 1, mathematical models can aid associated experimental and clinical studies by providing mechanistic insights about the disease and effects of the current drug administration regimes to subsequently revamp existing treatment methods. Towards this end, factors contributing to tumor initiation and development are to be investigated either at the intracellular level, that is the dynamics within a single cell or at the intercellular level, that is the interactions in the tumor micro-environment, or sometimes at the population level, that is the dynamics of various types of tumors in different populations (Fig. 1.1). The dynamics of the heterogeneous tumor micro-environment are highly complex and it involves the growth, decay, competition, and mutation of many cell populations and cell signaling biochemicals ((1.1)–(1.2)). Normal and cancer cells in the quiescent, proliferating, or necrotic stage and the cells that are resistive or sensitive to the drugs are some of the cell types (Fig. 1.2). Additionally, the influence of immune mechanism including the inherent feedback via biochemical signals (e.g. TGF-β, IL-2) and angiogenesis have major implications in cancer dynamics. In this section, the steps involved in building models that can reproduce the dynamics of various cell populations and biochemicals in the tumor micro-environment are discussed.

The first step in mathematical modeling is to adequately state the hypothesis or research question that needs to be substantiated or investigated (Fig. 2.1). The second step involves the identification of an experimental model with justifiable complexity that can contribute the required information regarding the research question. The third and fourth steps are data collection and parameter identification for the descriptive model of choice. These steps may include pre-processing of raw data (e.g. normalization/standardization, omitting outliers) to scale the data to a required range and to avoid data redundancy. After pre-processing of the data, parameter identification algorithms are used to find the parameter values for the descriptive model of our choice. One or more such algorithms can be used for a comparative assessment of the achieved fitting, or hybrid parameter fitting algorithm, which can offer improved parameter fitting against individual methods, can also be used [5]. The fifth step in the modeling process is the validation of the model against future data if any from the experimental model.

The choice of the descriptive models that represent functions $\mathscr{G}(\cdot)$, $\mathscr{A}(\cdot)$, $\mathscr{K}(\cdot)$, $\mathscr{C}(\cdot)$, and $\mathscr{M}(\cdot)$ and cells populations $C_{pi}, i = 1, 2, \ldots$ in (1.1)–(1.2) is made according to the question that is needed to be analyzed. According to the biological question that is investigated, the experiment is designed to investigate cancer dynamics in an intracellular, intercellular, or individual (patient) level. This can be an in vitro cell culture experiment using single or multiple cell types or a bit more complex one such as organ-on-chip or organoid model-based experiments [8–10]. In vivo experimental models include animal models established by injecting or inoculating tumor cells by a variety of techniques including transplantation of tumor cells, induction of tumor via a virus, radiation, or chemical agents.

Depending on the type of transplantations, it can be heterotopic/ectopic (not in proper place) or orthotopic (in proper place). Depending upon the animal (host) used, it can be syngeneic (genetically similar and immunocompatible) or allogeneic (genetically dissimilar and immunologically incompatible) [11]. Genetically modified animal models such as transgenic animals (with added gene(s)) and knockout animals (with removed gene(s)) are also used in cancer research. Xenograft is a term used to denote tissue transplants from a donor to different species (e.g. transplanting human cancer cells to mice) [11]. Clinical trials on human beings are also a major source of data for developing mathematical models. An illustrative timeline of experimental events for data collection for an in vivo experiment using an animal model is shown in Fig. 2.2.

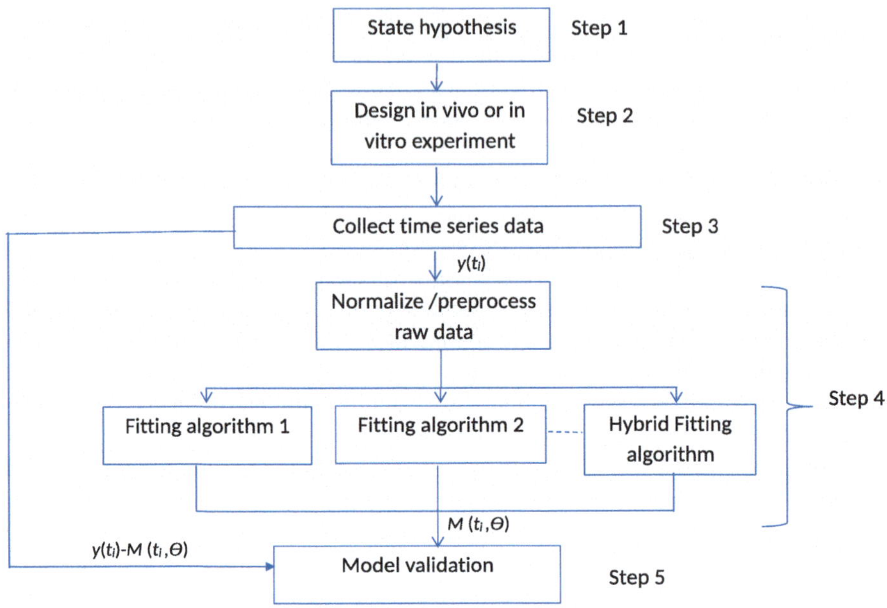

Fig. 2.1 Steps involved in modeling process; $y(t_i)$ is the observed data at N data points, where $1 < i \leq N$, and $M(t_i, \theta)$ denote the model, where θ is the parameter vector

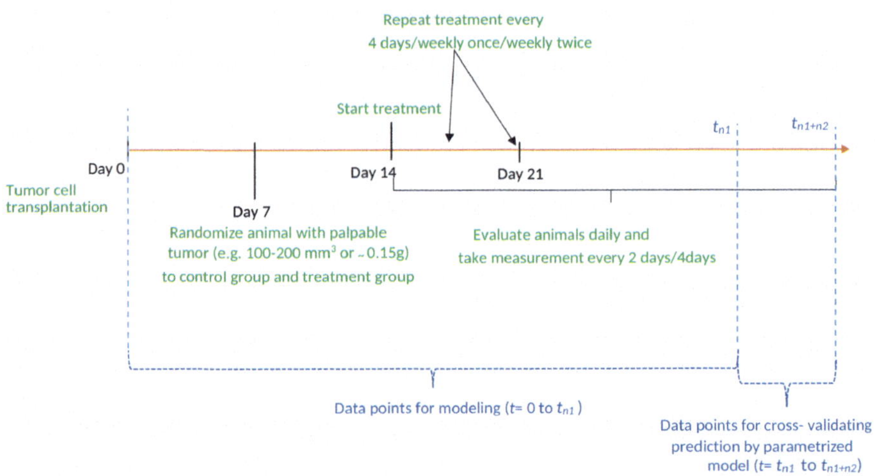

Fig. 2.2 An illustrative timeline of experimental events for data collection for an in vivo experiment using an animal model. The time period $(0, t_{n1})$ denotes the time during which data is collected for modeling and (t_{n1}, t_{n1+n2}) denotes the time interval during which data is collected for cross-validating the prediction by the parameterized model

2.2 Data Collection

Data collection methods should be rationally designed before conducting experiments to ensure the identifiability of parameters of the mathematical model. Due to the potential benefits of mathematical modeling, many ongoing clinical trials plan data collection to facilitate mathematical modeling (e.g. NCT03792529, NCT02028494, NCT03983538, NCT03381092) [9, 12, 13]. As shown in Fig. 2.2, the structure of the timeline of data collection is more or less the same for the in vivo and in vitro experiments. However, the total time duration of the experiment will be more for an in vivo experiment (animal models and clinical trials). In the case of in vivo experiment using animal models, tumor cells are transplanted on Day 0 and after sufficient days, say 7 d, animals with detectable (palpable) tumor are randomized to the control group and testing group (e.g. treated group). The animal may be evaluated every two to four days and measurements can be noted accordingly [14]. For instance, in [15], after tumor induction in mice models, tumor growth data are collected from 4 to 22 d in the case of lung cancer and 18 to 38 d in the case of breast cancer.

Similarly, in the case of in vitro models (e.g. 2D cell-culture, 3D spheroids, or organ-on-chip (OOC)), cancer cell lines are seeded on Day 0 and treated after 24 or 48 h and then, data collection (measurements) can be conducted on an hourly or daily basis. In Fig. 2.2, the time period $(0, t_{\mathrm{n1}})$ denotes the time interval during which data is collected for modeling and $(t_{\mathrm{n1}}, t_{\mathrm{n1+n2}})$ denotes the time interval during which data is collected for cross-validating the prediction by the parameterized model. In both cases (in vitro and in vivo), control and treated groups are maintained for model calibration.

Functional models that are devised based on the mechanistic insight about the disease rely on quantitative observations to estimate the parameter values of the model. Common quantitative measures include growth measurements, flow cytometry analysis, biochemical analysis, and immunological or histopathological biomarker-based assessment, to name few [16, 17]. For instance, to quantify a time-varying drug concentration, blood samples before and after treatment can be assessed using liquid chromatography or mass chromatography [18]. Calibrated images and time-lapse videos from various microscopes can be used for detecting fluorescence emitted by cells. Such 2D images and 3D time-lapse videos are commonly used in quantifying parameters required for modeling. For instance, in [19], the association of epithelial cells with endothelial cells that line the blood vessels is quantified using calibrated images to develop a mathematical model of metastasis. Similarly, in [20], fluorescence microscopy is used to quantify the effect of a drug on the internalization of HER2 (human epidermal growth factor receptor 2) in case of HER2 overexpressing breast cancer cells. In [21], treatment-induced reduction in the number of cells in a cell-culture plate is quantified using the time-resolved microscopy at a time resolution of 3 h for 4 d. Cell confluence data are converted into number of cells using an average cellular radius of 1.25×10^{-3} cm and plate area of $0.32\,\mathrm{cm}^2$.

2.3 Model Fitting

The fourth step in developing mathematical models is model fitting (Fig. 2.1). In this section, the details of data normalization, choosing appropriate descriptive models, types of growth models, types of treatment models, and various data fitting algorithms used for fitting individual or population data to the model parameters are presented.

2.3.1 *Normalization*

Normalization of data is a pre-processing step that is used to standardize or adjust the values of a data set in a meaningful way, sometimes to fit a common scale for comparison to make sense, or to bring the values of the parameters in the same range for comparison. For example, the min-max scaling is a normalization given by $y_N = \frac{y - y_{min}}{y_{max} - y_{min}}$, where y_N is the normalised version of the data point y, y_{min} and y_{max} are the minimum and maximum values of data. In the case of regression analysis, normalization is done using $y_N = \frac{y-\mu}{\sigma}$, where μ and σ are the mean and standard deviation of observed data, respectively. Normalization of data is important when computational tools are used to find numerical solutions to nonlinear ODEs. For instance, adding very small and very big numbers, and approximation of numbers by rounding off may pose errors in numerical solutions. Scaling of the data by using normalization methods facilitates easier and less erroneous use of numerical methods.

In the case of tumor growth data, often it is required to rescale measurements or convert growth measurements of a tumor to the number of cells in the tumor for easy interpretation and comparison. A common conversion factor is derived out of the relation $1\text{mm}^3 = 10^6$ cells [3, 22]. However, the number of cells per unit volume may be different for different cell types. The average cell size of various cell lines of cancers of breast, colon, kidney, and blood are reported to be in the range of 11.95–18.26, 11.09–14.48, 14.86–20.80, and 9.66–16.14 μm, respectively [23–25]. Hence, in [5], to compare data obtained from in vivo and in vitro experiments, first the volume of a single cell using the known initial number of cells and the initial tumor volume for each cancer cell lines are determined. For example, in the case of a cell line of pancreatic cancer, a multiplication ratio of 2.85×10^{-3} cells/μm^3 is used to convert the volume of the tumor to the number of cells in the tumor. If the measurement of the area of the tumor is available, the number of cells is obtained using the relation $\theta_r A_{area}\sqrt{A_{area}}$, where θ_r is the multiplication ratio, A_{area} is the area of the tumor to calculate the cell number from the volume conversion ratio. Similarly in [26], the tumor volume is calculated using $A_{vol} = \frac{1}{2}\phi_1^2\phi_2$, $\phi_1 < \phi_2$, where ϕ_1 and ϕ_2 are two perpendicular diameters. In [15], an ellipsoid shape is assumed for the tumor and its volume is calculated using $A_{vol} = \frac{\pi}{6}\phi_1^2\phi_2$.

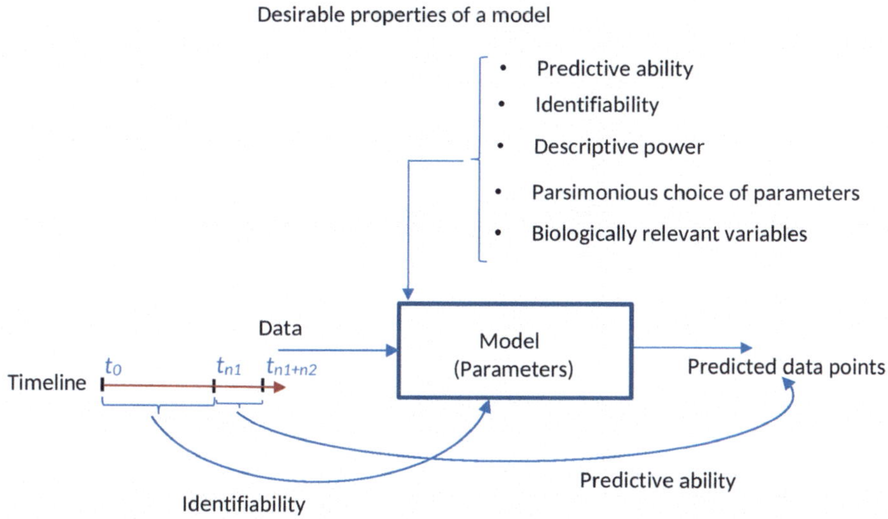

Fig. 2.3 Illustrative diagram showing the desirable properties of a model. Data should be rich enough for ensuring the identifiability of all parameters. The predictive ability assesses the capability of the model to predict any missing or future tumor dynamics that the model is representing. Data collected during the time period $(0, t_{n1})$ is used to estimate model parameters and (t_{n1}, t_{n1+n2}) is used to assess predictive ability. Descriptive power quantifies the goodness of fit of the model and data. A model with less number of (parsimonious) biologically relevant variables is desirable

2.3.2 *Choosing Descriptive Model*

Choosing an appropriate descriptive model is a very important step in developing a mathematical model. As shown in Fig. 2.1, $y(t_i) - M(t_i, \theta)$ shows the validity of a model in describing the cancer dynamics. Hence, choosing a biologically inappropriate or mathematically inadequate model description in place of $M(t, \theta)$ can affect the applicability and reliability of the mathematical model. Recall that mathematical models can accommodate a wide variety of biological mechanisms related to cancer. For instance, when some models represent the metastatic behavior of cancer cells, others study the behavior of drug-sensitive and drug-resistant cell types. As given in later chapters of this book, there exist models that characterize drug delivery and cancer annihilation mediated by oncolytic viruses and nanomedicines. Hence, according to the research hypothesis which is under investigation (Step 1 in Fig. 2.1), and based on the general understanding of the mechanism, an appropriate descriptive model should be selected to represent $M(t, \theta)$.

The experimental design for data collection should be planned according to the biological aspects that the model should account for. Figure 2.3 shows the desirable properties of a good model. A model with good descriptive power fitted appropriately to the observed data is expected to have a good predictive ability. Using a minimal (parsimonious) number of biologically relevant parameters is also a desirable prop-

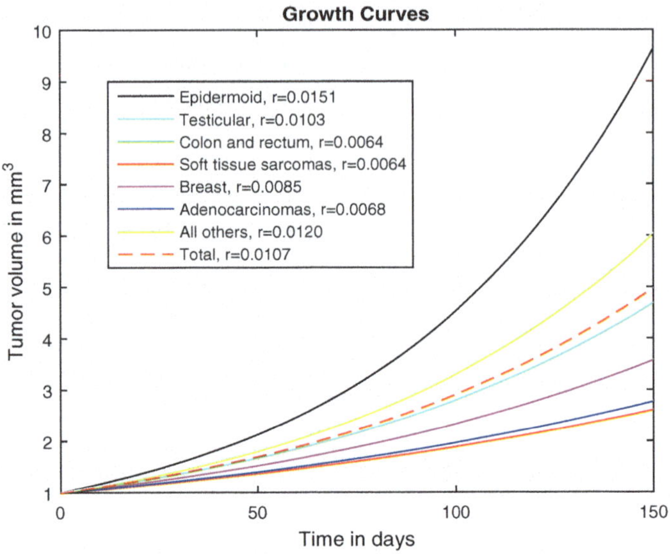

Fig. 2.4 Different growth rates for different types of cancers, where r is the growth rate calculated using Roentgenogram data [3, 22, 29]. In this figure, the tumor volume trajectory of cancer in colon and rectum and soft tissue sarcoma are plotted with the same r value

erty of a good model. Out of the desirable properties shown in Fig. 2.3, parameter parsimony and biological relevance can be decided by the appropriate choice of descriptive model. Identifiability, predictability, and goodness of fit of the model, and data can be assessed after the parameter estimation step.

2.3.3 *Types of Growth Models*

Attempts to study the tumor growth patterns have started in early 1930s [7, 27–29]. Initially, scientists modeled the tumor growth in terms of exponential model assuming a constant tumor volume-doubling time (TVDT). Figure 2.4 shows different growth rates of cancers using exponential constant r, $C_{\mathrm{p}}(t) = C_{\mathrm{p0}}e^{rt}$, $C_{\mathrm{p}}(0) = C_{\mathrm{p0}}$, calculated using the Roentgenogram data [3, 22, 29]. Using the data on TVDT, many research works emphasize that it can take 10–15 years for a tumor to grow to a detectable size $1\mathrm{cm}^3 \approxeq 10^9$cells [3, 22]. Many other clinical trials also support the fact that most of the lethal tumors are several years old at the time of detection or diagnosis. For many types of cancers, there is ample time between the tumor initiation to lethal period. This points out to the scope for improvement of treatment outcome by using better diagnostics tools for cancer. But unfortunately, very less is known about the initiation of a tumor which restricts diagnosis at an early stage.

Growth kinetics in tumors have been studied extensively using caliper based measurements and cellular level analysis. For instance, in [29] the growth kinetics of four types of breast cancer cells are analyzed using (1) growth curves, (2) thymidine labeling techniques, and (3) flow cytometric DNA analysis and it is reported that the growth rates of different types of cancer do not have similar patterns. Using the thymidine labeling technique, the mitotic index is calculated which is the ratio of cells undergoing mitoses to the total number of cells and it is shown that, even though the tumor growth is increasing, the mitotic index (the relative number of proliferating cells) is not increasing. Moreover, by using repeated flow cytometric DNA analysis on the cells aspirated from the tumors over time, it is confirmed that there is no change in cell-cycle characteristics of the tumor cells over the growth period [29]. However, many research works report the reduction in the number of proliferating cells in the tumor over time [22, 29–32]. The vigor of tumor growth may be different during different phases of tumor growth leading to different growth patterns. Similarly, in [15] it is pointed out that when the caliper measured data shows an exponential increase in the tumor volume, a bio-luminescence-based assay which only quantify living cells in a tumor shows a logistic pattern. Clinical observation based on Roentgenogram data also suggests that different types of cancers have different growth rates [3, 22, 29].

Over the last 70 years, numerous investigation have been conducted using various in vitro and in vivo experiments on different types of cancer and several reviews have been reported in this regard [3, 5–7, 15, 22, 29, 33–43]. These reviews identify (1) a different rate of tumor growth as the observed TVDT is different for different cancers, (2) a growth retardation factor is limiting the growth over time, hence simple exponential model cannot fit, (3) there is a threshold beyond which the growth pattern changes or switches from exponential to linear, (4) the net tumor growth reflects molecular interactions, genetic pathways, angiogenesis, and immune cell involvement, and (5) tumor cells in a single neoplasm display significant heterogeneity in morphological and physiological features such as proliferation rate, expression and types of cell surface receptors, and angiogenic potential. Characterizing these features are imperative in cancer modeling. Even though there is no universal law that fits growth patterns of all cancers, modeling cancer-specific growth can help in decision making regarding the choice of right drug dose and treatment schedules.

In the following part of this subsection, different types of growth models are presented that are used to represent the growth of various cell types ($C_{pi}(t), i = 1, 2, \ldots,$ in (1.1)) such as tumor cells, normal cells, immune cells, etc. in a tumor microenvironment. However, all of these models are primarily developed to explain tumor cell dynamics. Specifically, the exponential, Von Bertalanffy, logistic, Gompertz models, and a model that accounts for dynamic carrying capacity are explained.

2.3.3.1 Exponential and Exponential-Linear Models

As mentioned earlier, the exponential model of tumor growth is based on the assumption of a constant growth rate. This can be interpreted as all the cells taking a constant time to complete the cell-cycle (i.e. constant proliferation rate) from G_0 phase to the mitosis phase. The exponential model ($\mathrm{G_{Ex}}(r)$) is given by:

$$\frac{\mathrm{d}C_\mathrm{p}(t)}{\mathrm{d}t} = rC_\mathrm{p}(t), \tag{2.1}$$

where $C_\mathrm{p}(t) = C_{\mathrm{p}0}e^{rt}$, $C_\mathrm{p}(0) = C_{\mathrm{p}0}$, $C_\mathrm{p}(t)$ is the amount of tumor cells and r is the growth rate. Due to the heterogeneity of cells in the tumor micro-environment, proliferation rate may not be constant for all cells. Moreover, as mentioned earlier, all the cells in the tumor may not be undergoing cell division. Most of the tumors are identified to have a necrotic core that does not contribute to net tumor growth. Hence, an exponential-linear model ($\mathrm{G_{Ex-lin}}(r_0, r)$) as given by:

$$\frac{\mathrm{d}C_\mathrm{p}(t)}{\mathrm{d}t} = \begin{cases} r_0C_\mathrm{p}(t), & t \leq \tau \\ r, & t > \tau \end{cases}, \tag{2.2}$$

is also used [15, 44]. Here, r_0 is the proliferation of cells during $0 < t \leq \tau$, $\tau = \frac{1}{r_0}\log\left(\frac{r}{r_0C_{\mathrm{p}0}}\right)$ (to assure continuously differentiable solution), and r is the growth rate for linear part [15].

2.3.3.2 Power-Law Model

Power-law formula gives a relationship between the growth of the tumor and its geometrical features in terms of an exponent p. The increase in the overall tumor volume can be described with respect to the increasing tumor radius or in terms of the outer proliferative rim of the tumor. Mathematical model of the tumor growth that follows power-law ($\mathrm{G_{Po}}(r, p)$) is given by:

$$\frac{\mathrm{d}C_\mathrm{p}(t)}{\mathrm{d}t} = r(C_\mathrm{p}(t))^p, \tag{2.3}$$

where r is the growth rate and p is the exponent quantifying relative growth rate. Here, the proliferative tissue of the tumor is proportional to $(C_\mathrm{p}(t))^p$. When the tumor cell proliferation is limited to the outer rim of the tumor, the exponent value is set as $p = 2/3$. Assuming that the proliferative cells are uniformly distributed in the tumor, the value of the exponent becomes $p = 1$, which makes (2.3) same as (2.1). Any value of p, $0 < p < 1$, indicates a decreasing growth fraction or that the whole cell population is not contributing to the overall volume increase of the tumor. Similar case is when the vascular supply is limited to the outer area of the tumor. Hence, a modified form of the power-law is used in modeling tumor vasculature [45]. The solution of (2.3) when $p < 1$ is given by $C_\mathrm{p}(t) = \left(C_{\mathrm{p}0}^{(1-p)} + (1-p)rt\right)^{\frac{1}{1-p}}$ [46, 47].

2.3.3.3 Von Bertalanffy Model

The Von Bertalanffy growth model is based on the understanding that the overall growth of an organism is a result of a balance between constructive and destructive processes involved in its metabolism (anabolism and catabolism) [15, 38]. Von Bertalanffy equation is derived based on the allometric (growth-related to size, shape, physiology) observations related to the growth of the organism [1, 5, 15, 38]. Inspired from this, the net increase in the tumor volume is assumed to follow a similar pattern and hence is modeled using Von Bertalanffy ($G_{Vo1}(r, p, d)$) equation as:

$$\frac{\mathrm{d}C_{\mathrm{p}}(t)}{\mathrm{d}t} = r(C_{\mathrm{p}}(t))^{p} - dC_{\mathrm{p}}(t), \tag{2.4}$$

where r is the growth rate, p is the exponent that quantifies relative growth rate, and d accounts for the effect of destructive or growth-suppressive factors in the tumor micro-environment. The solution of (2.4) is given by:

$$C_{\mathrm{p}}(t) = \left(\frac{r}{d} + ((C_{\mathrm{p0}})^{1-p} - \frac{r}{d})e^{-d(1-p)t}\right)^{\frac{1}{1-p}}. \tag{2.5}$$

Under the assumption of the proliferative rim and necrotic core, a value of $p = 2/3$ is used in [46]. In [5], a two-parameter version of the Von Bertalanffy equation ($G_{Vo2}(r, k)$) such as:

$$\frac{\mathrm{d}C_{\mathrm{p}}(t)}{\mathrm{d}t} = r(k - C_{\mathrm{p}}(t)), \tag{2.6}$$

given in [48, 49] is used to make the number of parameters the same as that of the logistic model for ease of comparison of various models.

2.3.3.4 Generalized Logistic Law and Logistic Law

The experimentally observed decrease in the growth rate reported in many tumors made the researchers to think of a sigmoid model to describe the tumor growth. In this case, the assumption is that, as time progresses, the net tumor volume will converge to the carrying capacity. The generalized logistic law model ($G_{Glo}(r, k, p)$) is given by:

$$\frac{\mathrm{d}C_{\mathrm{p}}(t)}{\mathrm{d}t} = rC_{\mathrm{p}}(t)\left(1 - \left(\frac{C_{\mathrm{p}}(t)}{k}\right)^{p}\right), \tag{2.7}$$

where k is the carrying capacity and the solution of (2.7) is given by:

$$C_{\mathrm{p}}(t) = \frac{C_{\mathrm{p0}}k}{\left((C_{\mathrm{p0}})^p + (k^p - (C_{\mathrm{p0}})^p)e^{rpt}\right)^{1/p}}. \tag{2.8}$$

By setting $p = 1$, the model given in (2.7) is called as the logistic law ($G_{\mathrm{Lo}}(r, k)$) which accounts for the competition between different cell populations in the tumor micro-environment for nutrition and space [15].

2.3.3.5 Gompertz Law

Gompertz law accommodates the slow growth at the beginning and towards the end of the growth curve (sigmoid like) and there are generally many forms of Gompertz model. In [15], Gompertz model ($G_{\mathrm{Go1}}(r, \beta)$) is used as given by:

$$\frac{\mathrm{d}C_{\mathrm{p}}(t)}{\mathrm{d}t} = re^{\beta t}C_{\mathrm{p}}(t), \tag{2.9}$$

where r is the initial proliferation rate and β denotes the rate of decrease in the proliferation rate [15]. The solution of (2.9) is given by $C_{\mathrm{p}}(t) = C_{\mathrm{p0}}e^{\frac{r}{\beta}(1-e^{-\beta t})}$, and as $t \to \infty$, it follows that $C_{\mathrm{p}}(t) \to k$, where $k = C_{\mathrm{p0}}e^{r/\beta}$ [15]. The most popular form of the Gompertz model ($G_{\mathrm{Go2}}(r, k)$) is given by [5]:

$$\frac{\mathrm{d}C_{\mathrm{p}}(t)}{\mathrm{d}t} = r\log\left(\frac{k}{C_{\mathrm{p}}(t)}\right)C_{\mathrm{p}}(t), \tag{2.10}$$

where r is the growth rate, k is the carrying capacity, $C_{\mathrm{p}}(t) = ke^{\left(\log(C_{\mathrm{p0}}/k)e^{-rt}\right)}$, and as $t \to \infty$, it follows that $C_{\mathrm{p}}(t) \to k$.

2.3.3.6 Dynamic Carrying Capacity Model

This model ($G_{\mathrm{Dc}}(r, d, k_0)$) accounts for the varying carrying capacity due to the vascularization of the tumor and is given by:

$$\frac{\mathrm{d}C_{\mathrm{p}}(t)}{\mathrm{d}t} = rC_{\mathrm{p}}(t)\log\left(\frac{k(t)}{C_{\mathrm{p}}(t)}\right), \tag{2.11}$$

$$\frac{\mathrm{d}k(t)}{\mathrm{d}t} = d(C_{\mathrm{p}}(t))^{2/3}, \tag{2.12}$$

where $k(t)$ is the variable carrying capacity with intial value $k_0 = k(0)$. Even though this model is primarily used for quantifying anti-angiogenic therapy, in [15], this model is categorized as a type of tumor growth model. This model allows to account

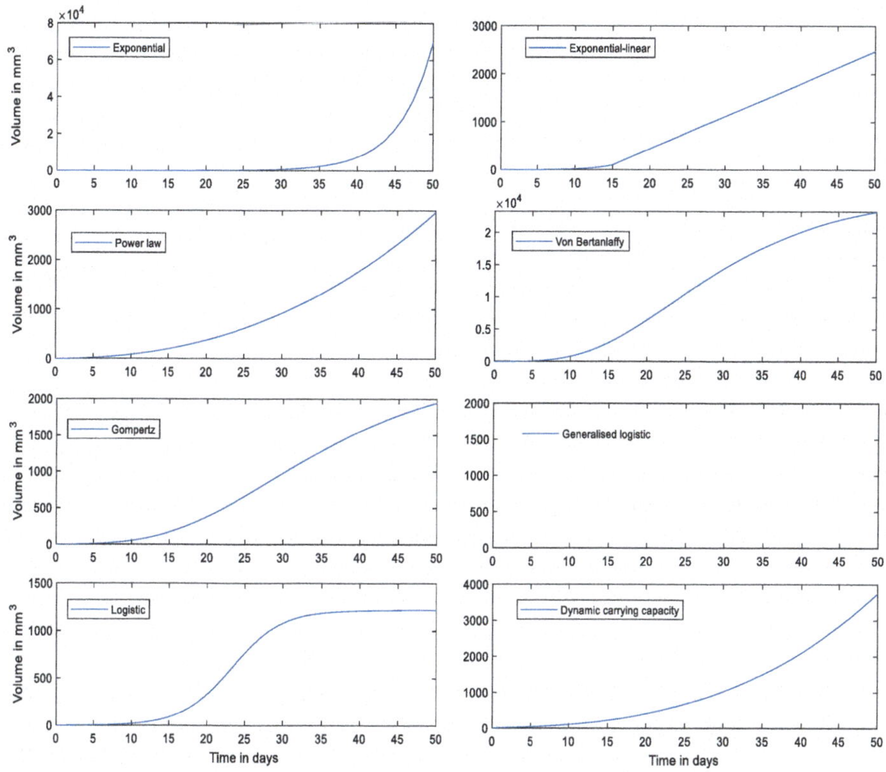

Fig. 2.5 Simulated plots for various types of growth models. Estimated parameter values of the breast cancer (population) data given in [15] are used to generate these plots. Model name, notation and parameter values of each model are given in order: exponential model, $G_{Ex}(r)$, $r = 0.223\,\text{day}^{-1}$; exponential-linear model, $G_{Ex-lin}(r_0, r), r_0 = 0.31\,\text{day}^{-1}, r = 67.8\,\text{mm}^3\,\text{day}^{-1}$, $\tau = 15$ days; power-law model $G_{Po}(r, p)$, $r = 1.32\ \text{mm}^{3(1-p)}\ \text{day}^{-1}$, $p = 0.58$; Von Bertalanffy model $G_{Vo1}(r, p, d)$, $r = 2.32\ \text{mm}^{3(1-p)}\ \text{day}^{-1}$, $p = 0.918$, $d = 0.808\ \text{day}^{-1}$; Gompertz model $G_{Go1}(r, \beta), r = 0.56\,\text{day}^{-1}, \beta = 0.0719\,\text{day}^{-1}$; Generalized logistic model $G_{Glo}(r, k, p), r = 2753$ day^{-1}, $k = 1964\ \text{mm}^3$, $p = 2.68 \times 10^{-05}$; Logistic model $G_{Lo}(r, k)$, $r = 0.305\ \text{day}^{-1}$, $k = 1221$ mm^3; Dynamic carrying capacity-based model $G_{Dc}(r, d, k_0)$, $r = 2.63\ \text{day}^{-1}$, $d = 0.829\ \text{mm}^{-2}$ day^{-1}, $k_0 = 12.7\ \text{mm}^3$ [15]. See Table 2.3 for model equations

for the effect of fully functional blood vessels that are limited to the surface of the tumor ($p = 2/3$ in (2.12)) on overall carrying capacity of the tumor.

Comparison of various types of growth models: Several works present comparative studies on various types of growth models using clinical and experimental data [5, 15, 26, 50]. These reviews point out that there is a high coefficient of variation in the parameters for each evaluated model fit. The reason for this high variation is attributed to the interpersonal change in the growth rate due to environmental and genetic factors, eating habits, and the extent of vascularization in the tumor. Figure 2.5 shows a comparison of various types of growth models.

In [5], an extensive study is conducted based on ten types of cancers such as cancers in bladder, breast, colon, head & neck, liver, lung, skin, ovary, pancreas, and kidney. Unit normalized form of the data published in 59 papers between the years 1983–2009 are used for this study which include both in vivo (in humans and mice) and in vitro data. Moreover, at least 5 or up to 10 sets of data are used for model fitting of each of the ten types of cancers. Similarly, in [15], a very detailed analysis of experimental mice models is conducted to compare various types of growth models in terms of goodness of fit, predictability, and identifiability. Tumor growth of induced lung and breast cancers in mice models are used for model fitting. Model fitting is done using 20 animals in case of lung cancer and 34 animals in case of breast cancer. In order to compare various growth models, the findings in [5] and [15] are summarized in Tables 2.3 and 2.4.

Comparing the descriptive power, identifiability, and predictability of eight types of models presented in Tables 2.3 and 2.4, it is clear that there is no single model that is suitable for all types of cancers. However, if one is looking for a model that fits not to all, but to most of the types of cancers, then based on the extensive analysis presented in [5] and [15] and summarized in these tables, Gompertz model shows reasonable goodness of fit for cancers in the lung, breast, head and neck, bladder, liver, and pancreas. Moreover, this model shows a reasonable predictive ability for breast cancer data as well. However, as stated in [15], $G_{Go1}(r, \beta)$ has better identifiability compared to $G_{Go2}(r, k)$.

Similarly, the logistic model $G_{Lo}(r, k)$ also shows a good fit for cancers in the breast, liver, lung, kidney, and skin. Based on breast cancer and lung cancer data, this model shows good identifiability [15] and exhibits a good fit in predicting the progression of lung cancer in human [50]. However, the logistic and generalized logistic model do not show acceptable predictive ability compared to all other models based on the breast and lung cancer data studied in [15]. Even though the generalized logistic model ($G_{Glo}(r, k, p)$) shows the best fitness characteristics for breast and lung data, however this model with three parameters has poor identifiability.

The power-law $G_{Po}(r, p)$ is the best fit (rank 1) for most of the types of cancers [5, 15, 26]. This model shows the best or a good fit for cancers in the bladder, colon, skin, ovary, pancreas, kidney, head and neck, and lungs. With respect to breast and lung cancer data, this model has good identifiability property as well. However, the power-law model is highly sensitive to changes in the values of r and p. Moreover, increasing the exponent p even by 10% results in a biologically unjustifiable increase in tumor growth. Hence, even though this model shows the best fit for most of the cancers (Table 2.3), it is not recommended due to its unstable nature. As it will be seen in the later chapters of this book, power-law is not commonly used to describe the tumor growth dynamics [5, 15].

It should be noted that, in Tables 2.3 and 2.4, the best fit refers to rank 1 and the good fit refers to rank 2 based on the used GFF metrics. Comparing the Gompertz and power-law models, while Gompertz shows good fit, power-law shows the best fit for most of the cancer data. However, due to its high sensitivity to parameters and biologically unjustifiable nature, Gompertz model or logistic model is preferred over the power-law model.

Table 2.3 Comparison of various types of growth models [5, 15]

Model	$\frac{dC_p(t)}{dt} =$	No. of parameters	Descriptive Power
(1) $G_{Ex}(r)$	$rC_p(t)$	1	Best fit for ovarian cancer data [5]
(2) $G_{Ex-lin}(r_0, r)$	$\begin{cases} r_0 C_p(t), & t \leq \tau \\ r, & t > \tau \end{cases}$	2	Best fit for breast cancer data in [15]
(3) $G_{Po}(r, p)$	$rC_p^p(t)$	2	Best fit for bladder, colon, melanoma, ovarian, pancreatic, and RCC and good fit for HNSCC and lung data [5]
(4) $G_{Vo1}(r, p, d)$ (5) $G_{Vo2}(r, k)$	$rC_p^p(t) - dC_p(t)$ $r(k - C_p^p(t))$	3 2	Good fit for colon data in [5] based on $G_{Vo2}(r, k)$
(6) $G_{Go1}(r, \beta)$ (7) $G_{Go2}(r, k)$	$re^{\beta t}C_p(t)$ $rC_p(t)\log\left(\frac{k}{C_p(t)}\right)$	2 2	Good fit for lung and breast data in [15] based model $G_{Go1}(r, \beta)$ Best fit for HNSCC and good fit for bladder, breast, liver, and pancreatic data in [5] based on model $G_{Go2}(r, \beta)$
(8) $G_{Glo}(r, k, p)$	$rC_p(t)\left(1 - \left(\frac{C_p(t)}{k}\right)^p\right)$	3	Best fit for breast and lung data in [15]
(9) $G_{Lo}(r, k)$	$rC_p(t)\left(1 - \frac{C_p(t)}{k}\right)$	2	Best fit for breast, liver, and lung and good fit for RCC and melanoma data in [5]
(10) $G_{Dc}(r, d, k_0)$	$rC_p(t)\log\left(\frac{k(t)}{C_p(t)}\right)$, $\frac{dk(t)}{dt} = d(C_p(t))^{2/3}$	3	–

[1] In [5], at least 5 data sets (in vitro, in mice, and in human) each on 10 different types of cancers (in bladder, breast, colon, head-neck, liver, lung, skin, ovary, pancreas, and kidney) are used to compare model numbers (1), (3), (5), (7), and (9). Normalized residuals of least-squares is the GFF metric used for model comparison. Best fit refers to the model with rank 1, and good fit refers to rank 2 based on GFF metric. RCC-renal cell carcinoma, HNSCC-head-neck squamous cell carcinoma

[2] In [15], data sets (in mice) on breast and lung cancers are used to compare model numbers (1), (2), (3), (4), (6), (8), (9) and (10). RMSE, R^2, and AIC are the GFF metrics used for model comparison

Table 2.4 Comparison of various types of growth models [5, 15]

Model	Identifiability	Predictability
(1) $G_{Ex}(r)$	Identifiable	–
(2) $G_{Ex-lin}(r_0, r)$	Identifiable	Best (83.8%) based on breast data
(3) $G_{Po}(r, p)$	Identifiable	Poor (42%) based on lung data and good (62.3%) based on breast data
(4) $G_{Vo1}(r, p, d)$ (5) $G_{Vo2}(r, k)$	Poor (44.5%) based on lung data	
(6) $G_{Go1}(r, \beta)$ (7) $G_{Go2}(r, k)$	Identifiable Poor identifiability	Good (59%) based on breast data
(8) $G_{Glo}(r, k, p)$	Poor identifiability	–
(9) $G_{Lo}(r, k)$	Identifiable	–
(10) $G_{Dc}(r, d, k_0)$	Poor identifiability	42% for the lung data and 63.3% for the breast data

In [15], it is emphasized that each model has a different percentage of predictive power for various cancer data. The exponential-linear model shows the highest value of predictive power (80%) for 12 d horizon for breast cancer data, and using the lung cancer data no model is able to achieve predictive power of (70%) for 1 day horizon. These values indicate the importance of using a cancer-specific growth pattern while modeling the tumor dynamics.

2.3.4 *Types of Treatment Models*

As mentioned in Sect. 1.3, various types of therapies such as chemotherapy, immunotherapy, radiotherapy, etc. are used to manage cancer. These therapies are classified according to the mode of action of the therapeutic agents. While some agents lead to cancer cell-lysis by inducing cell-cycle arrest, others mediate a drug-induced ligand-receptor binding that attracts immune cells to kill cancer cells. In general, the effect of therapy on the tumor micro-environment may not be direct cell-death and there can be drug-induced growth inhibition, cell mutation, and changes in the carrying capacity. For instance, the chemotherapeutic drug tamoxifen inhibits estrogen binding and thus restricts the progression of cell-cycle leading to the accumulation of cells in G_1 phase of the cell-cycle. Hence, tamoxifen does not induce apoptosis directly, instead cell stress due to cell-cycle arrest and cell accumulation in G_1 phase induces apoptosis [51, 52]. The following are some of the specific examples of treatment effects on the tumor dynamics:

- *Growth inhibition:* Many drugs cause the growth inhibition by mediating a cell-cycle arrest. For instance, cdk-inhibitor drugs such as palbociclib inhibit cells from passing the initial growth phase (G_1-phase) of cell-cycle and thus cannot proliferate further. Tubulin-targeting drug namely paclitaxel is an example of another agent that can bring about growth inhibition by blocking the progression of mitosis. Hormone deprivation therapy can inhibit the growth of hormone-dependent cancer cells. All these effects can be modeled as a reduction of the growth rate parameter r or using the drug effect parameter a in (1.1).
- *Direct cell-kill:* Oncovirotherapy can cause a direct cell-kill by increasing the viral burden in cancer cells. Most of the growth inhibitors which cause a cell-cycle arrest also lead to a cell death. Such effects can be modeled using the parameters r, d, or a in (1.1).
- *DNA damage:* Most of the alkylating agents used for cancer treatment cause cellular apoptosis by inducing DNA damage at various phases of cell-cycle (e.g. cisplatin). Radiation therapy can also cause DNA damage which later on leads to the cell death. Such effects can be modeled using the parameters r, d, or a in (1.1).
- *Antibody induced cell death:* Antibodies that specifically bind to the concerned receptor on the cancer cells are used to block intracellular signaling which leads to the growth inhibition and cell death (e.g. pertuzumab, trastuzumab). In this case, antibody specific drug effect can be modeled based on the number of receptors on the cancer cells and the time-varying amount of free and bound antibodies in the tumor micro-environment. Such effects can be modeled using the parameters r, d, or a in (1.1).
- *Enhanced predation by immune cells:* Most of the immunotherapeutic agents cause cancer cell lysis by this method. Several drug types such as immune checkpoint inhibitors, monoclonal antibodies, and immune-enhancing cytokines are used to boost the predation of cancer cells by the immune cells. For instance, monoclonal antibodies (e.g. trastuzumab) that bind with respective receptors on cancer cells can increase the immunogenicity of cancer. Such antibodies can attract immune cells to the tumor micro-environment, which in turn enhances the cancer cell lysis. All these effects can be modeled by increasing the competition term or predation term c or using the parameter a in (1.1).
- *Effect on carrying capacity:* Growth inhibition mediated by anti-angiogenic agents also induce tumor shrinkage. This effect of treatment can be modeled as a change in carrying capacity of tumor, i.e. in the parameters b, r, and d in (1.1).
- *Effect on mutation rate:* In the case of hormone deprivation, the drug effect reflects in cell mutation rate m as well. This is due to the mutation of hormone-dependent cells to independent cells. Similar is the case when cells mutate from drug-sensitive to drug-resistant variants under treatment.

Even though cancer management is facilitated through a wide variety of drugs with different mechanisms of action, most of the mathematical models that depict treatment effects are based on many simplifying assumptions. Moreover, many of the existing models reflect the effect of treatment rather than in vivo dynamics of the drugs. Next, some common types of cancer treatment models are discussed.

The model (1.1)–(1.2) can be rewritten as:

$$\frac{dC_{p1}(t)}{dt} = \overbrace{\mathscr{F}\left(r, d, b, c, m, C_{p1}(t, \tau), C_{p2}(t)\right)}^{\text{overall growth}} \pm \overbrace{\mathscr{D}\left(a, C_{p1}(t, \tau), U(t)\right)}^{\text{effect of therapy}}, \quad C_{p1}(0) = C_{p1_0}, \tag{2.13}$$

$$\frac{dU(t)}{dt} = \mathscr{D}_c\left(d_U, U(t, \tau), u(t)\right), \quad U(0) = U_0, \tag{2.14}$$

where $\mathscr{F}(\cdot)$ denotes a function representing the overall growth of the tumor, $\mathscr{D}(\cdot)$ is the effect of therapy, and $\mathscr{D}_c(\cdot)$ is the pharmacokinetics which includes circulation, metabolism, and elimination kinetics of the drug. As mentioned in Chap. 1, the function $\mathscr{D}(\cdot)$ may be added to or subtracted from the overall growth function $\mathscr{F}(\cdot)$ depending upon the type of therapy. For instance, while immune-boosting drugs increase the number of T cells and/or amount of cytokine, chemotherapeutic drugs reduce the overall cell growth.

2.3.4.1 Proportional Effect Model

In 1964, Skipper, Schabel, and Wilcox reported a chemotherapy treatment model that assumes that the cell-kill effect is proportional to tumor growth [53]. Specifically, early treatment models of cancer therapy are based on Skipper's first and second laws of cancer growth and treatment [54, 55]. The first law states that TVDT is constant and the second law states that the effect of the drug on the tumor growth follows a first-order kinetics. This implies that a fixed fraction of cancer cells is killed irrespective of the tumor size. Skipper-Schabel-Wilcox model of chemotherapy is also known as log-kill model [54, 55]. This model assumes that if the tumor grows exponentially with a constant TVDT (r), then due to a treatment, the tumor shrinks at a constant rate a. The log-kill model is given by:

$$\frac{dC_p(t)}{dt} = rC_p(t) - aC_p(t)U(t), \tag{2.15}$$

where $U(t)$ denotes the drug concentration (exposure). Note that, the log-kill model is originally defined for tumor cells that follow exponential growth. However, in many literature, a general, first-order cell-kill model as given by $\frac{dC_p(t)}{dt} = \mathscr{F}(C_p(t)) - aC_p(t)U(t)$ is termed as log-kill model [14, 40, 56].

Similar to the log-kill model which is defined based on exponential model of tumor growth and proportional cell-kill effect, Norton-Simon model is defined based on the Gompertzian model of tumor growth and proportional cell-kill effect [54, 57]. The Norton-Simon model is given by:

$$\frac{dC_p(t)}{dt} = r\log\left(\frac{k}{C_p(t)}\right)C_p(t) - aC_p(t)U(t). \tag{2.16}$$

Even though Norton-Simon model is defined with respect to Gompertz growth, in general, dose (exposure) dependent treatment effect are modeled as $\frac{dC_p(t)}{dt} = \mathscr{F}(C_p(t)) - aC_p(t)U(t)$ are called as Norton-Simon model [58, 59]. In some literature, the drug effect is modeled in terms of an additional damage cell compartment [40] given by:

$$\frac{dC_{p_s}(t)}{dt} = \mathscr{F}(C_{p_s}(t)) - aC_{p_s}(t)U(t), \tag{2.17}$$

$$\frac{dC_{p_d}(t)}{dt} = aC_{p_s}(t)U(t) - dC_{p_d}(t), \tag{2.18}$$

where $C_p(t) = C_{p_s}(t) + C_{p_d}(t)$, $C_{p_s}(t)$ and $C_{p_d}(t)$ are the drug sensitive cells and damaged cells, a and d are drug induced cell-kill rate and death rate, respectively. The concept of damage cell in modeling is useful in the case of radiotherapy which induces direct cell-death by double strand break and indirect cell-kill by single stand break in the DNA of the irradiated cells [60, 61].

2.3.4.2 Sigmoid Model

Michaelis–Menten equation: Michaelis-Menten form of equation, which is originally used to describe enzymatic kinetics in biochemical reactions are later on adapted to model treatment effect of cancer therapy. Specifically, in biochemistry, the enzyme-mediated chemical reactions are modeled in terms of the substrate-binding rate. Similarly, in cancer therapy, the immune cell-mediated tumor cell-kill is modeled in terms of the anti-tumor efficacy of immune cells. Michaelis-Menten equation is given by:

$$\mathscr{D}_1(a, C_p(t)) = \frac{I_{max} C_p(t)}{a + C_p(t)}, \tag{2.19}$$

where $C_p(t)$ denotes the cells on to which the effector cells or drug bind, a is the binding affinity (Michaelis-Menten constant), and I_{max} is the maximum interaction rate or maximum drug effect (limiting rate). Note that the effect of therapy in (2.13) is given by $\mathscr{D}(a, C_p(t), U(t)) = \mathscr{D}_1(a, C_p(t))U(t)$. This form is also used to accommodate the effect of the cytokines on the tumor-immune interactions [36, 62, 63]. For instance, in [64], the increase in immune cells due to the effect of cytokines (cell-signaling proteins) such as IL-12 and IL-2 are also modeled using Michaelis-Menten form.

Hill equation: Hill equation is another common nonlinear term used mainly to model the dose-dependent response of drugs including cytotoxic agents [65]. Drugs can act as ligands that bind to the receptors on the cells to mediate the drug effect. Hence, the drug effect which is proportional to the amount of ligand-bound receptors is modeled in terms of Hill equation as:

$$\mathscr{D}_1(a, U(t)) = \frac{1}{1 + \left(\frac{a}{U(t)}\right)^n}, \tag{2.20}$$

where $\mathscr{D}_1(a, U(t))$ denotes the ligand-receptor product, a is the half-saturation constant that models the ligand concentration resulting in half-occupancy of receptors, and n is the Hill-coefficient. Another form of Hill equation is:

$$\mathscr{D}_2(a, C_\mathrm{p}(t)) = \frac{I_{\max}(C_\mathrm{p}(t))^n}{a^n + (C_\mathrm{p}(t))^n}. \tag{2.21}$$

Note that the effect of therapy in (2.13) is given by $\mathscr{D}(a, C_\mathrm{p}(t), U(t)) = \mathscr{D}_1(a, U(t)) C_\mathrm{p}(t)$ or $\mathscr{D}(a, C_\mathrm{p}(t), U(t)) = \mathscr{D}_2(a, C_\mathrm{p}(t))U(t)$ based on the form of Hill equation.

Holling type equations: Holling types I, II, and II are functional response patterns commonly used in ecology for modeling the predator-prey dynamics in terms of the density of prey versus the number of prey that is consumed by the predator [66]. Holling type I accounts for linearly increasing consumption of prey by the predators. Type II models initially increasing and then decelerating consumption of the prey due to a limited capacity. Type III is similar to type II, however in type III, compared to type II the initial consumption of the prey by the predator is slightly lesser due to the initial learning time of predation and then increases and saturates as the number of prey increases. Holling type III is more like a sigmoid curve. The model equation for Holling types I, II, and III are given by ([67]):

$$\mathscr{D}_1(a, C_\mathrm{p}(t)) = aC_\mathrm{p}(t), \tag{2.22}$$

$$\mathscr{D}_2(a, C_\mathrm{p}(t)) = \frac{aC_\mathrm{p}(t)}{1 + C_\mathrm{p}(t)}, \tag{2.23}$$

$$\mathscr{D}_3(a, C_\mathrm{p}(t)) = a\frac{(C_\mathrm{p}(t))^2}{g + (C_\mathrm{p}(t))^2}, \tag{2.24}$$

where a is the drug effect and g is the concentration of therapeutic agent above which the effect increases quickly to saturation value (maximum effect). Note that the effect of therapy in (2.13) is given by $\mathscr{D}(a, C_\mathrm{p}(t), U(t)) = \mathscr{D}_i(a, C_\mathrm{p}(t))U(t)$, $i = 1, 2, 3$ based on the used Holling type.

In case of cancer modeling, competition between different cell populations such as the predator-prey type of interaction between cancer cells, host cells, and immune cells can be modeled using Holling type equations [68, 69]. Another example of a predator-prey type of interaction occurs in the case of oncovirotherapy. In the case of oncovirotherapy, the infection of cancer cells by the oncolytic virus can be modeled using the Holling type of equation [69]. Comparing the curves of Michaelis-Menten and Hill-equation, when the first type gives a rectangular hyperbola, the second one gives a sigmoid curve. Michaelis-Menten is a special case of the Hill model given by (2.21) with $n = 1$. Holling type III is similar to the Hill equation (sigmoid). Another form of sigmoid function that is used to model the drug effect is $\mathscr{D}_1(a, U(t)) = a\big(1 - e^{U(t)}\big)$, with $\mathscr{D}(a, C_p(t), U(t)) = \mathscr{D}_1(a, U(t))C_p(t)$ in (2.13).

When multiple drugs are used in combination, there can be a synergistic or additive drug interaction. Synergy is when one drug enhances the potency (effect) of another drug and additivity is when there is no interaction between the drugs, but the overall drug effect will be the sum of cell-kill due to individual drugs [70, 71]. As mentioned in the experimental design section, the data collected from the control group (untreated) can be used to calibrate the treatment independent parameters, and the data from the treated group can be used to calibrate treatment dependent parameters. In the case of treatment with drug combinations, there are two options (1) sequential doses, and (2) simultaneous doses. In the case of sequential treatment, after fixing general parameters $(\mathscr{G}, \mathscr{A}, \mathscr{K}, \mathscr{C})$, the drug effect term $(\mathscr{D}_1(a_1, \psi_1, C_{p1}(t), U_1(t))$, with ψ_1 as the drug synergy parameter, for the first drug can be calibrated. Then, fixing $\mathscr{D}_1(.)$ the parameters for $\mathscr{D}_2(a_2, \psi_1, C_{p1}(t), U_2(t))$ can be calibrated using the measurement data. In the case of combination treatment after fixing general parameters $(\mathscr{G}, \mathscr{A}, \mathscr{K}, \mathscr{C})$, the model parameters can be calibrated for the drug combination simultaneously [21]. Such parameter calibration strategies are used to develop mathematical models of cancer dynamics under combination treatment that is discussed in later chapters.

2.3.5 Drug Toxicity Effect

Drug-induced toxicity is a major concern in cancer therapy that is often graded from 1 to 5, where 1-mild, 2-moderate, 3-severe, 4-life-threatening, or 5-lethal [27]. Drug toxicity levels are decided by the cumulative effect of all enzymatic reactions between the toxic compounds in the drug and the intracellular components [120]. The cumulative drug toxicity in the body due to a drug (e.g. chemotherapy agent) can be modeled as ([120]):

$$\frac{\mathrm{d}T_x(t)}{\mathrm{d}t} = U_{cp}(t), \tag{2.25}$$

where $T_x(t)$ is the drug toxicity level and $U_{cp}(t)$ is the concentration of the drug in the blood plasma. Different drugs cause different kinds of toxic responses. In some cases, as the drug is metabolized and eliminated from the body, the toxicity level may decrease. This can be modeled as

$$\frac{\mathrm{d}T_x(t)}{\mathrm{d}t} = U_{cp}(t) - \eta_E T_x(t), \tag{2.26}$$

where the first term describes the increase in the toxicity with respect to increase in the drug concentration and the second term models the decrease in toxicity due to drug metabolism at a rate η_E. In order to account for the influence of the saturation of enzyme-catalyzed reactions in inducing drug toxicity, logistic and Gompertz model are also proposed in [120]. The logistic model is given by

$$\frac{\mathrm{d}T_{\mathrm{x}}(t)}{\mathrm{d}t} = \eta_{\mathrm{L}} T_{\mathrm{x}}(t)\left(1 - \frac{T_{\mathrm{x}}(t)}{2\theta_{\mathrm{Tx}}}\right), \tag{2.27}$$

and Gompertz model is given by

$$\frac{\mathrm{d}T_{\mathrm{x}}(t)}{\mathrm{d}t} = \eta_{\mathrm{G}} T_{\mathrm{x}}(t) \ln \frac{2\theta_{\mathrm{Tx}}}{T_{\mathrm{x}}(t)}, \tag{2.28}$$

where η_{L} and η_{G} are positive constants and θ_{Tx} is the maximal longanimous toxicity value.

In case of some drugs, the relation between drug toxicity and drug concentration remains linear for lower doses, however, shows an exponential response beyond a certain threshold value of drug concentration [27, 118]. In [27], initially linear and then exponentially increasing (with concentration) curve is chosen to represent the toxicity level. Since, the maximum level (grade) of toxicity is 5, the value of drug concentration that is slightly above the maximum tolerated dose (MTD) or maximum allowable dose ($U_{\mathrm{cp}}(t) = \mathrm{MTD} + 0.5\%$) is assigned a toxicity level of 5.

In [119], $T_{\mathrm{x}}(t) = \alpha U_{\mathrm{cp}}(t)$, where α is the slope of concentration-effect curve, $\alpha = 0.126\,\mu\mathrm{M}^{-1}$, is used to quantify the drug-induced toxicity on bone marrow cell proliferation (myelosuppression). Similar to [27], in [118], an illustrative graphical diagram is used to show that toxicity is low in low dose and it exponentially increases with high dose.

2.3.6 Model Fitting Approaches

Model fitting is the next important step in the development of mathematical models (Fig. 2.1). After choosing appropriate descriptive models for each of the functions in (1.1), model fitting can be done against experimentally observed data. Mathematically, the best fit of model parameters that can reproduce the observed data is required. Thus, the problem is to estimate θ such that

$$y(t_i) = M(t_i, \theta), \tag{2.29}$$

where $y(t_i)$ is the observed data at N data points, $1 < i \leq N, \theta \in \mathscr{R}^{\Gamma}$ is the parameter vector, and $M(t_i, \theta)$ is the model. There are many algorithms which use numerical and stochastic optimization methods to identify the best fit parameters for a given model and measured data [5, 15, 72, 73]. Some of the commonly used algorithms in the area of computational biology are Nelder-Mead algorithm [4, 15], Levenberg-Marquardt (LM) algorithm [74, 75], Markov-chain fitting with simulated annealing [5], Markov-chain Monte-Carlo method [76–78], stochastic approximation of expected maximization [15, 79, 80], interior-point-search algorithm [81], or combination of these algorithms [5, 15, 82]. All these algorithms basically implement two methods such as (1) least-square minimization or (2) likelihood maximization.

2.3.6.1 Least-Squares Approach

In the least-square curve fitting problem, the aim is to search for the parameter set θ that minimizes the least squared error, denoted as $S(\theta)$, given as:

$$S(\theta) = \sum_{i=1}^{N} \left[y_i - M(t_i, \theta) \right]^2, \tag{2.30}$$

and the weighted least square version is given by $S(\theta) = \sum_{i=1}^{N} w_i \left[y_i - M(t_i, \theta) \right]^2$, where w_i denotes weights. One of the caveat of least-square methods are its extreme sensitivity to outliers in the observed data which increase the residual, $y_i - M(t_i, \theta)$. Robust least square methods can be used to overcome this issue. Least absolute residual method and bisquare weighted methods are two robust least square methods [72, 83].

In the linear least-square problem, the model $M(t_i, \theta)$ (2.30) represents a linear model, while for nonlinear least-square problem, $M(t_i, \theta)$ is a nonlinear model. Gauss-newton method, gradient method, and direct search methods [84] are some of the techniques to solve the nonlinear least squared problem. Nelder-Mead algorithm (NMA) and Levenberg-Marquardt algorithm (LMA) are the most widely used nonlinear least-square algorithm to solve the parameter fitting problems pertaining to cancer dynamics [5, 15]. NMA is a heuristic numerical method that relies on a simplex direct search method to find an acceptable local optimal solution. LMA, which is also known as a damped least-square method is a type of Gauss-Newton method that uses the trust-region approach for solving the minimization problem. In [75], LMA is used to solve the nonlinear least-square problem. A nonlinear least-squares problem can also be formulated as a convex optimization problem with constraints. Such parameter estimation problems can also be solved using the LMA algorithm and interior-point algorithm [85, 86].

2.3.6.2 Stochastic Approaches

Nonlinear least-square methods that are based on probabilistic (stochastic) approaches are also used for solving parameter fitting problems [87, 88]. In this case, probability density function (PDF) is used to accommodate uncertainties associated with modeling. Note that, here the observed data (y_i), model function ($M(t_i, \theta)$), and parameters (θ) can have uncertainties that stem from the system-model mismatch, measurement errors, and noise. The stochastic approximation algorithm aims to identify the posterior PDF of the model parameters conditioned on the observed data so as to solve the parameter estimation problem given by (2.29). Thus, the problem here is to find the posterior PDF of the model, which is the conditional probability that can be assigned after considering the evidence (here measured data). Posterior PDF can be quantified using likelihood $\mathrm{p}(y|\theta)$ and prior probability $\mathrm{p}_{\mathrm{pr}}(\theta)$ such as:

$$\mathrm{p}_{\mathrm{po}}(\theta) = \theta_{\mathrm{k}}\mathrm{p}(y_i|\theta)\mathrm{p}_{\mathrm{pr}}(\theta) \tag{2.31}$$

where $\mathrm{p}_{\mathrm{po}}(\theta)$ is the posterior probability and θ_{k} is the normalization constant. The best fit model parameter can be obtained by maximizing the likelihood $\mathrm{p}(y_i|\theta)$, as given by:

$$M_{\mathrm{LS}} = \mathrm{argmax}_{\theta}\ \mathrm{p}(y_i|\theta), \tag{2.32}$$

where M_{LS} is the maximum likelihood solution and $\mathrm{p}(y_i|\theta)$ is the probability of y_i given the parameter θ [87, 88]. Note that there can be imperfection in the choice of the model function $M(t_i, \theta)$ which will also contribute to the residual error $(y_i - M(t_i, \theta))$. Hence, as mentioned earlier in Sect. 2.1, the choice of appropriate descriptive model is very important and should be revisited based on the new insights that are gained about cancer dynamics and treatment mechanism.

Deriving a complete analytical solution for the nonlinear least squared and stochastic approximation problems defined above is quite tedious and hence algorithms that are built-on well established numerical methods are used to find a solution [5, 15, 89]. There are several softwares such as MATLAB, R, Python, Monolix, Eureqa, JMP, etc. that have in-built toolboxes for solving curve-fitting problems defined above. As the stochastic estimation method accounts for the randomness in the model and measured data, algorithms used to solve the problem return estimated values of parameters as well as a measure of confidence on the estimated parameters with respect to the experimental data.

In [5], two algorithms, namely, Nelder-Mead simplex direct search function (e.g. *fminsearch* in MATLAB®) and Markov-chain fitting with simulated-annealing [5] are used to minimize the least-squared error between model prediction and data set. NMA is based on a local search method, in which the user needs to provide a good initial guess and the algorithm will search for the best-fit parameter in the bounded region in the parameter space around initial parameters. Hence, only an initial guess close to the global solution can provide a globally optimal solution. Otherwise, the algorithm can guarantee a local minimum solution only. Globally minimum solutions are desirable as they provide a better fit compared to local minimum solutions. Markov-chain Monte-Carlo (MCMC) is a stochastic fitting method that provides the global minimum as it can search in wider range of parameter space compared to NMA [76–78]. However, the algorithm converges to a global minimum with a higher number of iteration which may be computationally costly. For a lesser number of iterations, the algorithm gives different answers, which may be local minimal solutions.

In the case of simulated annealing, estimates of each iteration are used as the initial condition for the next iteration. Hence, as the number of iteration increases, the algorithm may converge to a solution that is closer to the global minimum. One advantage of the NMA method is that it is faster than MCMC. Hence, in [5], a hybrid of these two methods is also used. That is, first NMA is used to minimize the least square problem and then the results are used as initial conditions for MCMC which is repeated for a sufficient number of times to yield a good-fit. Note that even though MCMC often leads to the global minimum and is less likely to fall into a local minima, its convergence to the global minimum takes more time and computational steps. Hence, after running a sufficient number of MCMC and using the final result for running, one more round of NMA provides a better solution.

In [15], individual and population data-based parameter estimation problems are defined in the stochastic framework. The individual data-based approach is solved using the trust-region algorithm and Nelder-Mead algorithm to obtain the best estimate of parameter vector $\hat{\theta}$. In [14], a delayed-rejection adaptive metropolis (DRAM) based-bayesian inference method which involves an adaptive updation of the covariance matrix is used to solve the parameter estimation problem. DRAM is a reverse sampling method used in association with the MCMC method to improve the convergence of the algorithm [90]. In [26], the model parameters are estimated using Hooke and Jeeves optimization combining global and local search heuristics and least-squares curve-fitting [91]. Parameter sets achieving maximal model agreement with experimental training data are selected.

2.4 Model Validation

After deciding an appropriate model description $M(t, \theta)$, and estimating the parameter set $\hat{\theta}$ using any of the mentioned methods discussed earlier, the next step is to validate the model (Figs. 2.1, 2.2, and 2.3). Model validation is done using the measured data from the same experimental subjects used for parameter estimation or from a different set (separate training and validation data set) of experiments [15, 26, 92]. In general, a mathematical model is validated by assessing one or more of the following:

- Goodness of fit (GFF) metrics which assess how well the model $M(t, \hat{\theta})$ can reproduce observed data that are used for parameter estimation.
- Reliability of estimated parameters in terms of their confidence measures.
- Identifiability of parameter estimates from the available data.
- Predictability of individual or population behavior during t_i, $n_1 < i \leq n_2$, using estimated model $M(t, \hat{\theta})$.
- Standard errors pertaining to the range of values of the estimated parameter $\hat{\theta}$.

As shown in Fig. 2.3, a mathematical model that shows good fit, less standard errors of estimates, good reliability, identifiability, and predictability is desirable.

2.4.1 Goodness of Fit

There are many statistically motivated methods to assess GFF. Ideally, a model with a lesser number of parameters (parsimonious model) and acceptable GFF is appropriate. Trade-off between GFF and parameter parsimonious model is a balance to be achieved. The common measures of GFF are:

- Akaike information criterion (AIC)
- The root mean squared error (RMSE)
- Statistical test for normality of residuals (R^2, p-test), and
- Sum of squared error (SSE)

Akaike information criterion is a common estimator used to estimate the relative quality of various models [15, 93]. AIC is useful in comparing models with a different number of parameters. The model with lesser AIC value indicates better GFF and AIC penalizes models with more parameters thus favoring parsimonious models. RMSE is a classical GFF criterion that quantifies the error between observed value and model prediction. When RMSE quantifies the absolute fit between data and model, R^2 provides a relative measure of fit [26, 94]. Similar to AIC, lesser RMSE indicates better GFF. Ranking based on AIC is one of the important criteria used for model selection.

Apart from the criteria listed above, there are several statistical metrics used to assess GFF. Individual weighted residuals (IWRES) and visual predictive checks are used in [94] for model validation. Predictive models are mostly built based on probability theories such as in metastatic prediction, and relapse prediction [4, 94]. In [95], the mean squared error (MSE) and Schwarz Bayesian Criterion (SBC) are used to measure GFF of a mathematical model of prostate cancer that represents the dynamics of androgen deprivation therapy and prostate-specific antigen (PSA). Lower values of MSE and SBC indicate better goodness of fits. In [15], the reliability of the estimates ($\hat{\theta}$) is quantified using the nonlinear least squares (NLS) regression method in terms of standard errors and confidence intervals pertaining to the derived parameter vector $\hat{\theta}$ evaluated using the common metrics such as normalised mean square error (NMSE), coefficient of variation (CV), and normalized standard error (NSE).

2.4.2 Identifiability

Identifiability of parameters quantifies whether or not all the parameters can be estimated from the available experimental data. Identifying all the parameters of an overparameterized model may be difficult, hence it is imperative to judiciously choose an appropriate descriptive model for parameter estimation [4]. In a statistical framework, the parameters to be estimated is assumed as random variables, that has a distribution which accounts for uncertainty in the estimation according to the uncertainty in data. Thus, by using the Jacobian matrix derived from the error model and parameter sensitivity model, it is easy to determine the covariance matrix of the distribution [4, 73], and the standard errors related to parameter estimates are the square roots of the diagonals of the covariance matrix. This helps to assess the practical identifiability of estimated parameters of a model from a given data.

Similarly, the condition number obtained from Fisher-information matrix (FIM) can be used to assess the parameter identifiability [96, 97]. In the case of models with a large set of parameters and a limited set of data, FIM can be used to determine the identifiability of parameters from the available data. FIM along with estimates of the covariance matrix is used to assess the identifiability of parameters estimated using maximum likelihood approaches [97, 98]. In cases when the limitation in available data restricts the identifiability of parameters of a model, the ensemble Kalman filter may be used to provide a better estimation of the parameters.

2.4.3 *Predictability*

Predictability quantifies how well the model $M(t, \hat{\theta})$ is able to predict the behavior of the modeled dynamics. Prediction score can be calculated by quantifying the normalization error at each data points during the time interval $t_{n1} < t \leq t_{n1+n2}$ (Fig. 2.2). An estimated model with good predictability is expected to have less deviation from observed data, $y_i - M(t_i, \hat{\theta})$, $n_1 < i \leq (n_1 + n_2)$. In [96], the prostate cancer data is used to estimate the parameter values of a mathematical model. The ensemble Kalman filter is used to improve the identifiability and predictability of the model. Model parameters are estimated with respect to the observed prostate-specific antigen (PSA) level using *fmincon* in MATLAB which supports the interior-point algorithm and trust-region-reflective algorithm.

2.4.4 *Sensitivity Analysis*

In simple words, sensitivity analysis involves assessing the effect of small change in a parameter on the final outcome (e.g. tumor growth, cell-kill, immune cell influx) over a period of time. Sensitivity analysis is important to identify the parameters of the system that significantly influence the output of the system [75]. These sensitive parameters can influence the behavior of the system. For instance, in the case of tumor dynamics, a sensitive parameter can switch the system from a tumor-free state to a high tumor state or vice versa. On the other hand, insensitive parameters point to the redundant parameters which may be removed from the model for model simplification.

A common method to assess parameters of the model is by conducting fitting evaluation by following one-at-a-time method in which parameter sensitivity of one parameter is evaluated keeping others constant. However, a stronger sensitivity analysis is suggested for fitting evaluation of models with too many parameters [5, 21, 75]. In general, parameter sensitivity is assessed by varying each model parameter in a range, say 1–10% of its value and then corresponding changes in the final outcome are examined for the duration of about 10–50 days [5, 92]. For instance, in [92], parameters are perturbed by 1% to evaluate the corresponding changes for 25 d. A common sensitivity cutoff is 0.05, which indicates that the parameters cause less than 5% of variation in the output.

In [75], Sobol's global sensitivity method is used for sensitivity analysis. This method is based on analysis of variance (ANOVA) and it calculates sensitivity indices by randomly sampling the parameter space. In [14], a partial rank correlation coefficient (PRCC) analysis is used to investigate the sensitivity of parameters. The value of PRCC varies from -1 to 1, where a negative value is for an inverse relation. PRCC analysis studies the coefficient of correlation between input and output variables using the residual analysis. Sobol's sensitivity and PRCC can be evaluated using *sbiosobol* and *partialcorr* in Matlab software.

2.5 Equilibrium Points and Stability Analysis

As discussed in Chap. 1, the dynamics of the cell populations in a tumor microenvironment is influenced by several interlaced and nonlinear mechanisms represented mathematically using nonlinear dynamical equations. Deriving an analytical solution to study the long term behavioral of such heavily nonlinear system is quite tedious. Alternatively, stability of the linearized version of the original system can be analyzed to understand the approximate dynamics of the system around the equilibrium points. Similar to the parameter estimation and model validation steps discussed earlier, an equilibrium point analysis is a common technique that comes into picture while using mathematical models to analyze the cancer dynamics. This method can be used to check the compliance of the developed mathematical model with its real world counter part (cancer dynamics), i.e. in simple words, to know whether the mathematical model is able to show the commonly seen biological aspects of cancer with and without treatment. In order to illustrate the relevance of the equilibrium point analysis in deriving useful information about the system behavior, in this section, a nonlinear dynamical system of cancer dynamics with chemotherapy discussed in [99] is considered as an example. The model is given by

$$\frac{\mathrm{d}N(t)}{\mathrm{d}t} = r_2 N(t)\left(1 - b_2 N(t)\right) - c_4 N(t)A(t) - a_1\left(1 - e^{-U(t)}\right)N(t), \tag{2.33}$$

$$\frac{\mathrm{d}A(t)}{\mathrm{d}t} = r_1 A(t)\left(1 - b_1 A(t)\right) - c_2 E(t)A(t) - c_3 N(t)A(t) - a_2\left(1 - e^{-U(t)}\right)A(t), \tag{2.34}$$

$$\frac{\mathrm{d}E(t)}{\mathrm{d}t} = s + \frac{\rho E(t)A(t)}{\alpha + A(t)} - c_1 E(t)A(t) - d_1 E(t) - a_3\left(1 - e^{-U(t)}\right)E(t), \tag{2.35}$$

$$\frac{\mathrm{d}U(t)}{\mathrm{d}t} = -d_{\mathrm{U}} U(t) + u(t), \tag{2.36}$$

where $N(t)$ and $A(t)$ represent the normal and cancer cells, $E(t)$ and $U(t)$ represent the immune cells and drug concentration, and $u(t)$ is the drug input, respectively, r_i and b_i quantify the growth rate and the reciprocal carrying capacity, c_i and d_i are the competition rate and death rate, and a_i, s, and d_U denote the drug effect, immune cell influx, and drug decay rate, respectively. Note that, the model (2.33)–(2.36) is a special case of (1.1)–(1.2). More detailed description of this model with biological relevance of each term is presented in Chap. 3 of this book. In this section, the main focus is on the equilibrium point analysis.

First, consider the no-drug case, wherein $U(t) = 0$ in (2.33)–(2.35). Equilibrium point can be derived by setting $\frac{dN(t)}{dt} = \frac{dA(t)}{dt} = \frac{dE(t)}{dt} = 0$, in (2.33)–(2.35) as follows:

$$0 = r_2 N_E (1 - b_2 N_E) - c_4 N_E A_E, \tag{2.37}$$

$$0 = r_1 A_E (1 - b_1 A_E) - c_2 E_E A_E - c_3 N_E A_E, \tag{2.38}$$

$$0 = s + \frac{\rho E_E A_E}{\alpha + A_E} - c_1 E_E A_E - d_1 E_E, \tag{2.39}$$

where N_E, A_E, and E_E denote the equilibrium values. Solving (2.37)–(2.39) for non-trivial N_E, A_E, and E_E, it follows that:

$$N_E = \frac{1}{b_2} - \frac{A_E}{r_2 b_2}, \tag{2.40}$$

$$A_E = \frac{1}{b_1} - \frac{c_2}{r_1 b_1} E_E - \frac{c_3}{r_1 b_1} N_E, \tag{2.41}$$

$$E_E = \frac{s(\alpha + A_E)}{(c_1 A_E + d_1)(\alpha + A_E) - \rho A_E}, \tag{2.42}$$

where (2.40)–(2.42) represent three sets of null surfaces. Equilibrium points are at the intersection of these surfaces [99]. Three realistic equilibrium points are considered as follows ([99]):

(1) Tumor-free equilibrium is obtained by setting $A_E = 0$, in (2.40)–(2.42), to get:

$$(N_E, A_E, E_E) = \left(\frac{1}{b_2}, 0, \frac{s}{d_1}\right). \tag{2.43}$$

(2) Dead-equilibrium is obtained by setting $N_E = 0$, in (2.40)–(2.42). Dead-equilibrium can be of two types, first with $N_E = 0,\ A_E = 0$ as:

$$(N_E, A_E, E_E) = \left(0, 0, \frac{s}{d_1}\right). \tag{2.44}$$

The second dead-equilibrium is when $N_E = 0$ and $A_E = x$, where x denotes a small amount of tumor cells that survive. Accordingly, $E_E = f(x)$ and

$$(N_{\mathrm{E}}, A_{\mathrm{E}}, E_{\mathrm{E}}) = \big(0, x, f(x)\big). \tag{2.45}$$

Letting $A_{\mathrm{E}} = x$ and $E_{\mathrm{E}} = f(x)$ in (2.40)–(2.42), it follows that $f(x) = \frac{r_1 b_1}{c_2}(\frac{1}{b_1} - x)$.

(3) Co-existing equilibrium. In this case, there can be a nonzero population of normal cells and tumor cells that co-exist. For $A_{\mathrm{E}} = x'$ amount of tumor cells survive, there can be accordingly $g(x')$ amount of normal cells and $f(x')$ amount of immune cells. Letting

$$(N_{\mathrm{E}}, A_{\mathrm{E}}, E_{\mathrm{E}}) = \big(g(x'), x', f(x')\big) \tag{2.46}$$

in (2.40)–(2.42), it follows that

$$x' - \frac{1}{b_1} - \frac{c_2}{r_1 b_1} f(x') - \frac{c_3}{r_1 b_1} g(x') = 0, \tag{2.47}$$

where x' is a solution of (2.47). It is clear from (2.43)–(2.46) that the parameters value of the system decide the exact number and position of equilibrium points. Note that, the idea of therapy is to drive the system states (N, A, E) to an equilibrium point wherein the patient stays healthy.

That is, the used therapy should drive the system to a stable tumor-free equilibrium which forces $N_{\mathrm{E}} \to 1$ (healthy) and $A_{\mathrm{E}} \to 0$. Apart from the tumor-free equilibrium, a stable equilibrium state where there is negligibly small or harmless amount (x') of tumor cells is also acceptable. According to the co-existing equilibrium, (2.46) and (2.47), this implies that $x' \to \epsilon$, where ϵ is a very small value and $N_{\mathrm{E}} = g(x') \to 1$ (healthy).

In order to analyze the range of parameter values for which the tumor-free equilibrium is stable, the Jacobian matrix of (2.33)–(2.36) with $U(t) = 0$ can be obtained as:

$$J = \begin{bmatrix} r_2 - 2r_2 b_2 N - c_4 A & -c_4 & 0 \\ -c_3 A & r_1 - 2r_1 b_1 A - c_2 E - c_3 N & -c_2 A \\ 0 & \frac{\alpha\rho E}{(\alpha+A)^2} - c_1 E & \frac{\rho A}{\alpha+A} - c_1 A - d_1 \end{bmatrix}. \tag{2.48}$$

Using the tumor-free equilibrium $(N_{\mathrm{E}}, A_{\mathrm{E}}, E_{\mathrm{E}}) = \big(\frac{1}{b_2}, 0, \frac{s}{d_1}\big)$ in (2.48), it follows that:

$$J = \begin{bmatrix} -r_2 & -c_4 & 0 \\ 0 & r_1 - \frac{c_2 s}{d_1} - \frac{c_3}{b_2} & 0 \\ 0 & \frac{\rho s}{d_1 \alpha} - \frac{c_1 s}{d_1} & -d_1 \end{bmatrix}, \tag{2.49}$$

with eigenvalues $\lambda_1 = -r_2 < 0$, $\lambda_2 = r_1 - \frac{c_2 s}{d_1} - \frac{c_3}{b_2}$, and $\lambda_3 = -d_1 < 0$. The tumor-free equilibrium given by $(N_{\mathrm{E}}, A_{\mathrm{E}}, E_{\mathrm{E}}) = \big(\frac{1}{b_2}, 0, \frac{s}{d_1}\big)$ is locally stable as long as all the eigenvalues are negative (i.e. if $\lambda_2 = r_1 - \frac{c_2 s}{d_1} - \frac{c_3}{b_2} < 0$). Using $N_{\mathrm{E}} = 1$ for healthy state in $N_{\mathrm{E}} = \frac{1}{b_2}$, it follows that $b_2 = 1$, and hence for having $\lambda_2 < 0$, the following condition should holds:

$$r_1 < \frac{c_2 s}{d_1} + c_3. \tag{2.50}$$

This gives a relation between the tumor growth rate r_1 and its association with the immune cell influx rate (s), competition between tumor cells and immune cells (c_2), competition between tumor cells and normal cells (c_3), and the death rate of immune cells (d_1). From (2.50), it is clear that λ_2 can be negative for high value of s. The term $\frac{c_2 s}{d_1}$ is defined as a resistance coefficient and it quantifies the efficiency of the immune system to resist the tumor growth [99]. If this resistance is high enough to meet the condition (2.50), then λ_2 remains negative and thus the tumor-free equilibrium remains stable. Using a similar analysis, eigenvalues of dead equilibrium (2.44) are always unstable and the ones for (2.45) can be either stable or unstable according to the parameters values. Similarly, in the case of co-existing equilibrium (2.47), equilibrium points occur at the intersection of the null-surfaces given by (2.40)–(2.42) and the number of equilibrium points varies (zero to three) according to the parameter values. As mentioned earlier, the idea of therapy is to drive the system states (N, A, E) to an equilibrium point wherein the patient stays healthy with zero tumor cells or a harmlessly small amount of tumor cells.

2.5.1 *Non-dimensionalization*

Non-dimensionalization generalizes the model equations and reveals characteristic properties in the system dynamics and thus facilitates easy analysis of the model. New variables for non-dimensionalization is chosen such that the resulting equation is unitless and rescaled. Non-dimensionalization can be done by setting $\theta^* = \frac{\theta - \theta_{\mathrm{r}}}{\theta'_{\mathrm{s}}}$, where θ_{r} is a reference value, θ'_{s} is a scaling parameter which has the same unit as θ, and θ^* is the new dimensionless variable. Letting $\theta_{\mathrm{r}} = 0$, $\theta_{\mathrm{s}} = \frac{1}{\theta'_{\mathrm{s}}}$, then it follows that $\theta^* = \theta_{\mathrm{s}}\theta$.

In this subsection, non-dimensionalization of (2.33)–(2.35) is discussed to generate a non-dimensional form of the system which is then used to analyze the effect of treatment. First, consider the drug free version of (2.33)–(2.35) as given by:

$$\frac{\mathrm{d}N}{\mathrm{d}t} = r_2 N (1 - b_2 N) - c_4 N A, \tag{2.51}$$

$$\frac{\mathrm{d}A}{\mathrm{d}t} = r_1 A (1 - b_1 A) - c_2 E A - c_3 N A, \tag{2.52}$$

$$\frac{\mathrm{d}E}{\mathrm{d}t} = s + \frac{\rho E A}{\alpha + A} - c_1 E A - d_1 E. \tag{2.53}$$

where the argument t is removed for brevity. Here, the variables to be non-dimensionalized are t, N, A, and E. Using the relation $\theta = \frac{\theta^*}{\theta_s}$, and defining $t = \frac{t^*}{t_s}$, $N = \frac{N^*}{N_s}$, $A = \frac{A^*}{A_s}$, and $E = \frac{E^*}{E_s}$ in (2.51), it follows that:

$$\frac{t_s}{N_s}\frac{dN^*}{dt^*} = r_2\left(\frac{N^*}{N_s}\right)\left(1 - b_2\left(\frac{N^*}{N_s}\right)\right) - c_4\left(\frac{N^*}{N_s}\right)\left(\frac{A^*}{A_s}\right), \tag{2.54}$$

and letting $t_s = r_2$, $N_s = b_2$, $A_s = \frac{1}{\alpha}$, $E_s = \frac{r_2}{s}$, and $c_4^* = \frac{c_4\alpha}{r_2}$ in (2.54), it follows that:

$$\frac{dN^*}{dt^*} = N^*(1 - N^*) - c_4^* A^* N^*. \tag{2.55}$$

Similarly, substituting $t = \frac{t^*}{t_s}$, $E = \frac{E^*}{E_s}$, $A = \frac{A^*}{A_s}$, and $N = \frac{N^*}{N_s}$ in (2.52) and (2.53), and letting $N_s = b_2$, $A_s = \frac{1}{\alpha}$, $E_s = \frac{r_2}{s}$, and $t_s = r_2$, it follows that:

$$\frac{dA^*}{dt^*} = \frac{r_1}{r_2}A^*\left(1 - b_1\alpha A^*\right) - \frac{c_2 s}{r_2^2}E^*A^* - \frac{c_3}{r_2 b_2}N^*A^*, \tag{2.56}$$

$$\frac{dE^*}{dt^*} = 1 + \frac{\rho E^* A^*}{r_2(1 + A^*)} - \frac{c_1\alpha}{r_2}E^*A^* - \frac{d_1}{r_2}E^*. \tag{2.57}$$

Letting $r^* = \frac{r_1}{r_2}$, $b^* = b_1\alpha$, $c_2^* = \frac{c_2 s}{r_2^2}$, and $c_3^* = \frac{c_3}{r_2 b_2}$ in (2.56), $\rho^* = \frac{\rho}{r_2}$, $c_1^* = \frac{c_1\alpha}{r_2}$, and $d^* = \frac{d_1}{r_2}$ in (2.57), and dropping the star notation, the non-dimensionalized dynamics is obtained as:

$$\frac{dN}{dt} = N(1 - N) - c_4 NA, \tag{2.58}$$

$$\frac{dA}{dt} = rA(1 - bA) - c_2 EA - c_3 NA, \tag{2.59}$$

$$\frac{dE}{dt} = 1 + \frac{\rho EA}{1 + A} - c_1 EA - dE. \tag{2.60}$$

2.5.2 Analysis with Drug

The non-dimensionalized model (2.58)–(2.60) can be used to make easy interpretation about the effects of drug on the behavior of the system. Towards this end, first consider rewriting (2.58)–(2.60) as:

$$\frac{dN}{dt} = N(1 - N) - c_4 NA - \mathscr{D}_1(U, t)N, \tag{2.61}$$

$$\frac{dA}{dt} = rA(1 - bA) - c_2 EA - c_3 NA - \mathscr{D}_2(U, t)A, \tag{2.62}$$

$$\frac{dE}{dt} = 1 + \frac{\rho EA}{1 + A} - c_1 EA - dE - \mathscr{D}_3(U, t)E. \tag{2.63}$$

where $\mathscr{D}_1(U,t)$, $\mathscr{D}_2(U,t)$, and $\mathscr{D}_3(U,t)$ are $a_i(1-e^{U(t)})$, $i=1,2,3$, $U(t)=U_0e^{-d_U t}$, where $U_0=U(0)$ denotes some time after the termination of drug administration. The functions $\mathscr{D}_i(U,t), i=1,2,3$ are such that for any $\epsilon, 0<\epsilon\ll 1$ and $t>T_0$, $\mathscr{D}_i(U,t)$, $i=1,2,3$, are less than a small value ϵ. Here, T_0 denotes a sufficiently large time after the termination of drug input. For all, $t>T_0$, the system (2.61)–(2.63) is like a ϵ-perturbed system given by:

$$\frac{\mathrm{d}N}{\mathrm{d}t}=N(1-N)-c_4NA-\epsilon N, \tag{2.64}$$

$$\frac{\mathrm{d}A}{\mathrm{d}t}=rA(1-bA)-c_2EA-c_3NA-\epsilon A, \tag{2.65}$$

$$\frac{\mathrm{d}E}{\mathrm{d}t}=1+\frac{\rho EA}{1+A}-c_1EA-dE-\epsilon E. \tag{2.66}$$

The Jacobian matrix of no drug case ((2.58)–(2.60)) is obtained as:

$$J=\begin{bmatrix}1-2N-c_4A & -c_4N & 0\\ -c_3A & r-2brA-c_2E-c_3N & -c_2A\\ 0 & \frac{\rho E}{(1+A)^2}-c_1E & \frac{\rho A}{1+A}-c_1A-d\end{bmatrix}, \tag{2.67}$$

and that of the treated case ((2.64)–(2.66)) is obtained as:

$$J_{\text{drug}}=\begin{bmatrix}1-2N-c_4A-\epsilon & -c_4N & 0\\ -c_3A & r-2brA-c_2E-c_3N-\epsilon & -c_2A\\ 0 & \frac{\rho E}{(1+A)^2}-c_1E & \frac{\rho A}{1+A}-c_1A-d-\epsilon\end{bmatrix}, \tag{2.68}$$

where $J_{\text{drug}}=J-\epsilon I$, $I\in\mathbb{R}^{3\times 3}$ is an identity matrix. The linearized model of (2.58)–(2.60) and (2.64)–(2.66) can be derived by substituting $(N,A,E)=(N_{\mathrm{E}},A_{\mathrm{E}},E_{\mathrm{E}})$ in (2.67) and (2.68), respectively. It is clear that the number of eigenvalues of (2.67) and (2.68) are similar but slightly perturbed ($\mathrm{Re}(\lambda_i)-\epsilon$) and thus their signs remain same for sufficiently small ϵ [99]. Hence, the perturbed system (2.64)–(2.66) has similar stability conditions (Sect. 2.5) given as $\lambda_2<0$ which leads to $r_1<\frac{c_2s}{d_1}+c_3+\epsilon$, for sufficiently small ϵ. It can be seen that the drug effect also contributes to increase the resistance coefficient which is required to keep the tumor-free equilibrium stable. In [99], by analyzing the basin of attraction of the "with-drug" and "no-drug", it is concluded that chemotherapy can be stopped once a system trajectory is inside the basin of attraction of the tumor-free equilibrium.

As shown above, the equilibrium point analysis can be used to analyze conditions to reach and remain around the tumor-free equilibrium [14, 56]. Using perturbation analysis and bifurcation analysis, one can comment on the conditions by which the tumor goes to high tumor equilibrium. Similarly, with respect to parameter values, the basin of attraction for each mode can be analyzed to derive conditions for converging to a healthy state or diverge to an exponentially increasing tumor burden [75].

Apart from the equilibrium point analysis, several techniques can be used to analyze (not to solve) the characteristic behavior of the nonlinear system. Phase-plane method [91, 99, 100], Lyapunov stability analysis [101, 102], Popov criterion [103], circle criterion [103], center-manifold theorem [104, 105], small-gain theorem [103, 106], and singular perturbation method [107] are some of the techniques of nonlinear system analysis that are used to analyze cancer dynamics. As mentioned earlier, these methods do not lead to an analytical solution but provide critical insights into the system behavior. For instance, the phase portrait of the system is a graphical representation of a vector field and these plots qualitatively show the behavior of the system with respect to the solutions of the system equation from a given initial point. Elaborating on the mathematical basis of these methods is beyond the scope of this book. There are several mathematical software (e.g. Matlab, Mathematica) that have inbuilt toolboxes that can be used to deduce useful information for easily commenting on the behavior of the system.

2.6 Summary

In this chapter, various types of growth models, treatment and toxicity models, model fitting algorithms, metrics used for fitting assessment and model validation, and an example for equilibrium point analysis pertaining to mathematical modeling of cancer dynamics are reviewed. As summarised earlier, there is no single growth model that fits to the growth data of all types of cancers. Hence, cancer-specific growth models are imperative to conduct a more reliable theoretical analysis related to cancer. As stated in [5], very few data sets include growth data until the tumor reaches its carrying capacity. Similarly, growth kinetics during the early stages of cancer initiation is very less.

In ecology, the Allee effect refers to a relation between population size and individual fitness which are measured in terms of per capita growth rate of the species. This term is used in ecology to describe the effect of an increase in the population of the species if there are more number of species in close aggregation suggesting that aggregation can favorably influence survival rate. More specifically, if a population exhibits shrinkage in low densities, they are said to have a strong Allee effect. This ecological based effect inspires many researchers to study tumor growth in low cell densities to gain some insight about cancer initiation and related events [108–111]. In [110], using a basin of attraction of tumor-free equilibrium (tumor extinction), it is shown that combination therapy is more successful than monotherapy as it can drive the system to an Allee region wherein the cell-survival is further restricted due to the lack of aggregation. Moreover, it is stated that the feedback regulation in cancer stem cells can cause an Allee effect. More investigation in this area may help us to answer critical questions regarding tumor initiation, tumor persistence, spontaneous tumor remission, tumor invasion and metastasis, phenotypic plasticity, and feedback regulation in stem cells [108–111].

Very few mathematical models have accommodated the effects of drug interaction while modeling treatment effects on cancer dynamics [21]. Accounting for specific drug interaction effects (additive, synergistic, and antagonistic) while developing mathematical models of cancer is desirable. Most of the treatment models account for the effect of treatment based on the observed (measurable) cell-kill or growth inhibition effect. However, accounting for the mechanism of action of drugs can help to gain better insight into the influence of drugs on various cell populations in the tumor micro-environment. For instance enormous data about the detailed pharmacokinetics and pharmacodynamics of many anti-cancer drugs are available [112–115]. Making use of these knowledge to develop mathematical models of tumor regression with respect to drug-specific action kinetics in the tumor micro-environment such as that in [21, 52, 75, 116] is desirable.

As mentioned earlier, it is imperative to develop cancer-specific and treatment specific mathematical models of cancer dynamics. Such models when used for theoretical analysis can provide valuable insight regarding cancer dynamics. For instance, in [92], model validation and parameter sensitivity analysis are done to derive important conclusions regarding treatment. A tumor-immune interaction model is presented by highlighting the involvement of NK cells and $CD8^+$ T cells in facilitating tumor surveillance and anti-tumor activities. Importantly, using sensitivity analysis, it is shown that the model is highly sensitive to a patient-specific parameter (assessed by chromium release assay) which can be used to identify patients that will respond to specific immune-mediated treatment. This is the power of mathematical models, which if properly devised by incorporating measurable biological markers can be used to assess patient cohorts that will benefit from a particular type of treatment by conducting cost-effective and risk-free in silico analysis. Computationally expensive maximum likelihood estimation methods such as the one which includes extended Kalman filter can be also used to deduce more accurate estimates of model parameters with limited available observations [15, 117]. In Chaps. 3–9, different mathematical models under various treatment strategies are presented.

References

1. D. Pauly, G. Morgan, et al., *Length-Based Methods in Fisheries Research*, vol. 13 (WorldFish, 1987)
2. I. Somers et al., On a seasonally oscillating growth function. Fishbyte **6**(1), 8–11 (1988)
3. J.S. Spratt, J.S. Meyer, J.A. Spratt, Rates of growth of human neoplasms: Part II. J. Surg. Oncol. **61**(1), 68–83 (1996)
4. C. Serdjebi, A. Boyer, P. Tomasini, C. Pouypoudat, D. Barbolosi, F. Barlesi, F. Chomy, S. Benzekry, Quantitative mathematical modeling of clinical brain metastasis dynamics in non-small cell lung cancer. Sci. Rep. **9** (2019)
5. E.A. Sarapata, L. Depillis, A comparison and catalog of intrinsic tumor growth models. Bull. Math. Biol. **76** (2013)
6. P.M. Altrock, L.L. Liu, The mathematics of cancer: integrating quantitative models. Nat. Rev. Cancer **15**, 730–745 (2015)
7. H.M. Byrne, Dissecting cancer through mathematics: from the cell to the animal model. Nat. Rev. Cancer **10**(3), 221–230 (2010)
8. W. Sun, Z. Luo, J. Lee, H.J. Kim, K. Lee, P. Tebon, Y. Feng, M.R. Dokmeci, S. Sengupta, A. Khademhosseini, Organ-on-a-chip for cancer and immune organs modeling. Adv. Healthcare Mater. **8**(4), 1801363 (2019)
9. R. Padmanabhan, H. S. Kheraldine, N. Meskin, S. Vranic, and A.E. Al Moustafa, Crosstalk between HER2 and PD-1/PD-L1 in breast cancer: from clinical applications to mathematical models. Cancers **12**(3), 636 (2020)

10. A. Fatehullah, S.H. Tan, N. Barker, Organoids as an in vitro model of human development and disease. Nat. Cell Biol. **18**(3), 246–254 (2016)
11. B.A. Ruggeri, F. Camp, S. Miknyoczki, Animal models of disease: pre-clinical animal models of cancer and their applications and utility in drug discovery. Biochem. Pharmacol. **87**(1), 150–161 (2014)
12. A. Suresh, A. Ganju, E. Morgan, M. Palettas, J. A. Stephens, J. Liu, M. Berger, C. Vargo, A. Noonan, R. Reinbolt, et al., Efficacy of different dosing schedules of capecitabine for metastatic breast cancer: a single-institution experience. Investigat. New Drugs 1–7 (2020)
13. Clinical trials, *U.S. National library of medicine: Bethesda, MD, USA* (2019)
14. S. L. Elliott, E. Kose, A. L. Lewis, A. E. Steinfeld, E.A. Zollinger, Modeling the stem cell hypothesis: investigating the effects of cancer stem cells and TGF- β on tumor growth (2019)
15. S. Benzekry, C. Lamont, A. Beheshti, A. Tracz, J. Ebos, L. Hlatky, P. Hahnfeldt, Classical mathematical models for description and prediction of experimental tumor growth. PLoS Computat. Biol. **10**(8), e1003800 (2014)
16. M. Wu, T.D. Perroud, N. Srivastava, C.S. Branda, K.L. Sale, B.D. Carson, K.D. Patel, S.S. Branda, A.K. Singh, Microfluidically-unified cell culture, sample preparation, imaging and flow cytometry for measurement of cell signaling pathways with single cell resolution. Lab on a Chip **12**(16), 2823–2831 (2012)
17. W.J. Koopman, H.-J. Visch, J.A. Smeitink, P.H. Willems, Simultaneous quantitative measurement and automated analysis of mitochondrial morphology, mass, potential, and motility in living human skin fibroblasts. Cytom. Part A: J. Int. Soc. Anal. Cytol. **69**(1), 1–12 (2006)
18. N. Faisant, J. Siepmann, J. Richard, J. Benoit, Mathematical modeling of drug release from bioerodible microparticles: effect of gamma-irradiation. Eur. J. Pharm. Biopharm. **56**(2), 271–279 (2003)
19. Y. Connor, Y. Tekleab, S. Tekleab, S. Nandakumar, D. Bharat, S. Sengupta, A mathematical model of tumor-endothelial interactions in a 3D co-culture. Sci. Rep. **9**(1), 1–14 (2019)
20. M. Fehling Kaschek, D. B. Peckys, D. Kaschek, J. Timmer, N. de Jonge, Mathematical modeling of drug-induced receptor internalization in the HER2-positive SKBR3 breast cancer cell-line. Sci. Rep. **9**(1), 1–16 (2019)
21. A.M. Jarrett, A. Shah, M.J. Bloom, M.T. McKenna, D.A. Hormuth, T.E. Yankeelov, A.G. Sorace, Experimentally-driven mathematical modeling to improve combination targeted and cytotoxic therapy for HER2+ breast cancer. Sci. Rep. **9**(1), 1–12 (2019)
22. J.S. Spratt, J.S. Meyer, J.A. Spratt, Rates of growth of human solid neoplasms: Part I. J. Surg. Oncol. **60**(2), 137–146 (1995)
23. S.C. Dolfi, L.L.-Y. Chan, J. Qiu, P.M. Tedeschi, J.R. Bertino, K.M. Hirshfield, Z.N. Oltvai, A. Vazquez, The metabolic demands of cancer cells are coupled to their size and protein synthesis rates. Cancer Metabol. **1**(1), 20 (2013)
24. B. Shashni, S. Ariyasu, R. Takeda, T. Suzuki, S. Shiina, K. Akimoto, T. Maeda, N. Aikawa, R. Abe, T. Osaki et al., Size-based differentiation of cancer and normal cells by a particle size analyzer assisted by a cell-recognition PC software. Biol. Pharm. Bull. **41**(4), 487–503 (2018)
25. D. Kuksin, L.L. Chan, Analyzing NCI-60 cancer cell lines. Technical report. http://www.nexcelom.com/Applications/Cancer-Cells.html
26. M. Elishmereni, Y. Kheifetz, H. Søndergaard, R. V. Overgaard, Z. Agur, An integrated disease/pharmacokinetic/pharmacodynamic model suggests improved interleukin-21 regimens validated prospectively for mouse solid cancers. PLoS Comput. Biol. **7**(9) (2011)
27. W.V. Mayneord, On a law of growth of Jensen's rat sarcoma. Am. J. Cancer **16**(4), 841–846 (1932)
28. G. Steel, Growth and survival of tumor stem cells. Growth Kinet. Tumors 217–267 (1977)
29. M. Spang-Thomsen, K. Rygaard, L. Hansen, A.C. Halvorsen, L.L. Vindeløv, N. Brünner, Growth kinetics of four human breast carcinomas grown in nude mice. Breast Cancer Res. Treat. **14**, 235–243 (1989)
30. R. Sachs, L. Hlatky, P. Hahnfeldt, Simple ODE models of tumor growth and anti-angiogenic or radiation treatment. Math. Comput. Model. **33**(12), 1297–1305 (2001)
31. H. Byrne, M. Chaplain, Necrosis and apoptosis: distinct cell loss mechanisms in a mathematical model of avascular tumour growth. Comput. Math. Methods Med. **1**(3), 223–235 (1998)

32. H. Easwaran, H.C. Tsai, S.B. Baylin, Cancer epigenetics: tumor heterogeneity, plasticity of stem-like states, and drug resistance. Mol. Cell **54**(5), 716–727 (2014)
33. N. Bellomo, L. Preziosi, Modelling and mathematical problems related to tumor evolution and its interaction with the immune system. Math. Comput. Model. **32**(3), 413–452 (2000)
34. A. Friedman, A hierarchy of cancer models and their mathematical challenges. Discret. Contin. Dyn. Syst. Ser.-B **4**(1), 147–159 (2004)
35. A. Marusyk, K. Polyak, Tumor heterogeneity: Causes and consequences. Biochimica et Biophysica Acta-Reviews on Cancer **1805**(1), 105–117 (2010)
36. A. Rivaz, M. Azizian, M. Soltani, Various mathematical models of tumor growth with reference to cancer stem cells: a review. Iran. J. Sci. Technol. Trans. A: Sci. **43**(2), 687–700 (2019)
37. M. Chaplain, Mathematical modelling and simulation of aspects of cancer growth. J. Theor. Med. **4** (2002)
38. L. Von Bertalanffy, Quantitative laws in metabolism and growth. Q. Rev. Biol. **32**(3), 217–231 (1957)
39. C. Guiot, P.G. Degiorgis, P.P. Delsanto, P. Gabriele, T.S. Deisboeck, Does tumor growth follow a "universal law" ? J. Theor. Biol. **225**(2), 147–151 (2003)
40. A. Yin, D. J.A. Moes, J.G. van Hasselt, J.J. Swen, H.-J. Guchelaar, A review of mathematical models for tumor dynamics and treatment resistance evolution of solid tumors. CPT: Pharmacomet. Syst. Pharmacol. **8**(10), 720–737 (2019)
41. D. Hart, E. Shochat, Z. Agur, The growth law of primary breast cancer as inferred from mammography screening trials data. Br. J. Cancer **78**(3), 382–387 (1998)
42. H. Enderling, M. Chaplain, Mathematical modeling of tumor growth and treatment. Curr. Pharmaceut. Des. **20**(30), 4934–4940 (2014)
43. S. Weekes, B. Barker, S. Bober et al., A multicompartment mathematical model of cancer stem cell-driven tumor growth dynamics. Bull. Math. Biol. **76**(7), 1762–1782 (2014)
44. M. Simeoni, P. Magni, C. Cammia, G. De Nicolao, V. Croci, E. Pesenti, M. Germani, I. Poggesi, M. Rocchetti, Predictive pharmacokinetic-pharmacodynamic modeling of tumor growth kinetics in xenograft models after administration of anticancer agents. Cancer Res. **64**(3), 1094–1101 (2004)
45. P. Hahnfeldt, D. Panigrahy, J. Folkman, L. Hlatky, Tumor development under angiogenic signaling: a dynamical theory of tumor growth, treatment response, and postvascular dormancy. Cancer Res. **59**(19), 4770–4775 (1999)
46. P. Gerlee, The model muddle: in search of tumor growth laws. Cancer Res. **73**(8), 2407–2411 (2013)
47. A. Talkington, R. Durrett, Estimating tumor growth rates in vivo. Bull. Math. Biol. **77**(10), 1934–1954 (2015)
48. D. Brown, P. Rothery, et al. *Models in Biology: Mathematics, Statistics and Computing* (Wiley, 1993)
49. L. Von Bertalanffy, A quantitative theory of organic growth (inquiries on growth laws. II). Human Biol. **10**(2), 181–213 (1938)
50. V.G. Vaidya, F.J. Alexandro, Evaluation of some mathematical models for tumor growth. Int. J. Bio-Med. Comput. **13**(1), 19–35 (1982)
51. S.P. Robinson, S.M. Langan Fahey, D.A. Johnson, V.C. Jordan, Metabolites, pharmacodynamics, and pharmacokinetics of tamoxifen in rats and mice compared to the breast cancer patient. Drug Metabol. Disposit. **19**(1), 36–43 (1991)
52. J.A. Florian Jr., J.L. Eiseman, R.S. Parker, Nonlinear model predictive control for dosing daily anticancer agents using a novel saturating-rate cell-cycle model. Comput. Biol. Med. **38**(3), 339–347 (2008)
53. H.E. Skipper, Experimental evaluation of potential anticancer agents XIII, on the criteria and kinetics associated with" curability" of experimental leukemria. Cancer Chemother. Rep. **35**, 3–111 (1964)
54. L. Norton, The Norton-Simon hypothesis revisited. Cancer Treat. Rep. **70**(1), 163–169 (1986)

55. A. Stein, W. Wang, A.A. Carter, O. Chiparus, N. Hollaender, H. Kim, R.J. Motzer, C. Sarr, Dynamic tumor modeling of the dose-response relationship for everolimus in metastatic renal cell carcinoma using data from the Phase 3 RECORD-1 trial. BMC Cancer **12**(1), 311 (2012)
56. L.G. de Pillis, W. Gu, A.E. Radunskaya, Mixed immunotherapy and chemotherapy of tumors: Modeling, applications and biological interpretations. J. Theor. Biol. **238**(4), 841–862 (2006)
57. H. Moradi, M. Sharifi, G. Vossoughi, Adaptive robust control of cancer chemotherapy in the presence of parametric uncertainties: a comparison between three hypotheses. Comput. Biol. Med. **56**, 145–157 (2015)
58. A. Ouerdani, H. Struemper, A. Suttle, D. Ouellet, B. Ribba, Preclinical modeling of tumor growth and angiogenesis inhibition to describe pazopanib clinical effects in renal cell carcinoma. CPT: Pharmacom. Syst. Pharmacol. **4**(11), 660–668 (2015)
59. O. Majid, A. Gupta, L. Reyderman, M. Olivo, Z. Hussein, Population pharmacometric analyses of eribulin in patients with locally advanced or metastatic breast cancer previously treated with anthracyclines and taxanes. J. Clin. Pharmacol. **54**(10), 1134–1143 (2014)
60. E. Ollier, P. Mazzocco, D. Ricard, G. Kaloshi, A. Idbaih, A. Alentorn, D. Psimaras, J. Honnorat, J.Y. Delattre, E. Grenier et al., Analysis of temozolomide resistance in low-grade gliomas using a mechanistic mathematical model. Fundam. Clin. Pharmacol. **31**(3), 347–358 (2017)
61. B. Ribba, G. Kaloshi, M. Peyre, D. Ricard, V. Calvez, M. Tod, B. Čajavec-Bernard, A. Idbaih, D. Psimaras, L. Dainese et al., A tumor growth inhibition model for low-grade glioma treated with chemotherapy or radiotherapy. Clin. Cancer Res. **18**(18), 5071–5080 (2012)
62. D. Kirschner, J.C. Panetta, Modeling immunotherapy of the tumor-immune interaction. J. Math. Biol. **37**(3), 235–252 (1998)
63. S. Banerjee, R.R. Sarkar, Delay-induced model for tumor-immune interaction and control of malignant tumor growth. Biosystems **91**(1), 268–288 (2008)
64. E. Nikolopoulou, L.R. Johnson, D. Harris, J.D. Nagy, E.C. Stites, Y. Kuang, Tumour-immune dynamics with an immune checkpoint inhibitor. Lett. Biomath. **5**(sup1), S137–S159 (2018)
65. A.W. El-Kareh, T.W. Secomb, Two-mechanism peak concentration model for cellular pharmacodynamics of doxorubicin. Neoplasia (New York, NY) **7**(7), 705 (2005)
66. C.S. Holling, The components of predation as revealed by a study of small-mammal predation of the European pine sawfly. Can. Entomol. **91**(5), 293–320 (1959)
67. J. Dawes, M. Souza, A derivation of Holling's Type I, II and III functional responses in predator-prey systems. J. Theor. Biol. **327**, 11–22 (2013)
68. S.T.R. Pinho, D.S. Rodrigues, P.F.A. Mancera, A mathematical model of chemotherapy response to tumour growth. Can. Appl. Math. Q. **19**, 369–384 (2011)
69. S. Chakraborty, X. Cao, S. Bhattyacharya, P. Roy, The role of HPV on cervical cancer with several functional response: a control based comparative study. Comput. Math. Model. **30**(4), 439–453 (2019)
70. W.H. Carter Jr., G.L. Wampler, Review of the application of response surface methodology in the combination therapy of cancer. Cancer Treat. Rep. **70**(1), 133–140 (1986)
71. C.F. Minto, T.W. Schnider, T.G. Short, K.M. Gregg, A. Gentilini, S.L. Shafer, Response surface model for anesthetic drug interactions. Anesthesiol.: J. Am. Soc. Anesthesiol. **92**(6), 1603–1616 (2000)
72. J. Marzec, L. Marzec, P. Martus, D. Zips, A.-C. Müller, Matlab®-based fitting method to evaluate survival fractions after multimodal treatment. Clin. Transl. Radiat. Oncol. **10**, 36–41 (2018)
73. G.A. Seber, C.J. Wild, *Nonlinear Regression* (Wiley-Interscience, 2003)
74. M. Marušić, S. Vuk-Pavlovic, J.P. Freyer et al., Tumor growth in vivo and as multicellular spheroids compared by mathematical models. Bull. Math. Biol. **56**(4), 617–631 (1994)
75. A.M. Jarrett, M.J. Bloom, W. Godfrey, A.K. Syed, D.A. Ekrut, L.I. Ehrlich, T.E. Yankeelov, A.G. Sorace, Mathematical modelling of trastuzumab-induced immune response in an in vivo murine model of HER2+ breast cancer. Math. Med. Biol.: A J. IMA **36**(3), 381–410 (2019)
76. M. Nagase, S. Aksenov, H. Yan, J. Dunyak, N. Al Huniti, Modeling tumor growth and treatment resistance dynamics characterizes different response to gefitinib or chemotherapy in non-small cell lung cancer. CPT: Pharmacom. Syst. Pharmacol. (2020)

77. P.K. Newton, J. Mason, K. Bethel, L. Bazhenova, J. Nieva, L. Norton, P. Kuhn, Spreaders and sponges define metastasis in lung cancer: a Markov chain Monte Carlo mathematical model. Cancer Res. **73**(9), 2760–2769 (2013)
78. M.R. dos Santos, J.A. Achcar, E.Z. Martinez, Bayesian and maximum likelihood inference for the defective Gompertz cure rate model with covariates: An application to the cervical carcinoma study. Ciência e Natura **39**(2), 244–258 (2017)
79. M. C. Pigatto, R. M. Roman, L. Carrara, A. Buffon, P. Magni, T. Dalla Costa, Pharmacokinetic/pharmacodynamic modeling of etoposide tumor growth inhibitory effect in Walker-256 tumor-bearing rat model using free intratumoral drug concentrations. Eur. J. Pharm. Sci. **97**, 70–78 (2017)
80. C. Vaghi, A. Rodallec, R. Fanciullino, J. Ciccolini, J.P. Mochel, M. Mastri, C. Poignard, J.M. Ebos, S. Benzekry, Population modeling of tumor growth curves and the reduced Gompertz model improve prediction of the age of experimental tumors. PLoS Comput. Biol. **16**(2), e1007178 (2020)
81. F. Hoffman, D. Gavaghan, J. Osborne, I. Barrett, T. You, H. Ghadially, R. Sainson, R. Wilkinson, H. Byrne, A mathematical model of antibody-dependent cellular cytotoxicity (ADCC). J. Theor. Biol. **436**, 39–50 (2018)
82. M. Marušić, Mathematical models of tumor growth. Math. Commun. **1**(2), 175–188 (1996)
83. E. Enerly, I. Steinfeld, K. Kleivi, S.-K. Leivonen, M.R. Aure, HG. Russnes, J.A. Rønneberg, H. Johnsen, R. Navon, E. Rødland, et al. miRNA-mRNA integrated analysis reveals roles for miRNAs in primary breast tumors. PloS One **6**(2) (2011)
84. C.T. Kelley, *Iterative methods for optimization* (SIAM, 1999)
85. K.M. Brown, J. Dennis, Derivative free analogues of the Levenberg-Marquardt and gauss algorithms for nonlinear least squares approximation. Numer. Math. **18**(4), 289–297 (1971)
86. J.J. Moré, The Levenberg-Marquardt algorithm: Implementation and theory, in *Numerical Analysis* (Springer, 1978), pp. 105–116
87. T.K. Moon, The expectation-maximization algorithm. IEEE Signal Process. Mag. **13**(6), 47–60 (1996)
88. W.J. Roberts, S. Furui, Maximum likelihood estimation of K-distribution parameters via the expectation-maximization algorithm. IEEE Trans. Signal Process. **48**(12), 3303–3306 (2000)
89. H. Motulsky, A. Christopoulos, *Fitting models to biological data using linear and nonlinear regression: A practical guide to curve fitting* (Oxford University Press, 2004)
90. A. Mira, On Metropolis-Hastings algorithms with delayed rejection. Metron **59** (2001)
91. V.A. Kuznetsov, I.A. Makalkin, M.A. Taylor, A.S. Perelson, Nonlinear dynamics of immunogenic tumors: parameter estimation and global bifurcation analysis. Bull. Math. Biol. **56**(2), 295–321 (1994)
92. L.G. de Pillis, A.E. Radunskaya, C.L. Wiseman, A validated mathematical model of cell-mediated immune response to tumor growth. Cancer Res. **65**(17), 7950–7958 (2005)
93. K.P. Burnham, D.R. Anderson, Multimodel inference: understanding aic and BIC in model selection. Sociol. Methods Res. **33**(2), 261–304 (2004)
94. N. Hartung, S. Mollard, D. Barbolosi, A. Benabdallah, G. Chapuisat, G. Henry, S. Giacometti, A. Iliadis, J. Ciccolini, C. Faivre et al., Mathematical modeling of tumor growth and metastatic spreading: validation in tumor-bearing mice. Cancer Res. **74**(22), 6397–6407 (2014)
95. T. Portz, Y. Kuang, J.D. Nagy, A clinical data validated mathematical model of prostate cancer growth under intermittent androgen suppression therapy. AIP Adv. **2**(1), 011002 (2012)
96. Z. Wu, T. Phan, J. Baez, Y. Kuang, E.J. Kostelich, Predictability and identifiability assessment of models for prostate cancer under androgen suppression therapy. Math. Biosci. Eng. **16**(5), 3512–3536 (2019)
97. M.C. Eisenberg, M.A. Hayashi, Determining identifiable parameter combinations using subset profiling. Math. Biosci. **256**, 116–126 (2014)
98. P.A. Vanrolleghem, M. Van Daele, D. Dochain, Practical identifiability of a biokinetic model of activated sludge respiration. Water Res. **29**(11), 2561–2570 (1995)
99. L.D. Pillis, A. Radunskaya, The dynamics of an optimally controlled tumor model: a case study. Math. Comput. Model. **37**(11), 1221–1244 (2003)

100. N. Tsur, Y. Kogan, M. Rehm, Z. Agur, Response of patients with melanoma to immune checkpoint blockade-insights gleaned from analysis of a new mathematical mechanistic model. J. Theor. Biol. **485**, 110033 (2020)
101. D. Kirschner, A. Tsygvintsev, On the global dynamics of a model for tumor immunotherapy. Math. Biosci. Eng. **6**(3), 573–583 (2009)
102. B. Mukhopadhyay, R. Bhattacharyya, A nonlinear mathematical model of virus-tumor-immune system interaction: deterministic and stochastic analysis. Stoch. Anal. Appl. **27**(2), 409–429 (2009)
103. H. Özbay, C. Bonnet, H. Benjelloun, J. Clairambault, Stability analysis of cell dynamics in leukemia. Math. Model. Nat. Phenom. **7**(1), 203–234 (2012)
104. S. Khajanchi, S. Banerjee, Stability and bifurcation analysis of delay induced tumor immune interaction model. Appl. Math. Comput. **248**, 652–671 (2014)
105. Y. Chang, X. Wang, Z. Feng, W. Feng, Bifurcation analysis in a cancer growth model. Int. J. Bifurc. Chaos **30**(02), 2050024 (2020)
106. H. Ozbay, C. Bonnet, J. Clairambault, Stability analysis of systems with distributed delays and application to hematopoietic cell maturation dynamics, in *2008 47th IEEE Conference on Decision and Control* (IEEE, 2008), pp. 2050–2055
107. T. Hillen, H. Enderling, P. Hahnfeldt, The tumor growth paradox and immune system-mediated selection for cancer stem cells. Bull. Math. Biol. **75**, 11 (2012)
108. Z. Neufeld, W. von Witt, D. Lakatos, J. Wang, B. Hegedus, A. Czirok, The role of Allee effect in modelling post resection recurrence of glioblastoma. PLoS Comput. Biol. **13**(11), e1005818 (2017)
109. L. Sewalt, K. Harley, P. van Heijster, S. Balasuriya, Influences of Allee effects in the spreading of malignant tumours. J. Theor. Biol. **394**, 77–92 (2016)
110. A. Konstorum, T. Hillen, J. Lowengrub, Feedback regulation in a cancer stem cell model can cause an Allee effect. Bull. Math. Biol. **78**(4), 754–785 (2016)
111. K. Böttger, H. Hatzikirou, A. Voss-Böhme, E.A. Cavalcanti-Adam, M.A. Herrero, A. Deutsch, An emerging Allee effect is critical for tumor initiation and persistence. PLoS Comput. Biol. **11**(9) (2015)
112. S.S. De Buck, A. Jakab, M. Boehm, D. Bootle, D. Juric, C. Quadt, T.K. Goggin, Population pharmacokinetics and pharmacodynamics of BYL 719, a phosphoinositide 3-kinase antagonist, in adult patients with advanced solid malignancies. Br. J. Clin. Pharmacol. **78**(3), 543–555 (2014)
113. A. Ouerdani, S. Goutagny, M. Kalamarides, I.F. Trocóniz, B. Ribba, Mechanism-based modeling of the clinical effects of bevacizumab and everolimus on vestibular schwannomas of patients with neurofibromatosis Type 2. Cancer Chemother. Pharmacol. **77**(6), 1263–1273 (2016)
114. B.C. Bender, E. Schindler, L.E. Friberg, Population pharmacokinetic-pharmacodynamic modelling in oncology: a tool for predicting clinical response. Br. J. Clin. Pharmacol. **79**(1), 56–71 (2015)
115. E. Hansson, M. Amantea, P. Westwood, P. Milligan, B. Houk, J. French, M.O. Karlsson, L.E. Friberg, PK-PD modeling of VEGF, sVEGFR-2, sVEGFR-3, and sKIT as predictors of tumor dynamics and overall survival following sunitinib treatment in GIST. CPT: Pharmacom. Syst. Pharmacol. **2**(11), 1–9 (2013)
116. T. Chen, N.F. Kirkby, R. Jena, Optimal dosing of cancer chemotherapy using model predictive control and moving horizon state/parameter estimation. Comput. Methods Prog. Biomed. **108**(3), 973–983 (2012)
117. S. Patmanidis, A.C. Charalampidis, I. Kordonis, G.D. Mitsis, G.P. Papavassilopoulos, Tumor growth modeling: parameter estimation with maximum likelihood methods. Comput. Methods Prog. Biomed. **160**, 1–10 (2018)
118. J. Pinheiro, S. Vinga, A nonlinear MPC approach to minimize toxicity in HIV-1 infection multi-drug therapy, in *CONTROLO'2012* (2012)
119. J. Zhu, R. Liu, Z. Jiang, P. Wang, Y. Yao, Z. Shen, Optimization of drug regimen in chemotherapy based on semi-mechanistic model for myelosuppression. J. Biomed. Inform. **57**, 20–27 (2015)
120. Y. Liang, K.S. Leung, T.S.K. Mok, Evolutionary drug scheduling models with different toxicity metabolism in cancer chemotherapy. Appl. Soft Comput. **8**(1), 140–149 (2008)

Chapter 3
Chemotherapy Models

Chemotherapy is a standard treatment method used for managing many types of cancers. Chemotherapy involves the use of different types of drugs or drug combinations that can reduce the abnormal proliferation of cancer cells and lead to cell death. Cancer cell-lysis is achieved either by inducing cell-cycle arrest, manipulating the structure of DNA that is necessary for replication, or altering metabolic pathways [1, 2]. Chemotherapeutic drugs are also called as antineoplastics or cytotoxic agents. A recent statistical analysis on the use of various therapeutic measures for cancer points out the prevalent use ($\approx$70% on average) of chemotherapy for the treatment of acute myeloid leukemia (AML), acute lymphocytic leukemia (ALL), classical Hodgkin's lymphoma (CHL), as well as different types of cancers including breast cancer, rectal cancer, and lung cancer [3].

Noticeably, depending upon the site of the target, there are many side effects for chemotherapy such as impaired fertility, premature menopause, increased risk of osteoporosis, myalgia, arthralgia, secondary cancer such as endometrial cancer, thromboembolic disease, neuropathy, bowel and bladder dysfunction, infection, anemia, dry mucous membranes, etc. [3]. Compared to other cancer therapy methods such as surgery or radiation therapy which can be localized to the area of interest, in the case of chemotherapy, treatment is facilitated by cytotoxic agents, which are transported via the circulatory system and hence the side effects are not localized. This considerably increases the concern regarding the type and amount of drugs used in this context. The potential side effects that come along with the excessive use of chemotherapeutic drugs call for more vigilant investigations on the drug dosing strategies so as to ensure optimal use of drugs which will minimize side effects and maximize desired effects due to treatment.

Even though the cytotoxic agent can annihilate many of the cancer cells, some drug-resistant cells remain unaffected (Fig. 3.1). Moreover, the drug used can also affect some of the normal cells (side-effect). Other factors that affect the growth of the tumor and efficacy of drugs used are the immune response and vascular delivery (which supplies oxygen, nutrients, and drug) to the tumor. As mentioned in Chap. 1,

R. Padmanabhan et al., *Mathematical Models of Cancer and Different Therapies*, Series in BioEngineering, https://doi.org/10.1007/978-981-15-8640-8_3

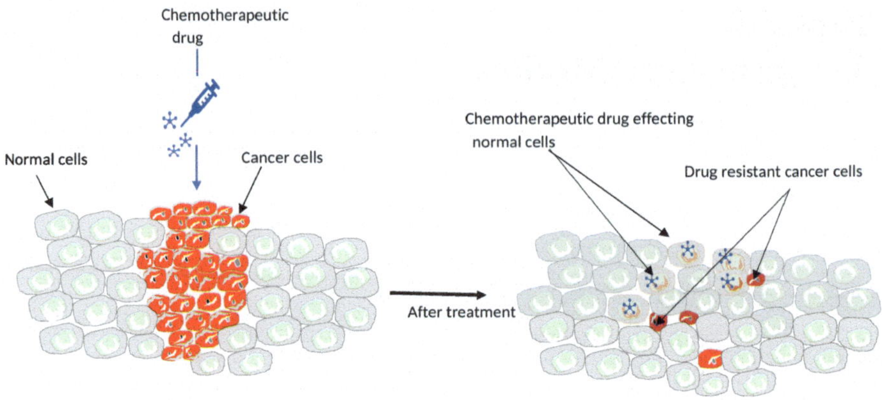

Fig. 3.1 Illustrative diagram showing the effect of a chemotherapeutic drug on cancer cells and normal cells

the overall mechanism involved in the progression of cancer and its management using chemotherapeutic drugs involves highly complex and nonlinear dynamics of various cell populations and biochemicals. However, the cell populations and biochemicals that are included in a mathematical model varies according to the mechanism under study. Hence, the following special cases of the general model (1.1)–(1.2) are discussed that account for the dynamics of different cell populations and biochemicals under chemotherapy, namely:

1. Three cell-based model of tumor dynamics under chemotherapy,
2. Model of tumor dynamics that accounts for the drug resistance of cells due to chemotherapy,
3. Model of tumor dynamics that accounts for cell transition under chemotherapy,
4. Model of tumor dynamics that accounts for metastasis under chemotherapy,
5. Cell-cycle-based compartment model of tumor dynamics under chemotherapy, and
6. Model for leukemia under chemotherapy.

Even though the cell populations involved in these models vary, the underlying mechanism in the tumor growth and regression is more or less the same. The main difference between these models lies in the assumptions involved in the development of the model, type of the cell growth or depletion pattern used, and inclusion of some specific parameters that are relevant to the cell population under study. Tables 3.1 and 3.2 summarize the notations used in this chapter.

Table 3.1 Parameter notations used in chemotherapy

Param.	Description	Param.	Description
a	Fractional cell-kill rate due to therapy	b	Reciprocal carrying capacity
c	Competition rate	d	Death rate or depletion rate
r	Growth rate	m	Mutation (cell transition) rate
s	Immune cell influx rate	α	Immune threshold rate
ρ	Immune response rate	η	Metabolic rate
U^{th}	Drug concentration threshold	m_0	Maximum cell transition rate per day
Q^{50}	Quiescent cell population at which nonlinear transition rate is half	n	Sensitivity of $m(\cdot)$
g	Combination rate of the therapeutic agent	b_{d}	Carrying capacity without therapeutic intervention
b_{c}	Carrying capacity in the absence of competition		

3.1 Three Cell-Based Model of Tumor Dynamics Under Chemotherapy

In Chap. 1, Sect. 1.2, some basic mechanisms involved in the tumor growth and tumor-immune interaction are discussed and also various cell populations that are important related to cancer dynamics are listed. The growth of the normal cells, tumor cells, immune cells, cancer stem cells, and drug-resistant cells and concentration of drugs used play a role in deciding the overall cell-dynamics in a tumor micro-environment. Recall that the influx of various effector cells (immune cells) into the tumor micro-environment and competition between various cells are also important ((1.1)–(1.2)). The vascular delivery to the tumor site is another vital factor that influences the carrying capacity of the tumor micro-environment and the pharmacokinetics of the drug. In this section, one of the most widely investigated three cell-based model of cancer dynamics under chemotherapy given in [4] is presented. The main advantage of this model compared to its single-cell and two cell-based predecessors is that this model accounts for the interaction between the normal cells, cancer cells, and immune cells in the presence of a chemotherapeutic agent [5–10]. The model is given by [4, 11]:

Table 3.2 Different types of cells and biochemicals in chemotherapy

Var.	Description	Var.	Description
$N(t)$	Normal (host) cells	$N_{\mathrm{p}}(t)$	Normal cells at the primary site
$N_{\mathrm{s}}(t)$	Normal cells at the secondary site	$A(t)$	Abnormal (cancer) cells
$A_{\mathrm{p}}(t)$	Cancer cells at the primary site	$A_{\mathrm{s}}(t)$	Cancer cells at the secondary site
$E(t)$	Effector cells used as general representative of attacking immune cells	$Q(t)$	Quiescent (resting) cells
$S(t)$	Cell population sensitive to therapy	$R(t)$	Cell population resistant to therapy
$R_{\mathrm{m}}(t)$	Resistant cell population developed via mutation	$R_{\mathrm{p}}(t)$	Resistant cell population developed via phenotype switching
$A_{\mathrm{Pl}}(t)$	Proliferating cells (leukemia)	$A_{\mathrm{L}}(t)$	Mature red blood cells (leukemia)
$A_{\mathrm{Q}}(t)$	Population of red blood cells in quiescence (leukemia)	$T_{\mathrm{X}}(t)$	Toxicity of therapy
$u(t)$	Drug input	$u_{\mathrm{p}}(t)$	Drug infusion to the primary site
$u_{\mathrm{p}}(t)$	Drug infusion to the secondary site	$U(t)$	Intensity (concentration) of therapy (drug) at the tumor site
$U_{\mathrm{p}}(t)$	Concentration of the drug at the primary site	$U_{\mathrm{s}}(t)$	Concentration of the drug at the secondary site
$V(t)$	Total cell count	$MCV(t)$	Mean corpuscular volume

$$\frac{\mathrm{d}E(t)}{\mathrm{d}t} = s + \frac{\rho E(t)A(t)}{\alpha + A(t)} - d_1 E(t) - c_1 E(t)A(t) - a_1\left(1 - e^{-U(t)}\right)E(t), \tag{3.1}$$

$$\frac{\mathrm{d}A(t)}{\mathrm{d}t} = r_1 A(t)\,(1 - b_1 A(t)) - c_2 E(t)A(t) - c_3 N(t)A(t) - a_2\left(1 - e^{-U(t)}\right)A(t), \tag{3.2}$$

$$\frac{\mathrm{d}N(t)}{\mathrm{d}t} = r_2 N(t)\,(1 - b_2 N(t)) - c_4 N(t)A(t) - a_3\left(1 - e^{-U(t)}\right)N(t), \tag{3.3}$$

$$\frac{\mathrm{d}U(t)}{\mathrm{d}t} = -d_{\mathrm{U}}U(t) + u(t), \tag{3.4}$$

where $E(t)$ and $A(t)$ denote the number of immune cells and cancer cells, and $N(t)$ and $U(t)$ denote the number of normal cells and drug concentration, respectively.

Comparing (3.1)–(3.4) to the general model given by (1.1)–(1.2) sheds light on the important biological mechanisms accommodated by this model and simplifying assumptions involved. Note that the general cell population notation $C_{pi}(t)$, $i = 1, 2, 3$, are replaced by $E(t)$, $A(t)$, and $N(t)$ in (3.1)–(3.3). The first two terms in (3.1) account for our body's immune surveillance mechanism and apparent recruitment of the effector cells $E(t)$ to the site of abnormality. Presence of cancer cells above the immune threshold rate α triggers the immune system response and the number of immune cells increases in a nonlinear fashion. This nonlinear growth is captured by the function $\mathscr{G}(\rho, s, \alpha, A(t), E(t)) = s + \frac{\rho E(t)A(t)}{\alpha + A(t)}$ in (3.1), where ρ is the immune response rate, s denotes the rate of inflow of effector cells to the tumor site, and α is the immune threshold rate. Next, the decrease in the immune cell population due to normal death (apoptosis) is captured by $\mathscr{A}(d_1, E(t)) = -d_1 E(t)$, where d_1 denotes the per capita depletion rate of the immune cells from the tumor site [4, 11, 12].

The overall progression and regression of normal cells, tumor cells, and effector cells are all interdependent as they share available resources and threaten the existence of each other. In (3.1)–(3.3), the competition between these cells for existence is captured using the competition term, c_i, $i = 1, \ldots, 4$. For instance, in (3.1), the competition function ($\mathscr{C}(\cdot)$) is modeled as $c_1 E(t)A(t)$, where the cell population involved in competition are $E(t)$ and $A(t)$, with c_1 as the associated competition term. Similarly, in (3.2) it can be seen that, there are two competition terms such as $c_2 E(t)A(t)$ and $c_3 N(t)A(t)$, where the first term represents a predator-prey style competition between effector cells and tumor cells and the second term accounts for the competition for resources between tumor cells and normal cells. The competition terms c_1 and c_2 in (3.1) and (3.2) quantify how much damaging is the competition between immune cells and cancer cells to each other. Similarly, c_3 and c_4 in (3.2) and (3.3) quantify the effect of competition between normal cells and cancer cells on each other.

The cell-killing effect of the chemotherapeutic drug ($\mathscr{D}(\cdot)$) on each of the cell population is captured by $a_i\left(1 - e^{-kU(t)}\right)C_{pi}(t)$, where $C_{pi}(t)$, $i = 1, 2$, and 3, are $E(t)$, $A(t)$, and $N(t)$, respectively, $a_i, i = 1, 2, 3$, represent their respective fractional cell-kill rates, and k is a parameter that accounts for the pharmacokinetics of the drug. In (3.1)–(3.3), the value of k is assumed to be 1 for simplicity.

It can be seen that the general growth function defined in (1.1) is given by $\mathscr{G}(r_1, A(t)) = r_1 A(t)$ and $\mathscr{G}(r_2, N(t)) = r_2 N(t)$ in (3.2) and (3.3) for the cancer cells and normal cells, respectively. It is apparent that the increase in each cell population is limited by the carrying capacity of the tumor micro-environment and hence in this model the function $\mathscr{K}(b_1, A(t)) = r_1 b_1 A^2(t)$ and $\mathscr{K}(b_2, N(t)) = r_2 b_2 N^2(t)$ capture the reciprocal carrying capacities of the cancer cells and normal cells, respectively. Here, the growth of the tumor is modeled using the realistic and popular logistic growth pattern.

Next, compared to the drug dynamics function $\mathscr{D}_c(d_U, U(t, \tau), u(t))$ in (1.2), this term is given as $\mathscr{D}_c(d_U, U(t), u(t)) = -d_U U(t) + u(t)$ in (3.4), where $u(t)$ is the drug infusion rate and d_U represents the per capita depletion rate of the drug. Note that the delay involved in drug dynamics (τ) is assumed to be negligible in (3.4).

In (3.1), as the concentration $U(t)$ increases, the value of the term $\left(d_1 + a_1\left(1 - e^{-U(t)}\right)\right)E(t)$ increases and thus the number of immune cells decreases. This term is included to model the reduced immunity of the patient as a side effect of chemotherapy [13]. Similarly, as $U(t)$ increases, the net growth of cancer cells decreases. This desired effect of drug is modeled in (3.2) using the term $\left(r_1 - a_2\left(1 - e^{-U(t)}\right)\right)A(t)$.

Note that, in general, the competition functions $\mathscr{C}(\cdot)$ in (3.1)–(3.3), are modeled as the product of the cell populations $\left(c, C_{p1}(t), C_{p2}(t)\right)$ involved. The assumption that every cell type is equally likely to compete with each other makes sense in the case of leukemia, however, it is not true in case of solid tumors in which the boundary between the normal cells and tumor cells decides the competition pattern. Moreover, clinical experiments hint the possibility of changes in the competition patterns between different cell populations at different time [14, 15]. Hence, investigating the efficacy of model that accounts for the stochasticity in the model parameter is important. Similarly, as noted in [16], it is important to account for the transition of a cell population to another to explain clinically seen phenomenon such as asynchronous oscillations in the tumor volume with chemotherapy.

The nonlinear four-state model (3.1)–(3.4) given in [4] is an extension of the lower-dimensional model presented in [12]. The model originally given in [12] is validated using the data set derived from chimeric mice with lymphoma in the spleen [17]. This model accounts for many clinically observed mechanisms in tumor dynamics such as sneaking through, tumor dormancy, etc. that arise as a consequence of the interaction between tumor and immune system. Some of the other lower-dimensional models that motivated the development of the three cell-based model in [4] are those discussed in [5–10]. In [4], it is suggested to study the effect of drug in the important stage of cell-cycle such as mitosis as a possible extensions for the model given by (3.1)–(3.4). Table 3.3 summarizes the parameter values of the rescaled and non-dimensionalized model of (3.1)–(3.4) [11]. The initial conditions for the variables in (3.1)–(3.4) are $E(0) = s/d_1$, $A(0) = 10^{-5}$, and $N(0) = 1$. The units are rescaled (normalized) so that carrying capacity of normal cells is 1. Accordingly, the values of parameters, say r_1 and r_2 represent per unit growth rates.

Table 3.3 Parameter values of the chemotherapy model (3.1)–(3.4) [11]

Param.	Value	Param.	Value	Param.	Value	Param.	Value
s	0.33	ρ	0.01	α	0.3	c_1, c_3, c_4	1
d_1	0.2	a_1	0.2	r_1	1.5	c_2	0.5
b_1, b_2	1	r_2	1	a_2	0.3	a_3	0.1
d_U	1						

3.2 Model of Tumor Dynamics That Accounts for the Drug Resistance in Cells

A tumor micro-environment is believed to accommodate heterogeneous cells with different degrees of response to therapeutic intervention (Fig. 3.1). In this section, the overall tumor dynamics is investigated with respect to different cell populations that are categorized according to their response to chemotherapeutic drugs.

One of the important problem associated with chemotherapy is that the tumor cells often develop resistance to chemotherapeutic drugs used for treatment while the normal (host) cells still remain susceptible to lethal effects of the drugs [18]. In order to combat the complications related to the development of drug resistance due to cancer treatment, it is often recommended to use multiple drugs concurrently. Consequently, several mathematical models have been developed to analyze the drug response dependent dynamics of cell population in the heterogeneous tumor micro-environment [9, 19, 20]. In [19], compartmental representation of sub-populations is used to analyze the concomitant infusion of multiple drugs. Specifically, instead of identifying different cells according to their location or function, tumor cells are segregated into different sub-populations according to whether the cells are sensitive or resistant to one or more of the drugs used. When it comes to the modeling of drug sensitivity, an important parameter that comes into the picture is the mutation rate of each cell population to a drug-resistant variant. The mutation rate of cells varies according to the site, grade, and stage of the tumor.

In [19], patient data on advanced stage of lung cancer is used to discuss the response to three drugs. The associated parameters are denoted by using the subscript $i = 1, 2, 3$. Depending upon the drug response of the cell populations to different drug combinations, there can be 8 sub-populations of tumor cells and thus the model involves 8 ODEs. Cells that are sensitive to the first drug ($i = 1$) may mutate or transform to cells sensitive to the second or third drugs ($i = 2$ or $i = 3$), spontaneously. However, as the cell mutation probability is not readily known, the mutation rates for cells residing in the same site of the tumor are assumed to be the same in many literature. Other main assumptions pertaining to this model are: (1) drug effect is instantaneous, (2) all population have the same growth rate, (3) drugs are assumed to be non-cross-resistant (will not develop resistance to an unrelated drug), and (4) cell-kill rate of drugs are assumed to have an additive effect, i.e. cell-kill rate when i number of drugs are administrated concurrently is equal to the cell-kill rate of each drug when applied alone. As per the model discussed in [19], the dynamics of the cell population that are sensitive to all the three drugs is given by:

$$\begin{aligned}\frac{\mathrm{d}S(t)}{\mathrm{d}t} &= r\left[(1-m_1-m_2-m_3)\,S(t)\right] - a_1\left(U_1(t)-U_1^{\mathrm{th}}\right)F\left(U_1(t)-U_1^{\mathrm{th}}\right)S(t)\\ &\quad - a_2\left(U_2(t)-U_2^{\mathrm{th}}\right)F\left(U_2(t)-U_2^{\mathrm{th}}\right)S(t)\\ &\quad - a_3\left(U_3(t)-U_3^{\mathrm{th}}\right)F\left(U_3(t)-U_3^{\mathrm{th}}\right)S(t), \quad S(0)=S_0,\end{aligned} \tag{3.5}$$

where $S(t)$ represents the cells that are sensitive to all drugs, r denotes the rate of exponential growth, m_i, $i = 1, 2, 3$, denotes the rate of mutation of sensitive sub-population to resistive sub-population, $U_i(t)$, $i = 1, 2, 3$, denotes the concentration of the ith drug, a_i, $i = 1, 2, 3$, denotes the cell-kill rate of the ith drug per drug concentration, and U_i^{th}, $i = 1, 2, 3$, denotes the drug concentration threshold above which drug effect is identified in each sub-population. Note that, for each of the drug, $i = 1, 2, 3$, $U_i(t) > U_i^{\text{th}}$ is essential for the drug to be effective.

Compared to (1.1), in (3.5) the growth function $\mathscr{G}(\cdot)$ involves a single linear term $rS(t)$ which models an exponential progression of cells. Apart from the cell growth, this model mainly accounts for the cell transition dynamics $\mathscr{M}(m, S(t))$ and the reduction in the number of cells due to the cell-killing effect $\mathscr{D}\left(U(t), a, U^{\text{th}}\right)$. Specifically, in (3.5), the reduction in the number of drug-sensitive cell population ($S(t)$) due to the mutation of some of its cells to other sub-population is modeled. This mutation can be due to the effect of drug 1, drug 2, and/or drug 3 and is quantified as $\mathscr{M}(m, S(t)) = -m_i S(t)$, $i = 1, 2, 3$. The Heaviside step function $F(x)$ in (3.5) is given by:

$$F(x) = \begin{cases} 1, & \text{if } x \geq 0, \\ 0, & \text{otherwise.} \end{cases} \tag{3.6}$$

Next, the dynamics of the cells that are resistant to one drug is given by:

$$\begin{aligned} \frac{\mathrm{d}R_i(t)}{\mathrm{d}t} &= r\left[(1 - m_j - m_k) R_i(t) + m_i S(t)\right] - \left(a_j \left(U_j(t) - U_j^{\text{th}}\right) F\left(U_j(t) - U_j^{\text{th}}\right)\right. \\ &\quad \left. + a_k \left(U_k(t) - U_k^{\text{th}}\right) F\left(U_k(t) - U_k^{\text{th}}\right)\right) R_i(t), \quad R_i(0) = R_{i0}, \end{aligned} \tag{3.7}$$

where $R_i(t)$ represents the cells that are resistant to one drug. The dynamics of the sub-population resistant to first, second, or third drugs is obtained by replacing ($i = 1, j = 2, k = 3$), ($i = 2, j = 1, k = 3$), and ($i = 3, j = 1, k = 2$) in (3.7), respectively. Similarly, the dynamics of the sub-population that are resistant to two drugs are given by:

$$\begin{aligned} \frac{\mathrm{d}R_{ij}(t)}{\mathrm{d}t} &= r\left[(1 - m_k) R_{ij}(t) + m_j R_i(t) + m_i R_j(t)\right] \\ &\quad - a_k \left(U_k(t) - U_k^{\text{th}}\right) F\left(U_k(t) - U_k^{\text{th}}\right) R_{ij}(t), \\ &\quad R_{ij}(0) = R_{ij0}, \end{aligned} \tag{3.8}$$

where i and j represent the two drugs for which the sub-population $R_{ij}(t)$ is resistant and k represents the third drug for which the sub-population is sensitive. Finally, the dynamics of the sub-population resistant to all the three drugs is given by:

$$\frac{\mathrm{d}R_{ijk}(t)}{\mathrm{d}t} = r\left[m_i R_{jk}(t) + m_j R_{ik}(t) + m_k R_{ij}(t)\right], \quad R_{ijk}(0) = R_{ijk0}, \tag{3.9}$$

Table 3.4 Parameter values used for chemotherapy model (3.5)–(3.11) [19]

Parameter	Value (unit)	Parameter	Value (unit)
r	0.0099 (days^{-1})	m_1	0.008
m_2	0.01	m_3	0.014
a_1	0.0084 (days^{-2}D^{-1})	a_2	0.0074 (days^{-2}D^{-1})
a_3	0.0092 (days^{-2}D^{-1})	$U_1^{\text{th}}, U_2^{\text{th}}, U_3^{\text{th}}$	10 (days D)
d_{U_1}	0.32 (days^{-1})	d_{U_2}	0.27 (days^{-1})
d_{U_3}	0.25 (days^{-1})	η_1	0.4 (days^{-1})
η_2	0.5 (days^{-1})	η_3	0.45 (days^{-1})

where the sub-population $R_{ijk}(t)$ which is resistant to all drugs are assumed to be derived from other sub-population by mutation. In [19], a model of drug toxicity reported in [21] is also used to study the response of the tumor population under chemotherapy as given by

$$\frac{\mathrm{d}U_i(t)}{\mathrm{d}t} = -d_{\text{U}i}U_i(t) + u_i(t), \quad i = 1, 2, 3, \tag{3.10}$$

$$\frac{\mathrm{d}T_{\text{X}i}(t)}{\mathrm{d}t} = -\eta_i T_{\text{X}i}(t) + U_i(t), \quad i = 1, 2, 3, \tag{3.11}$$

where $U_i(t)$ denotes the drug concentration, $u_i(t)$ denotes the drug infusion rate, and $T_{\text{X}i}(t)$ denotes the drug toxicity for each of the three drugs. Here, the depletion or decay of each drug occurs at a half-life of $d_{\text{U}i}$. It should be noted that the net drug toxicity of chemotherapy increases with an increase in drug concentration $U_i(t)$, $i = 1, 2, 3$, and decreases with respect to the metabolic rate of each drug in the body denoted by η_i, $i = 1, 2, 3$. The drug kinetics given by (3.10) is same as in (3.4) [4]. Table 3.4 summarizes the parameter values of the chemotherapy model (3.5)–(3.11) [19] where the unit D in Table 3.4 denotes the dosage unit of the used drug. The initial conditions for the variables in (3.5)–(3.11) are $S(0) = 4.605 \times 10^{11}$ and $R_i(0)$, $R_{ij}(0)$, $R_{ijk}(0) = 0$. The range of value for drug concentration is $U_i(t) = [0, 50]$ (D) and toxicity is $T_{\text{X}i}(t) = [0, 100]$.

Note that the dynamics given in (3.5)–(3.11) models the cell transition dynamics involved in the drug-sensitive and drug-resistant cell populations. However, the mechanisms that lead to the development of drug-resistant cell population is much more complex and according to the root cause behind it, several subclasses of resistant cell population ($R(t)$) can be identified. Typically, cell populations that are resistant to a drug may be developed from [20, 22]:

- A group of pre-existing cells via resistant cell selection mechanism (pre-existing drug resistance),
- A group of drug-sensitive cells via spontaneous nongenetic phenotype switching or random genetic mutation (acquired drug resistance), and
- Due to the induction of drug resistance by the chemotherapeutic agent itself (induced drug resistance).

Similar to (3.5)–(3.9), in [22] the drug dependent cell dynamics is modeled as:

Table 3.5 Parameter values of the chemotherapy model (3.12)–(3.13) [22]

Parameter	Value	Parameter	Value
r	0.2	m_a	10^{-6}
m_d	0, 10^{-2}	a	1

$$\frac{\mathrm{d}S(t)}{\mathrm{d}t} = \left(1 - \left(S(t) + R(t)\right)\right)S(t) - (m_a + m_d u(t))S(t) - au(t)S(t), \quad (3.12)$$

$$\frac{\mathrm{d}R(t)}{\mathrm{d}t} = r\left(1 - \left(S(t) + R(t)\right)\right)R(t) + (m_a + m_d u(t))S(t), \quad (3.13)$$

where $S(t)$ and $R(t)$ denote sensitive and resistant cell populations, respectively, r, $0 \leq r < 1$, denotes the relative proliferation rate of resistant cell population with respect to sensitive cell population, and $u(t)$ denotes the effective drug dose. The condition $r < 1$ implies that the growth of $R(t)$ is less than that of $S(t)$ [23]. The term $m_a S(t)$ in (3.12) and (3.13) models the acquired drug resistance mechanism which facilitates the transition of drug-sensitive cells to drug resistive cells via genetic mutations as well as drug independent epigenetic events. Here, m_a denotes the cell transition rate associated with acquired drug resistance. The term $m_d u(t)S(t)$ in (3.12) and (3.13) models the induced drug resistance mechanism, where m_d denotes the drug dependent cell transition rate.

In (3.12), the effect of therapy on the cell population is modeled using the term $au(t)S(t)$, where a is the cell-kill rate due to the therapeutic intervention and $u(t)$ is assumed to be a measurable parameter which is related to the drug dosage. In this model, it is assumed that the drug has no cell-kill effect on the resistant cell population whereas a log-kill effect is considered for the sensitive cells. As per log-kill hypothesis, while the size of the tumor increases exponentially, a constant fraction of tumor cells are annihilated due to the effect of chemotherapeutic drug. More details on the log-kill hypothesis are presented in Chap. 2. Table 3.5 summarizes the parameter values of the chemotherapy model (3.12)–(3.13) [22]. The initial conditions for the variables in (3.12)–(3.13) are $S(0) = 0.01$ (dimensionless) and $R(0) = 0$.

In [20], the irreversible and reversible mutation of drug sensitive cells to drug resistant cells in the tumor micro-environment is modeled. Figure 3.2 illustrates such cell transitions in a heterogeneous tumor micro-environment.

Similar to the model discussed in [19, 22], in [20], the model dynamics of three cell populations is as given by:

$$\begin{aligned}\frac{\mathrm{d}S(t)}{\mathrm{d}t} &= r_1\left(1 - bV(t)\right)S(t) - \left(m_1 + m_2\right)S(t) - \left(m_3 + m_4\right)u(t)S(t) \\ &\quad - au(t)S(t) + m_5 R_p(t),\end{aligned} \quad (3.14)$$

$$\frac{\mathrm{d}R_m(t)}{\mathrm{d}t} = r_2\left(1 - bV(t)\right)R_m(t) + m_1 S(t) + \alpha_m u(t)S(t) - a_m u(t)R_m(t), \quad (3.15)$$

$$\frac{\mathrm{d}R_p(t)}{\mathrm{d}t} = r_3\left(1 - bV(t)\right)R_p(t) + m_2 S(t) + \alpha_p u(t)S(t) - m_5 R_p(t) - a_p u(t)R_p(t), \quad (3.16)$$

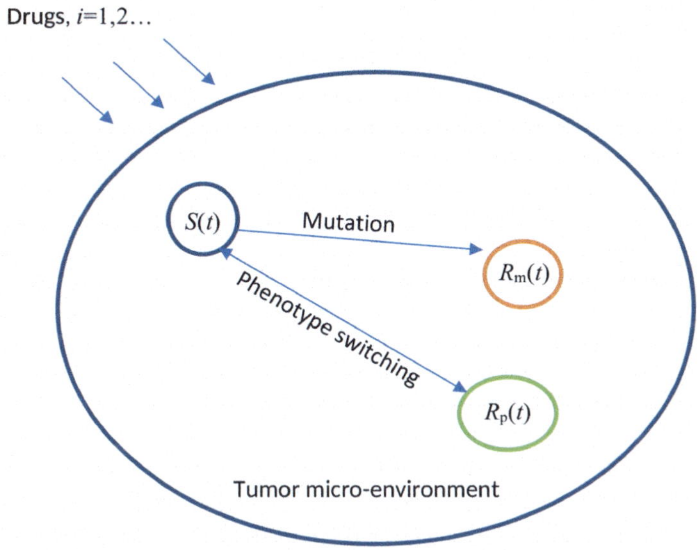

Fig. 3.2 Illustrative diagram showing drug induced and/or random cell transitions in a tumor micro-environment. Drug sensitive cells can change to irreversible (by mutation) or reversible (by phenotype switching) drug resistant cell variant

where $S(t)$ denotes the sensitive cell population, $R_m(t)$ is the resistive cell population developed via mutation, $R_p(t)$ represents the resistive cell population developed via phenotype switching, $V(t)$ denotes total cell count and is given by $V(t) = S(t) + R_m(t) + R_p(t)$, r_1, r_2, and r_3 are the growth rates of $S(t)$, $R_m(t)$, and $R_p(t)$, respectively, m_1 and m_2 are the cell transition rates that result in cells with acquired drug resistance via genetic mutation and phenotype switching, and $u(t)$ denotes effective drug dose. Note that, compared to a genetic mutation which involves irreversible changes in the genes, phenotype switching involves only epigenetic changes which are reversible and hence these cell populations may turn back to sensitive cells. This cell transition is modeled in (3.14) and (3.16) using the term $m_5 R_p(t)$, where m_5 denotes the rate at which the resistant cell population transition to sensitive cell population (resensitize). The growth rates follow the relation $0 \leq r_3 < r_1$ and b^{-1} represents the carrying capacity of $V(t)$.

3.3 Model of Tumor Dynamics That Accounts for Cell Transition Delay

In this section, a special case of the general model (1.1) and (1.2) is discussed that accounts for the delay involved in the transition of cells from one type to another with respect to chemotherapy. Various delays involved in the mechanism related to cancer are:

- Time-delay involved in metastasis (the time lapsed after which the cancer cells start leaving the primary site to metastasize),
- Time taken by the immune cells ($E(t)$) to identify a cancer cell and facilitate cytolytic immune response,

- Drug mixing delay,
- Time taken for the drug to show desired drug effect(s) or drug response, etc.

In [24], the effect of delay involved in the conversion of the typical immune cells such as T helper cells to transform into cytolytic T lymphocytes (hunting cells) is investigated. In simple words, the time taken by the resting immune cells to switch to active hunting cells is analyzed in [24]. In [25], the predator-prey model that depicts delay-induced tumor-immune dynamics discussed in [24] is further extended by adding the effect of chemotherapeutic drug as given by:

$$\frac{\mathrm{d}E(t)}{\mathrm{d}t} = m_1 E(t) Q(t-\tau) - d_1 E(t) - c_1 A(t) E(t) - \frac{a_1 E(t)}{b_{\mathrm{d}1} + E(t)} U(t), \tag{3.17}$$

$$\frac{\mathrm{d}Q(t)}{\mathrm{d}t} = r_1 Q(t)\,(1 - b_1 Q(t)) - m_1 E(t) Q(t-\tau) - \frac{a_2 Q(t)}{b_{\mathrm{d}2} + Q(t)} U(t), \tag{3.18}$$

$$\frac{\mathrm{d}A(t)}{\mathrm{d}t} = r_2 A(t)\,(1 - b_2 A(t)) - c_2 A(t) E(t) - \frac{a_3 A(t)}{b_{\mathrm{d}3} + A(t)} U(t), \tag{3.19}$$

$$\frac{\mathrm{d}U(t)}{\mathrm{d}t} = u(t) - \left(d_{\mathrm{U}} + \frac{g_1 E(t)}{b_{\mathrm{d}1} + E(t)} + \frac{g_2 Q(t)}{b_{\mathrm{d}2} + Q(t)} + \frac{g_3 A(t)}{b_{\mathrm{d}3} + A(t)} \right) U(t), \tag{3.20}$$

where $E(t)$ denotes the active hunting immune (effector) cells, $Q(t)$ denotes the resting (quiescent) immune cells, $A(t)$ denotes the cancer cells, and $U(t)$ represents the drug dynamics.

In (3.17), the increase in $E(t)$ due to the transition of $Q(t)$ to $E(t)$ and the time delay τ involved in the conversion of the resting cells to hunting cells is modeled by the term $m_1 E(t) Q(t-\tau)$. The function $\mathscr{A}(\cdot)$ involves the term $-d_1 E(t)$ which accounts for the apoptosis or natural death of the hunting cells. When a hunting immune cell encounters with the tumor cell, either the tumor cell is killed or the immune cell is deactivated [11]. These two losses are captured using the terms $-c_1 A(t) E(t)$ and $-c_2 A(t) E(t)$ in (3.17) and (3.19). The effect of chemotherapeutic drug on immune cells and cancer cells is assumed to obey Michaelis–Menten saturation function, where a_i, $i = 1, 2, 3$, denote the cell-kill rates or predation coefficients of the chemotherapeutic agent on hunting cells, quiescent cells, and tumor cells, respectively. See Sect. 2.3.4 in Chap. 2 for more details on Michaelis–Menten saturation function.

The growth pattern $\mathscr{G}(\cdot)$ of the quiescent cells and tumor cells are modeled using the terms $r_1 Q(t)$ and $r_2 A(t)$, in (3.18) and (3.19), respectively. From (3.18) and (3.19), it is clear that the resting and tumor cells follow a logistic growth pattern, with b_i, $i = 1, 2$ as reciprocal carrying capacities, respectively.

Finally, with respect to the general Eq. (1.2), and the model Eq. (3.4), it can be seen that the function $\mathscr{D}_c(\cdot)$ is different and involves $u(t)$ as the drug infusion rate, d_{U} as the drug elimination rate, $b_{\mathrm{d}i}, i = 1, 2, 3$, representing the rate at which hunting, quiescent, and tumor cells reach carrying capacities when no drug is infused, and g_i, $i = 1, 2, 3$, quantifying the combination rates of the chemotherapeutic agent with the hunting, quiescent, and tumor cells, respectively.

Except for the additional time-delay part and the drug dynamics part, the model discussed in [25] is similar to that given in [4, 11]. However, compared to the models in [4, 11], in [25], the hunting and quiescent types of immune cells where separately considered but the dynamics of the normal cell population is ignored. Compared to the growth function $\mathscr{G}(\cdot)$ in (3.1), it can be seen that in (3.17), the growth of hunting cells due to the constant influx of immune cells to the tumor micro-environment and nonlinear growth of effector cells due to active proliferation and differentiation of immune cells are ignored. Instead, this model ((3.17)–(3.20)) assumes that the hunting cells originate solely by cell transition of quiescent cells and hence modeled as $m_1 E(t) Q(t-\tau)$ similar to the function $\mathscr{M}(m, C_{\mathrm{p}1}(t))$ in (1.1).

Table 3.6 summarizes the parameter values of the non-dimensionalized chemotherapy model (3.17)–(3.20) [24, 25]. The initial conditions for the variables in the model (3.17)–(3.20) are $E(0) = 0.01$, $A(0) = 0.18$, $Q(0) = 0.48$, and $U(0) = 0$. The range of value for the infusion rate is $u(t) = [0, 0.03]$.

Table 3.6 Parameter values of the chemotherapy model (3.17)–(3.20) [24, 25]

Param.	Value	Param.	Value	Param.	Value
m_1	9.3×10^{-2}	d_1	0.0412	c_1	5.133×10^{-3}
r_1	0.0245	b_1	1.5	a_i	1×10^{-3}
r_2	0.18	b_2	3	c_2	1.6515
τ	45.6	b_{di}	1×10^{-4}	d_U	0.2
g_i	0.1				

3.4 Mathematical Model That Accounts for Tumor Metastasis

Malignant tumors often metastasize after a period of time. Hence, apart from modeling the proliferation, competition, and survival of cancer cells, it is important to analyze the dynamics involved in the detrimental process of tumor metastasis. Main factors that should come into picture are

- Cell dynamics in the primary and secondary sites,
- Threshold values of parameters beyond which metastasis is detected, and
- Mechanisms that foster metastasis such as,
  - Epithelial to mesenchymal transition (EMT),
  - Limitation due to carrying capacity of the tumor micro-environment,
  - Influence of malformed vasculature in tumor.

In [26], a model is proposed to illustrate the tumor metastasis using 6 differential equations. Three equations are used to represent the interactions between the normal host cells, tumor cells and the chemotherapy agent at the primary site and the other three equations provide interactions at the secondary site. The model also accounts for the time delay involved in the migration of these tumor cells from the current site (primary site) to a new site (secondary site) as given by [26]:

$$\frac{dN_p(t)}{dt} = r_1 N_p(t)\left(1 - b_1 N_p(t)\right) - c_1 N_p(t) A_p(t) - \frac{a_1 N_p(t) U_p(t)}{b_{c1} + N_p(t)}, \tag{3.21}$$

$$\frac{dA_p(t)}{dt} = r_2 A_p(t)\left(1 - b_2 A_p(t)\right) - c_2 N_p(t) A_p(t) - \frac{a_2 A_p(t) U_p(t)}{b_{c2} + A_p(t)} - \delta A_p(t), \tag{3.22}$$

$$\frac{dU_p(t)}{dt} = u_p(t) - \left[d_{U1} + \frac{g_1 N_p(t)}{b_{c1} + N_p(t)} + \frac{g_2 A_p(t)}{b_{c2} + A_p(t)}\right] U_p(t), \tag{3.23}$$

$$\frac{dN_s(t)}{dt} = r_3 N_s(t)\left(1 - b_3 N_s(t)\right) - c_3 N_s(t) A_s(t) - \frac{a_3 N_s(t) U_s(t)}{b_{c3} + N_s(t)}, \tag{3.24}$$

$$\frac{dA_s(t)}{dt} = r_4 A_s(t)\left(1 - b_4 A_s(t)\right) - c_4 N_s(t) A_s(t) - \frac{a_4 A_s(t) u_s(t)}{b_{c4} + A_s(t)} + \varepsilon\delta A_p(t-\tau), \tag{3.25}$$

$$\frac{dU_s(t)}{dt} = u_s(t) - \left[d_{U2} + \frac{g_3 N_s(t)}{b_{c3} + N_s(t)} + \frac{g_4 A_s(t)}{b_{c4} + A_s(t)}\right] U_s(t), \tag{3.26}$$

where $N_p(t)$ and $A_p(t)$ denote the number of normal and tumor cells, respectively, $U_p(t)$ denotes the concentration of chemotherapeutic drug at the primary site, $N_s(t)$, $A_s(t)$, and $U_s(t)$ denote that of the secondary site, respectively, τ is the time taken by the tumor cells in the primary site to move to a new site and initiate the secondary tumor growth, δ is the rate at which the cells leave the primary site, ϵ is the fraction of cancer cell which reaches the secondary site and starts interacting with the new environment to initiate tumor growth, r_i and b_i, $i = 1, 2$, denote the growth rate and the reciprocal carrying capacity of the normal and tumor cells at the primary site, respectively. Similarly, r_i and b_i, $i = 3, 4$, denote the growth rate and the reciprocal carrying capacity of the normal and tumor cells at the secondary site, respectively. The parameter b_{ci}, $i = 1, \dots 4$, denotes the speed at which the normal and tumor cells reach the carrying capacity in the absence of competition and predation at the primary and secondary sites, $u_p(t)$ and $u_s(t)$ are the rate of drug infusion to the primary and secondary sites, and respectively, and d_{U1} and d_{U2} are the rate of elimination of the chemotherapy agent from the primary and secondary sites, respectively. Finally, g_i, $i = 1, \dots, 4$, are the combination rates of the chemotherapy agent with the respective cells, which are proportional to respective predation coefficients of the drug given by a_i, $i = 1, \dots, 4$. A logistic growth pattern is used to model the normal and cancer cells at both sites.

To make the model more realistic, inequalities such as $r_2 > r_1$ and $r_4 > r_3$ are imposed to account for the increased growth rate of cancer cells compared to the normal ones. Similarly, in the absence of treatment, typically the cancer cells outcompete the normal cells irrespective of initial conditions. Furthermore, the pharmacodynamics of the chemotherapy agent is such that the drug is more effective in killing cancer cells than in killing normal cells. These drug dependent dynamics are captured by the inequalities, $a_2 \gg a_1$ and $a_3 \gg a_4$. The response to chemotherapy killing action on both normal and cancer cells is assumed to obey Michaelis–Menten saturation function.

With respect to (1.1), it can be seen that each cell population in the primary site involves growth function $\mathscr{G}(\cdot)$, the reduction in cell numbers due to competition $\mathscr{C}(\cdot)$, the limitation in growth due to carrying capacity of the environment $\mathscr{K}(\cdot)$, and the reduction of cells due to chemotherapeutic drug $\mathscr{D}(\cdot)$. In the secondary site of tumor, additional term $\varepsilon\delta A_p(t - \tau)$ is added to account for the movement of the abnormal cells from the primary site to secondary site after a delay of τ. Also note that the model given by (3.21)–(3.26) are more or less similar to the cell transition model given by (3.17)–(3.20). The cells that detach from the primary site have to overcome several natural barriers that prevent intravasation and extravasation of such invading cells so as to successfully metastasize. It is not clear whether it is appropriate to model such cell movements as a continuous transfer of cells from the primary site to secondary site. Further analysis is required in this regard.

Table 3.7 summarizes the parameter values of the non-dimensionalized chemotherapy model (3.21)–(3.26) [26]. The range of initial conditions for the variables in (3.21)–(3.26) are $N_p(0) > 0$, [124,1460], $A_p(0) >= 0$, [0,165], $U_p(0) >= 0$ [0,1000], $N_s(0) > 0$, [100,1750], $A_s(0) >= 0$, and $U_s(0) >= 0$, [0,1000]. The range of value for $u_p(t)$ and $u_s(t)$ is [0,650].

Table 3.7 Parameter values of the chemotherapy model (3.21)–(3.26) [26]

Param.	Value	Param.	Value	Param.	Value	Param.	Value
r_1	1.5	b_1	0.00068	c_1	0.0075	a_1	0.0008
r_2	10	b_2	0.00047	c_2	0.005	a_2	0.08
r_3	2	b_3	0.00057	c_3	0.002	a_3	0.0006
r_4	12	b_4	0.00043	c_4	0.001	a_4	0.1
g_1	0.0024	g_2	0.24	g_3	0.0018	g_4	0.3
ϵ	0.0001	τ	1	d_{U_i}	20	b_{ci}	1
δ	0.1						

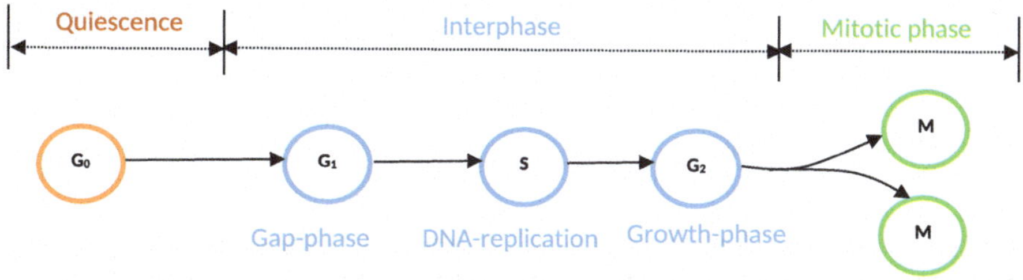

Fig. 3.3 Illustrative diagram showing different phases in cell-cycle

3.5 Cell-Cycle-Based Compartmental Model of Tumor Dynamics

As suggested in [11], studying cancer dynamics with respect to cell-cycle kinetics can give more insight about the factors that contribute to the uncontrolled growth of cancer cells. Moreover, as mentioned in the introduction of this chapter, many chemotherapeutic drugs (e.g. doxorubicin, paclitaxel) bring about tumor regression by delaying cell-cycle or inhibiting cell division and thereby inducing cell death. Such a model is discussed in [27], in which each cell population in a particular phase of cell-cycle is considered as a compartment. As shown in Fig. 3.3, there are mainly 5 phases identified between cell birth and cell division, namely:

- G_0 phase or quiescent phase,
- G_1 phase which denotes the initial growth phase of a cell,
- S phase which marks the DNA synthesis phase,
- G_2 phase which accounts for the period during which the cell grows prior to mitosis, and
- M is the mitotic phase wherein cell divides into two daughter cells.

After mitosis (cell-division), some of the new daughter cells enter to a dormant cell phase or resting phase (G_0 phase). The rest of the daughter cells enter directly to G_1 phase to go through the next phase of proliferation. It is apparent that a drug that can limit the mitotic division can reduce the abnormal multiplication of cells. Some chemotherapeutic drugs can slow down the DNA synthesis phase of the cell division, others can recruit cells in the dormant stage G_0 and initiate cell-cycle so that these cells can be killed later by a killing agent.

In [27], three models in which the cell populations are categorized into different compartments based on their response to various chemotherapeutic drugs are reviewed. First one is a 2-compartment model as given by:

$$\frac{\mathrm{d}A_1(t)}{\mathrm{d}t} = -\lambda_1 A_1(t) + 2\lambda_2 A_2(t) - 2\lambda_2 u(t), \tag{3.27}$$

$$\frac{\mathrm{d}A_2(t)}{\mathrm{d}t} = \lambda_1 A_1(t) - \lambda_2 A_2(t), \tag{3.28}$$

where $A_1(t)$ denotes the cell population in G_0, G_1, and S phases, and $A_2(t)$ denotes the cell population in G_2 and M phases, $u(t)$ denotes a cell-killing agent, and the λ_i, $i = 1, 2$ are positive coefficients whose values are related to the average transit times of cells through the ith compartment. The 3-compartment model is given by:

$$\frac{dA_1(t)}{dt} = -\lambda_1 A_1(t) + 2\lambda_3 A_3(t) - 2\lambda_3 u_1(t), \tag{3.29}$$

$$\frac{dA_2(t)}{dt} = \lambda_1 A_1(t) - \lambda_2 A_2(t) + \lambda_2 u_2(t), \tag{3.30}$$

$$\frac{dA_3(t)}{dt} = \lambda_2 A_2(t) - \lambda_3 A_3(t) - \lambda_2 u_2(t), \tag{3.31}$$

where $A_1(t)$ denotes the cell population in G_0 and G_1 phases, $A_2(t)$ denotes the cell population in S phase, and $A_3(t)$ denotes the cell population in G_2 and M phases. Here, two cell-killing agents $u_1(t)$ and $u_2(t)$ are considered, where the first agent is active during G_0 and G_1 phases and the second one is active during S, G_2, and M phases. Here, $u_2(t)$ denotes a blocking agent which slows the transit time of cancer cells during the S phase, and λ_i, $i = 1, 2, 3$ are positive coefficients whose value is related to the average transit times of cells through the ith compartment.

One more 3-compartment model given by:

$$\frac{dA_0(t)}{dt} = -\lambda_0 A_1(t) + 2b_0\lambda_2 A_2(t) - 2b_0\lambda_2 u_1(t) - \lambda_0 v_1(t), \tag{3.32}$$

$$\frac{dA_1(t)}{dt} = \lambda_0 A_1(t) - \lambda_1 A_2(t) + 2b_1 a_2 A_2(t) - 2b_1\lambda_2 u_2(t) + \lambda_0 v_1(t), \tag{3.33}$$

$$\frac{dA_2(t)}{dt} = \lambda_1 A_2(t) - \lambda_2 A_3(t), \tag{3.34}$$

is discussed in [27] where the main difference compared to the one discussed earlier is that, here the dormant phase (G_0) is considered as a separate compartment denoted by $A_0(t)$. $v_1(t)$ is a recruiting agent used to reduce the average stay time in the dormant phase. The term $A_1(t)$ includes cells in G_1 and S phases, and $A_2(t)$ denotes cells in G_2 and M phases. A closer look at (3.27)–(3.34) reveals that this model is also a special case of the general model given by (1.1)–(1.2) with cell growth, cell transition, and drug response terms. However, the three cell-cycle-based models discussed in this section does not directly account for the apoptosis rate and cell loss due to cell-cell competition or predation. Moreover, the time delay involved in cell transition is assumed to be negligible. Tables 3.8 and 3.9 summarize the parameter values of the chemotherapy models (3.27)–(3.31) and (3.32)–(3.34) [27]. The state variables $A_i(t)$, $i = 1, 2, 3$ denote the average number of cancer cells in respective compartments and $\lambda_i(t)$, $i = 0, 1, 2, 3$ are transit time. The initial conditions for the variables in (3.29)–(3.31) are $A_1(0) = 15$, $A_2(0) = 3.8$, and $A_3(0) = 0.8$. The initial conditions for the variables in (3.32)–(3.34) are $A_0(0) = 6.5$, $A_1(0) = 0.2$, and $A_2(0) = 0.1$.

Table 3.8 Parameter values of the chemotherapy model (3.27)–(3.31) [27]

Param.	Value	Param.	Value	Param.	Value
λ_1	0.197	λ_2	0.395	λ_3	0.107

Table 3.9 Parameter values of the chemotherapy model (3.32)–(3.34) [27]

Param.	Value	Param.	Value	Param.	Value
λ_0	0.05	λ_1	0.5	λ_2	1
b_0	0.9	b_1	0.1		

3.6 Mathematical Model for Leukemia

Mathematical models for tumor progression and regression are more or less similar for all types of cancer except for the cancers in blood tissues. As mentioned in Sect. 1.2.2 and shown in Fig. 1.3, different types of cells that constitute the blood tissue are generated by the hematopoietic stem cells (HSC). HSCs can be found in peripheral blood and bone marrow. Leukemia is a type of cancer which is characterized by the increased production of abnormal white blood cells (WBCs). These abnormal WBCs can impair the ability of the bone marrow to generate red blood cells (RBCs) and platelets. There are mainly 4 types of leukemia namely (1) acute myelogenous leukemia (AML), (2) acute lymphocytic leukemia (ALL), (3) chronic myelogenous leukemia (CML), and (4) chronic lymphocytic leukemia (CLL).

In case of cancers in blood, apart from the rate of growth, apoptosis, and competition of cells involved, there are few more significant mechanisms that need to be considered while developing mathematical models. Compared to the tumor-immune interactions in a solid tumors, additional factors that a mathematical model for leukemia should address are as follows:

- Various types of cell differentiation and cell transitions involved in the formation of mature red blood cells and white blood cells,
- Influx of cells from bone marrow, and
- Dynamics of the specialized cells called hematopoietic stem cells.

In [28], the hematopoietic stem cell-based basic model presented in [29] is extended by incorporating additional parameters to account for the simultaneous proliferation and differentiation phases of these cells as well as the movement of differentiated reticulocytes (immature RBCs) into the bloodstream.

Dynamics involved in the cell-cycle of the red blood cells (RBCs) and the effects of the chemotherapeutic drug 6-mercaptopurine (6 thioguanine nucleotide (6TGN)) on these cells are modeled as [28]:

$$\frac{\mathrm{d}A_{\mathrm{L}}(t)}{\mathrm{d}t} = r_1 A_{\mathrm{Q}}(t) - d_1 A_{\mathrm{L}}(t-120), \tag{3.35}$$

$$\frac{\mathrm{d}A_{\mathrm{Q}}(t)}{\mathrm{d}t} = -r_1 A_{\mathrm{Q}}(t)\left(2e^{a_1\tau}-1\right) m(A_{\mathrm{Q}}(t))A_{\mathrm{Q}}(t), \tag{3.36}$$

$$\frac{\mathrm{d}A_{\mathrm{P}l}(t)}{\mathrm{d}t} = -a_1 A_{\mathrm{PI}}(t) + \left(1-e^{-a_1\tau}\right) m\left(A_{\mathrm{Q}}(t)\right) A_{\mathrm{Q}}(t), \tag{3.37}$$

$$\frac{\mathrm{d}MCV(t)}{\mathrm{d}t} = \Bigg((g_1 U(t) + MCV_0) r_1 A_{\mathrm{Q}}(t) - 0.85 MCV(t-120) d_1 A_{\mathrm{L}}(t-120) - 0.15 MCV(t) d_1 A_{\mathrm{L}}(t) \Bigg) \frac{1}{A_{\mathrm{L}}(t)}, \tag{3.38}$$

where $A_{\mathrm{L}}(t)$ is the mature RBCs, $A_{\mathrm{Q}}(t)$ is the population of RBCs in the quiescent state, $A_{\mathrm{PI}}(t)$ is the population of RBCs in the proliferating or differentiating stage, $MCV(t)$ is the mean corpuscular volume, and r_1 and d_1 are the per day rate of cell differentiation (growth) and deterioration (death), respectively [28]. In the above model equations, $(t-120)$ accounts for the fact that a mature cell has an average life span of 120 days.

In this model, the cell transition pattern $\mathscr{M}(\cdot)$ of the resting cells to proliferating cells which follows a Hill-type equation is given by $m(A_{\mathrm{Q}}(t)) = \left(\frac{m_0 (Q^{50})^n}{(Q^{50})^n + (A_{\mathrm{Q}}(t))^n}\right)$. Here, m_0 is the maximum transition rate per day, Q^{50} is the quiescent state population at which $m(A_{\mathrm{Q}}(t))$ is half of m_0, and n denotes sensitivity of $m(A_{\mathrm{Q}}(t))$ to changes in size of the population in resting phase. Note that, in this model the effect of chemotherapeutic drug is modeled in the terms of a_1 and τ, where

Table 3.10 Parameter values of the chemotherapy model (3.35)–(3.38) [28]

Parameter	Value (unit)	Parameter	Value (unit)
r_1	0.00139 (days^{-1})	d_1	0.00710 (days^{-1})
a_0	0.00022 (days^{-1}pMol^{-1} per 8 × 10^{8}RBCs)	τ_h	0.68 (days)
MCV_h	85 (fL)	MCV_0	85 (fL)
g_1	0.0317 (fL pMol^{-1} per 8 × 10^8 RBCs)	d_1	0.00710 (days^{-1})
m_0	1.01 (days^{-1})	Q^{50}	2.70×10^{10} (cells kg^{-1})
n	1		

a_1 and τ are the drug induced death rate and cell-cycle time, respectively. Here, $a_1 = a_0 U(t)$ and $\tau = (g_1 U(t) + MCV_0)\frac{\tau_h}{MCV_h}$, where a_0 is a coefficient that describes the linear relationship between the drug (6TGN) and death rate, τ_h is the cell-cycle time of healthy cells, and MCV_h is healthy MCV [29].

Dynamics of $MCV(t)$ includes the rate of change of blood volume due to in and out movement of RBCs in periphery as well as the changes in the size of RBCs due to aging. The parameter g_1 is a coefficient that quantifies the linear relationship between the concentration of 6TGN (chemotherapeutic drug) which is denoted by $U(t)$ and ΔMCV. The value of g_1 is derived using the clinical trial discussed in [30]. More details about the clinical as well as experimental data sources that are used for the estimation of the parameters involved in this model are given in [28].

Compared to the general model (1.1), here the growth function involves $\mathscr{M}\left(m, C_{p1}(t)\right)$ which is actually the quiescent cells that transition to mature RBC. In (3.35), one can identify the growth function $\mathscr{G}(\cdot)$ and the reduction in the cell number due to apoptosis $\mathscr{A}(\cdot)$. Similarly, in (3.37) there is no explicit growth function $\mathscr{G}(\cdot)$, instead the increase in the cell number due to transition of quiescent cells ($A_Q(t)$) to proliferating cells ($A_{Pl}(t)$) is modeled using the term $\left(1 - e^{-a_1\tau}\right) m\left(A_Q(t)\right) A_Q(t)$. Note that, this model assumes that the drug has no effect on mature RBCs ($A_L(t)$). However, the drug induced ($\mathscr{D}(\cdot)$) cell-kill effect on the quiescent and proliferation phases of cell growth are accounted for in this model. In [28], this model is used to derive drug dose for achieving a target value of MCV. The patient data from the clinical trials reported in [30, 31] are used for the development and validation of the model (3.35)–(3.38) [28].

Table 3.10 summarizes the parameter values of the chemotherapy model (3.35)–(3.38) [28]. In model (3.35)–(3.38), the unit of the variables $A_L(t)$, $A_Q(t)$, and $A_{Pl}(t)$ is cells kg^{-1}, the unit of $MCV(t)$ is fL, and that of $U(t)$ is pMol per 8 × 10^8 RBCs. The steady state ratio of proliferating cells ($A_{Pl}(t)$) to quiescent cells ($A_Q(t)$) is given by $\frac{0.71\times10^8}{6.43\times10^8}$. The value of $U(t)$ is in the range [158,1000] units and the steady-state values of $A_L(t)$ is in the range [3.1×10^{12}, 3.9×10^{12}].

3.7 Summary

In Sects. 3.1–3.6, six mathematical models are discussed that depict different aspects of cancer dynamics under chemotherapy. Analysis of these models reveals that the dynamics of various cell populations basically involves the mechanisms such as birth, death, competition, and cell transition

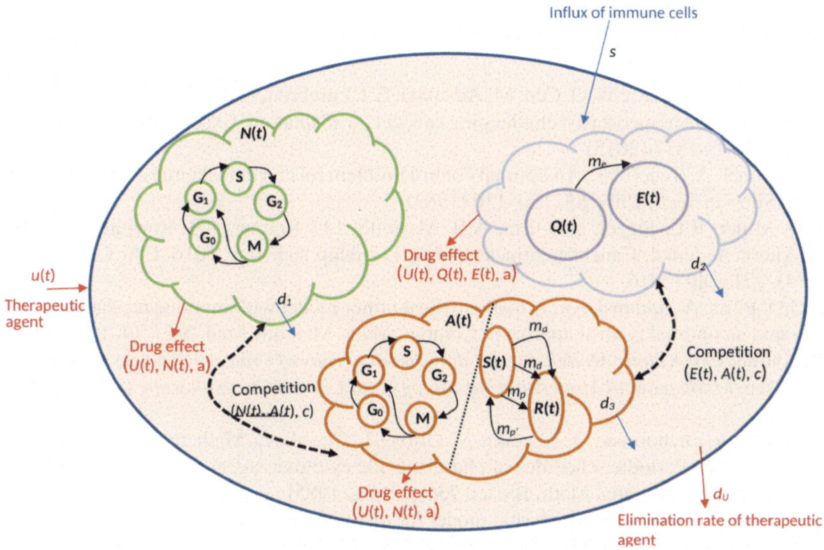

Fig. 3.4 Illustrative diagram showing dynamics in a tumor micro-environment. Normal cells-$N(t)$, cancer cells-$A(t)$, quiescent immune cells-$Q(t)$, hunting immune cells-$E(t)$, drug sensitive cells-$S(t)$, drug resistant cells-$R(t)$, drug concentration-$U(t)$, competition rate-c, drug effect-a, death rates-$d_i, i = 1, 2, 3$, cell transition rate of quiescent cell to hunting cells-m_e, acquired mutation rate of drug sensitive cells to drug resistant cells-m_a, drug induced mutation rate of drug sensitive cells to drug resistant cells-m_d, reversible phenotype switching rate of drug sensitive cells to drug resistant cells-m_p, reversible phenotype switching rate of drug resistant cells to drug sensitive cells-$m_{p'}$, and cells in G_0, G_1, S, G_2, and M phase of cell-cycle

as listed in the general model (1.1)–(1.2). However, several simplifying assumptions are used in each model. Figure 3.4 is an illustrative diagram which brings together different cell populations in a tumor micro-environment, the interaction between them, cell transitions, and the effect of chemotherapeutic drug on each cell population.

As shown in Fig. 3.4, the heterogeneous cell populations in the tumor micro-environment ($A(t)$, $N(t)$, $E(t)$) compete with each other for resources and survival. A common trend to account for the effect of the chemotherapeutic drug is to model the cell-kill effect of the drug on each cell population using a nonlinear term as discussed in Sects. 3.1, 3.3, and 3.4. Instead of analysing the effect of drug on all cell populations in the tumor micro-environment, in Sect. 3.5, the effect of drug on the particular cell cycle phase of cancer cells ($A_0(t)$, $A_1(t)$, $A_2(t)$) is modeled. The dynamics of cell-cell competition, cell-transition (mutation), and immune response on cancer cells are ignored in Sect. 3.5. In Sect. 3.6, the drug dynamics of the quiescent and proliferating red blood cells while treating leukemia is modeled.

Looking at Fig. 3.4 and the models discussed in this chapter, it can be seen that most of the models focus on one or two aspects of tumor dynamics and neglect the effect of other factors. Hence, a more general mathematical model that brings together most of the significant mechanisms involved in cancer dynamics is desirable. For instance, along with the dynamics of cell-cell competition, cell-transition (mutation), and immune response on cancer cells, dynamics related to drug resistance and drug toxicity such as that discussed in Sect. 3.2 should also be added while devising mathematical models of chemotherapy.

References

1. M. Moschovi, E. Critselis, O. Cen, M. Adamaki, G.I. Lambrou, G.P. Chrousos, S. Vlahopoulos, Drugs acting on homeostasis: challenging cancer cell adaptation. Expert Rev. Anticancer Ther. **15**(12), 1405–1417 (2015)
2. M. Kimmel, A. Świerniak, An optimal control problem related to leukemia chemotherapy. Sci. Bull. Silesian Tech. Univ. **65**, 120–130 (1983)
3. K.D. Miller, R.L. Siegel, C.C. Lin, A.B. Mariotto, J.L. Kramer, J.H. Rowland, K.D. Stein, R. Alteri, A. Jemal, Cancer treatment and survivorship statistics, 2016. CA: Cancer J. Clin. **66**(4), 271–289 (2016)
4. L.G.D. Pillis, A. Radunskaya, A mathematical tumor model with immune resistance and drug therapy: an optimal control approach. Comput. Math. Methods Med. **3**(2), 79–100 (2001)
5. H. Knolle, *Cell Kinetic Modelling and the Chemotherapy of Cancer* (Springer, Berlin, 1988)
6. M. Eisen, *Mathematical Models in Cell Biology and Cancer Chemotherapy* (Springer, Berlin, 1979)
7. B. Dibrov, A. Zhabotinsky, Y. Neyfakh, M. Orlova, L. Churikova, Mathematical model of cancer chemotherapy. Periodic schedules of phase-specific cytotoxic-agent administration increasing the selectivity of therapy. Math. Biosci. **73**(1), 1–31 (1985)
8. A. Coldman, J. Goldie, A stochastic model for the origin and treatment of tumors containing drug-resistant cells. Bull. Math. Biol. **48**(3), 279–292 (1986)
9. R. Martin, K.L. Teo, *Optimal Control of Drug Administration in Cancer Chemotherapy* (World Scientific, Singapore, 1993)
10. J. Murray, Optimal control for a cancer chemotheraphy problem with general growth and loss functions. Math. Biosci. **98**(2), 273–287 (1990)
11. L.D. Pillis, A. Radunskaya, The dynamics of an optimally controlled tumor model: a case study. Math. Comput. Model. **37**(11), 1221–1244 (2003)
12. V.A. Kuznetsov, I.A. Makalkin, M.A. Taylor, A.S. Perelson, Nonlinear dynamics of immunogenic tumors: parameter estimation and global bifurcation analysis. Bull. Math. Biol. **56**(2), 295–321 (1994)
13. R.A. Kempf, M.S. Mitchell, Effects of chemotherapeutic agents on the immune response. I. Cancer Investig. **2**(6), 459–466 (1984)
14. E. Moreno Lampaya, Is cell competition relevant to cancer?. Nat. Rev. Cancer **8**, 141–147 (2008)
15. M.M. Merino, R. Levayer, E. Moreno, Survival of the fittest: essential roles of cell competition in development, aging, and cancer. Trends Cell Biol. **26**(10), 776–788 (2016)
16. M. Baar, L. Coquille, H. Mayer, M. Hölzel, M. Rogava, T. Tueting, A. Bovier, A stochastic model for immunotherapy of cancer. Sci. Rep. **6**, 24169 (2016)
17. H. Siu, E. Vitetta, R.D. May, J.W. Uhr, Tumor dormancy. I. Regression of BCL1 tumor and induction of a dormant tumor state in mice chimeric at the major histocompatibility complex. J. Immunol. **137**, 1376–1382 (1986)
18. R.S. Kerbel, A cancer therapy resistant to resistance. Nature **390**(6658), 335 (1997)
19. S.M. Tse, Y. Liang, K.S. Leung, K.H. Lee, T.S.K. Mok, A memetic algorithm for multiple-drug cancer chemotherapy schedule optimization. IEEE Trans. Syst. Man Cybern. Part B (Cybern.) **37**(1), 84–91 (2007)
20. J.M. Greene, J.L. Gevertz, E.D. Sontag, Mathematical approach to differentiate spontaneous and induced evolution to drug resistance during cancer treatment. JCO Clin. Cancer Inform. **3**, 1–20 (2019)
21. Y. Liang, K.S. Leung, T. Mok, A novel evolutionary drug scheduling model in cancer chemotherapy. IEEE Trans. Inf. Technol. Biomed. **10**(2), 237–245 (2006)
22. J.M. Greene, C. Sanchez-Tapia, E.D. Sontag, Mathematical details on a cancer resistance model. BioRxiv, 475533 (2018)
23. W.P. Lee, The role of reduced growth rate in the development of drug resistance of HOB1 lymphoma cells to vincristine. Cancer Lett. **73**(2), 105–111 (1993)

24. S. Banerjee, R.R. Sarkar, Delay-induced model for tumor-immune interaction and control of malignant tumor growth. Biosystems **91**(1), 268–288 (2008)
25. F. Borges, K. Iarosz, H. Ren, A. Batista, M. Baptista, R. Viana, S. Lopes, C. Grebogi, Model for tumour growth with treatment by continuous and pulsed chemotherapy. Biosystems **116**, 43–48 (2014)
26. S. Pinho, H. Freedman, F. Nani, A chemotherapy model for the treatment of cancer with metastasis. Math. Comput. Model. **36**(7), 773–803 (2002)
27. A. Świerniak, U. Ledzewicz, H. Schättler, Optimal control for a class of compartmental models in cancer chemotherapy. Int. J. Appl. Math. Comput. Sci. **13**(3), 357–368 (2003)
28. S.L. Noble, E. Sherer, R.E. Hannemann, D. Ramkrishna, T. Vik, A.E. Rundell, Using adaptive model predictive control to customize maintenance therapy chemotherapeutic dosing for childhood acute lymphoblastic leukemia. J. Theor. Biol. **264**(3), 990–1002 (2010)
29. M. Mackey, Unified hypothesis for the origin of aplastic anemia and periodic hematopoiesis. Blood **51**(5), 941–956 (1978)
30. G. Decaux, F. Prospert, Y. Horsmans, J. Desager, Relationship between red cell mean corpuscular volume and 6-thioguanine nucleotides in patients treated with azathioprine. J. Lab. Clin. Med. **135**(3), 256–262 (2000)
31. F. Innocenti, R. Danesi, C. Favre, M. Nardi, M. Menconi, A. Di Paolo, G. Bocci, S. Fogli, C. Barbara, S. Barachini, G. Casazza, P. Macchia, M. Del Tacca, Variable correlation between 6-mercaptopurine metabolites in erythrocytes and hematologic toxicity: implications for drug monitoring in children with acute lymphoblastic leukemia. Ther. Drug Monit. **22**, 375–382 (2000)

Chapter 4
Immunotherapy Models

Immunotherapy is a treatment strategy that uses external adjuvants to boost our immune system and thus make use of our body's inherent mechanisms to fight cancer [1]. An increased incidence and development of cancer in immunodeficient animals and in human beings who take immune suppressive agents are reported in several literature [2–4]. Even though, early stages of tumorigenesis and possible regression of tumor by immune system is not documented in human beings, such evidences are collected from experimental models [5, 6]. All these evidences substantiate the capability of immune system to eradicate some of the tumors but not all. In other words, it is apparent that the process of tumorigenesis can progress only when tumor cells successfully override our body's immunosurveillance to certain extent. Hence, immunotherapy is a promising method that can contribute to cancer management.

The use of immunotherapy for cancer management is becoming more and more popular recently, mainly due to the fact that it is a biological strategy that can enhance specific anti-tumor functionalities of our immune system [7, 8]. Parallel to this, several related mathematical models have also been developed to analyze various therapeutic options, and to derive optimal treatment protocols [9–11]. In this chapter, five mathematical models are presented which are categorized based on the immunotherapy strategies adopted in Sects. 4.1–4.5. In order to follow this categorization, it is imperative to understand the related biological aspects. Hence, first, a very short note is provided on some of the related terms and mechanisms and the classification of immunotherapy. In Chap. 1, the general cell dynamics in a tumor micro-environment and tumor-immune interactions is discussed in Sects. 1.2 and 1.4. However, in this chapter, further elaboration on some of the components and mechanisms pertaining to tumor dynamics are provided which are significant in facilitating immunotherapy in particular.

Tumor micro-environment: In the case of solid tumors, various elements in the tumor micro-environment includes: (1) host cells such as epithelial cells or endothelial cells, (2) extracellular matrix (ECM) which plays a key role in cell adhesion, proliferation, migration, and differentiation, (3) stromal cells which are involved

R. Padmanabhan et al., *Mathematical Models of Cancer and Different Therapies*, Series in BioEngineering, https://doi.org/10.1007/978-981-15-8640-8_4

in the synthesis of extracellular matrix, (4) various types of immune cells, (5) signaling molecules such as cytokines, and (6) growth factors. Typically, the immune cells (lymphocytes) which have left the bloodstream and migrated into the site of the tumor are called as tumor-infiltrating lymphocytes (TILs). The tumor-infiltrating lymphocytes can be of different types according to the type of antigen receptors that are present on their surface. As mentioned earlier, the tumor-immune interaction is a complex mechanism, which involves numerous cell types and cell signaling proteins. The cell types from the immune system include natural killer cells, macrophages, cytotoxic T, helper T, regulator T, memory T, dendritic, helper B, effector B, and memory B cells [2]. It can be seen from Fig. 1.3 that all these cells are derived from myeloid progenitors and lymphoid progenitors by cell differentiation.

Types of immune system: It is well known that the immune system is capable of differentiating between the healthy host cells, abnormal cells, or external invaders by identifying the antigens present on the surface of these cells. Once a pathogen (abnormal or invader cell) is identified, then the immune system either counteracts using its non-specific fighters such as phagocytotic leukocytes and natural killer cells (e.g. monocytes, neutrophils, mast cells, and macrophages), or using pathogen-specific fighters such as B and T cells. The general response of the immune system which is not specific to a particular pathogen is called as nonspecific immune response (innate immunity) while the specific immune response is the one that particularly looks for the type of the pathogen and acts accordingly (adaptive immunity).

Identification, activation, and hunting: The overall actions involved in the specific immune response involve several co-inhibitory and co-stimulating pathways to make sure that only the harmful pathogens are attacked and host cells are spared (avoid autoimmunity). Even though these mechanisms are quite complex, in simple terms these actions can be categorized into the following 3 steps:

- Step 1: identification of the type of pathogens according to the antigen present on them,
- Step 2: activation of associated antigen-specific immune cells (helper, effector, and memory cells) using signaling molecules, and
- Step 3: hunting of the pathogen by active immune cells (effector cells).

Dendritic cells and macrophages are antigen presenting cells (APC) which help to connect innate (natural) and adaptive (acquired) immune systems. The process of pathogen identification by the APCs, presentation of antigens by the APCs to respective immune cells, and hunting of pathogens by immune cells is illustrated in Fig. 4.1. Even though there are many types of APCs such as macrophages, dendritic cells, and B cells in the immune system, dendritic cells are selected for illustration as they are one of the important immunotherapeutic target (DC vaccination) and many mathematical models discussed in the later sections of this chapter are built on the dynamics of the dendritic cell-mediated immune response.

As shown in Fig. 4.1, the immune cells such as dendritic cells interact with the tumor cells to process the antigen on the tumor cell surface. This is marked as the pathogen identification phase (Step 1) in Fig. 4.1. After processing the tumor-specific antigen (protein), the dendritic cells present (express) the antigen on the major histo-

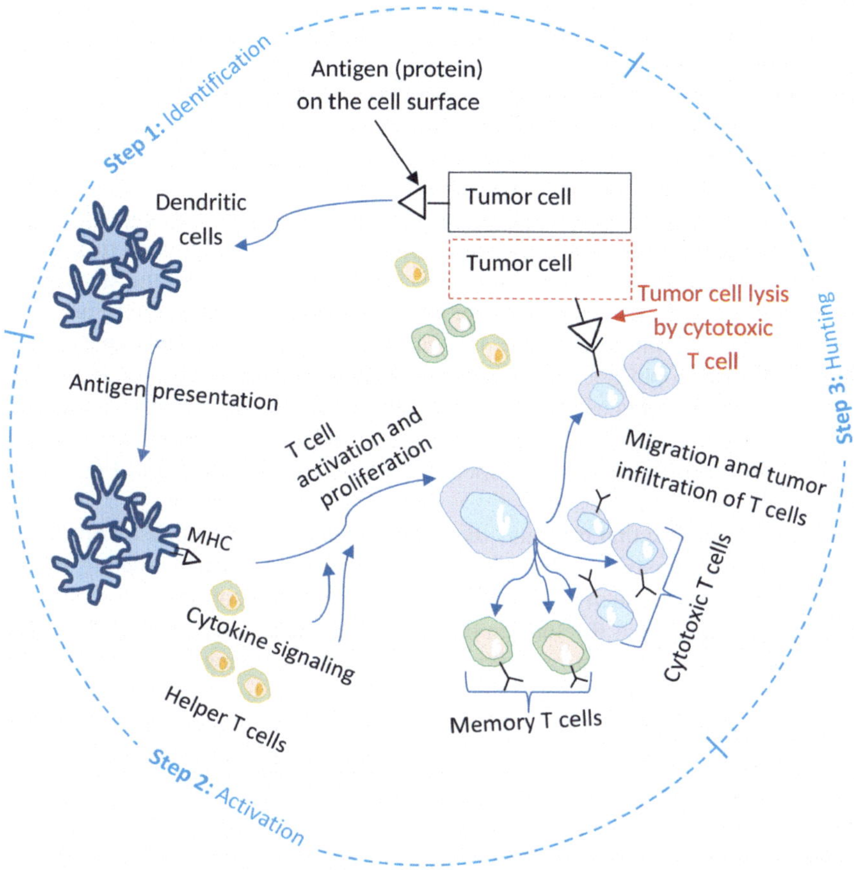

Fig. 4.1 Simplified illustration of antigen presentation, T cell activation, and tumor cell lysis. Step 1: Identification: Upon experiencing antigens on the tumor cell surface, dendritic cells get activated (licensed) and they present antigen via MHC (major histocompatibility complex), which attracts helper T cells. Step 2: Activation: The helper T cells initiate T cell activation and proliferation via cytokine signaling. Some of the activated T cells differentiate to form memory T cells. Step 3: Hunting: The cytotoxic T cells migrate/infiltrate to the tumor micro-environment. Antigen experienced cytotoxic T cells interact with tumor cells and facilitate tumor cell lysis

compatibility complex (MHC). Typically, a fragment of the tumor-specific antigen (i.e. peptide) is expressed on the surface of dendritic cells in the form of MHC peptide. This is marked as antigen presentation in Fig. 4.1. On identifying the pathogen labels (tumor labels) on the dendritic cells, the helper T cells get activated and differentiate to type 1 and type 2 helper T cells which will activate macrophages, killer T cells, and B cells [12]. For instance, the helper T cells mediate cytokine secretion and signal the T cell precursors (naive T cells). The helper T cells ($CD4^{+}$) induce secretion of cytokine IL-2, a specific signaling protein that can activate the killer

T cells ($CD8^+$). The naive form of major hunting cells of the immune system is capable of identifying these MHC peptides and once they experience tumor-specific antigen, they get activated (Step 2) and start proliferating. Some of the daughter cells of these antigen-experienced T cells turn to memory T cells and others mature to cytotoxic T cells to facilitate lysis of pathogens and abnormal cells (Step 3). In most cases, both the newly formed (by proliferation) cytotoxic T cells and memory T cells are equipped with toxic granules or antibodies that can counteract the tumor-specific antigen. Hence, if the same type of pathogen happens to invade our body again, these memory T cells are more effective in attacking and destroying them. This process of memorizing earlier attacks involves immune editing and thus facilitates adaptive immunity. Recall that the antigen-presenting cells such as the dendritic cells, macrophages, and B cells can mediate this memorizing process and hence these cells are often called as the link between innate and adaptive immunity. Even though various other cell types, cytokines, and receptor-ligand pairs play a key role in mediating the immune response, such details are omitted in Fig. 4.1 for brevity.

Another mechanism that mediates the annihilation of invading cells is opsonization. Similar to the antigen-presenting process that helps in the labeling of the pathogens and increases their visibility to the immune system, opsonization involves identifying and tagging of the foreign particles to facilitate phagocytosis. Once the pathogen is marked using an opsonin molecule (e.g. immunoglobulin G-IgG) by the macrophages or dendritic cells, the phagocytotic cells (e.g. natural killer cells, macrophages) engulf and digest the abnormal cells or foreign particles. There exist several therapeutic agents that utilize opsonization pathways to facilitate anti-cancer activities [13–16]. In [17], an artificially synthesized protein is tested for its potency to enhance opsonization using experimental mouse model. Such proteins are used in anti-cancer antibodies which mediate phagocytosis of opsonized target cells (tumor cells) [18].

Immune regulation: The immune response is a strictly regulated process that involves both co-inhibitory and co-stimulatory pathways [19, 20]. The immune system maintains a balance between these opposing pathways for its normal functioning. Breaching any of the regulator mechanisms of the system leads to an impaired immune response. Co-stimulatory (activatory) pathways are also called as immunogenic pathways as they facilitate immune response actions. For instance, completion of the T cell activation process requires two signals, one antigen-specific signal via MHC molecules and second a co-stimulatory signal between the T cell receptor (eg. CD28) and its ligand (CD80) on the APCs. Hindering any of these signals reduces the immunogenicity of the tumor which in turn restricts the immune response. In fact, tumor cells trick the immune system and escape from being recognized by the immune surveillance team by manipulating such handshaking immunogenic signals.

Co-inhibitory pathways are also called as tolerogenic pathways as they suppress the immune response. CTLA-4 is an immune checkpoint protein receptor that is capable of downregulating the immune response. Cancer cells express CTLA-4 and block the immune response [21]. Similar blocking of T cell activation and proliferation via binding of PD-1 receptor with its ligand PD-L1 is another example of a co-inhibitory pathway. Evidence suggests that cancer cells are capable of taking advantage of these tolerogenic immune response pathways to evade the immune response [21–23].

As shown in Fig. 4.2, upon identifying the tumor-specific antigen, the co-stimulatory pathways promote the immune response. This involvement of co-stimulatory signals is important to foster the transition of naive immune cells to active immune cells so as to facilitate the tumor regression. On the other hand, the co-inhibitory pathways inhibit such immune responses and facilitate the tumor progression. Immune functionality of the T regulator cells and cytokine TGF-β are other examples of immune system components that favor the tumor progression.

Immune evasion: It is apparent that the tumor cells are capable of altering and overriding most of the immune mechanisms that are in place for maintaining a healthy status. The tumor cells accomplish this by creating a metabolically unfavorable condition for the immune cells by means of one or more of the mechanisms listed below ([24, 25]):

1. Interfering and altering the antigen-presenting mechanism and thus hindering the recognition and elimination of tumor cells.
2. Enriching the regulatory immune cells such as T regulator cells, immune inhibitory B cells, etc., which are actively involved in suppressing immune responses.
3. Deteriorating immunoglobulin (antibody) mediated opsonization.
4. Upregulating the co-inhibitory lymphocyte signals.
5. By inducing a tolerogenic immune response.
6. Epigenetic silencing, which involves non-mutational inactivation of genes associated with recognition and elimination of tumor cells.

Signaling molecules or cytokines: Along with various types of immune cells, signaling molecules play a significant role in stimulating or inhibiting the immune response. Due to the role of the cytokines in mediating the anti-tumor activity, their presence and absence are correlated with various aspects related to disease prognosis and response to treatment [26–28]. Figure 4.3 shows different signaling proteins (collectively called as cytokines) which are often discussed in the context of tumor dynamics. Even though cytokines are identified to regulate various functions of the immune system, many of these signaling molecules are multi-functional. It is interesting to note that these molecules work independently, together, or against each other. Moreover, it is important to mention that the information on the types of cytokines and their role in cancer dynamics is updated now and then and hence the list shown in Fig. 4.3 is not meticulous.

Three main classes of cytokines include chemokines, interferons, and interleukins. Since chemokines are responsible for cell movement, they are said to mediate chemotaxis. For instance, increased expression of the CXC chemokine ligands such as CXCL9 and CXCL10 is correlated with the presence of higher levels of cytotoxic T cells ($CD8^+$ T cells) in the tumor micro-environment [29, 30]. Similarly, CXCR4 is believed to have a role in the tumor metastasis [31]. The expression of chemokines is regulated intrinsically by genetic pathways. External factors such as hypoxia, metabolic indications, and the microbiota can also influence the expression

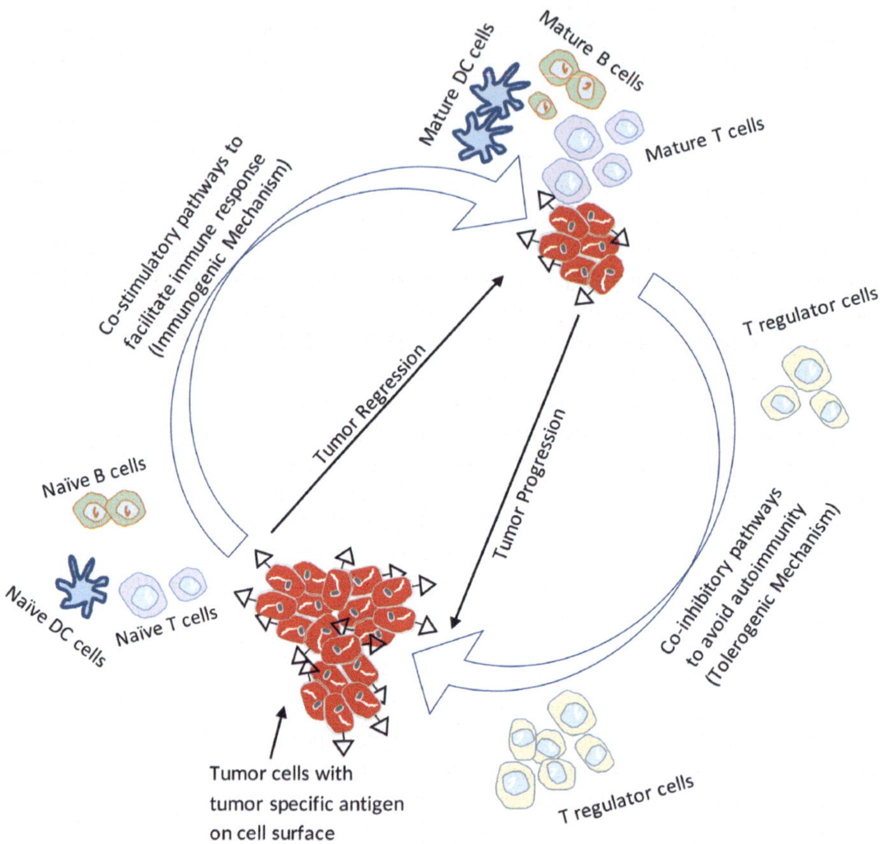

Fig. 4.2 Simplified illustration of the immune response and immune regulation facilitated by the co-stimulatory and co-inhibitory pathways, respectively. While immunogenic mechanisms facilitate the tumor regression by activating naive DC cells, B cells, and T cells to their mature counterparts, tolerogenic mechanisms hinder the immune response. Tumor-specific antigens (TAA) are simply the proteins present on the surface of tumor cells. Some of the immune cells are capable of identifying the TAA on cancer cells and act accordingly to facilitate tumor regression. However, cancer cells utilize tolerogenic pathways to evade (escape) from the immune response and thus facilitate the tumor progression

of chemokines [29]. The four main subclasses of chemokines are the CC-chemokines, CXC-chemokines, C-chemokines, and CX3C-chemokines [29]. Many chemokines are believed to have a role in metastasis, angiogenesis, stemness, and proliferation-related to the tumor dynamics [29].

Interferons (IFNs) are another type of cytokines released by the host cells to initiate protective functions (e.g. anti-viral) of our immune system. These signaling molecules are identified to have a role in anti-tumor activities as well [6]. The serum concentration of interferons is found to have a link with the tumor, grade, lymph node involvement, and metastasis [32, 33]. Interleukins (ILs) are another important

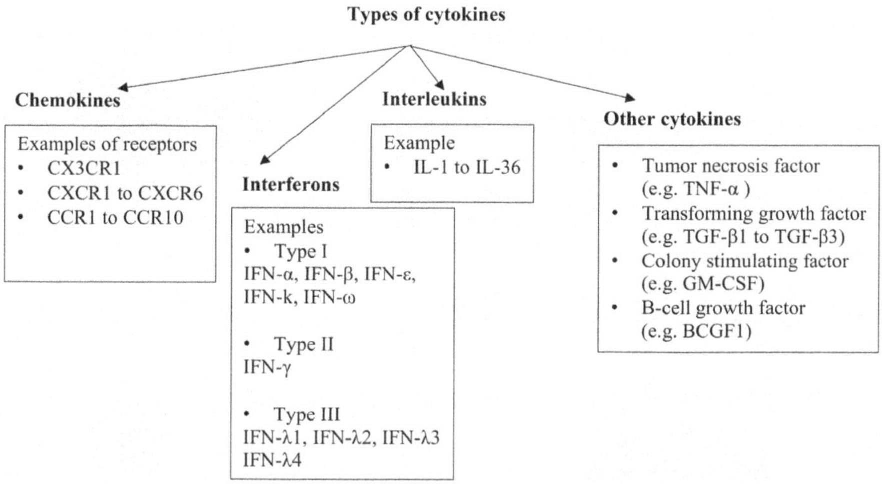

Fig. 4.3 Types of cytokines. Chemokines, interferons (IFN), and interleukins (ILs) are the three main types of cytokines. Tumor necrosis factor (TNF), transforming growth factor (TGF), granulocyte-macrophage colony-stimulating factor (GM-CSF), and B-cell growth factor (BCGF) are some other examples for cytokines. Even though there exist many more examples of cytokines, the cytokines frequently discussed in the context of cancer dynamics and considered in the existing mathematical models of tumor dynamics are listed

cytokine secreted by the immune system. For instance, T cells, macrophages, monocytes, and endothelial cells secrete various interleukins which promote the growth and differentiation of T cells, B cells, hematopoietic cells and play a key role in immune functions.

Apart from the three main types of cytokines, there are other cytokines such as tumor necrosis factor (TNF), transforming growth factor or tumor growth factor (TGF), colony-stimulating factor (CSF), and B-cell growth factor. Tumor necrosis factor sometimes called as TNF-α is a cytokine that is mainly produced by macrophages. Other immune cells that secrete TNF include CD4$^+$ cells, neutrophils, eosinophils, and mast cells.

The cytokine TGF-β is identified to have a key role in the cellular homeostasis and carcinogenesis [34]. Specifically, TGF-β is a tumor suppressor, and hence inhibition of signaling pathway mediated by TGF-β can induce carcinogenesis. In contrast to its tumor suppressor function, TGF-β is identified to play tumor promoter role by inducing remodeling of extracellular matrix (ECM) and epithelial to mesenchymal transition (EMT) so as to facilitate cell migration. Favoring tumor growth, the cytokine TGF-β promotes tumor cell proliferation, migration, and angiogenesis and block apoptosis and immune surveillance [34]. Evidence suggests that tumor cells can secrete TGF-β and inhibit the activation of naive CD8$^+$ cells [34–36]. Similar to the contradicting role of TGF-β in tumor progression, most of the cytokines are multi-functional and their exact involvement in tumor progression is yet to be understood clearly.

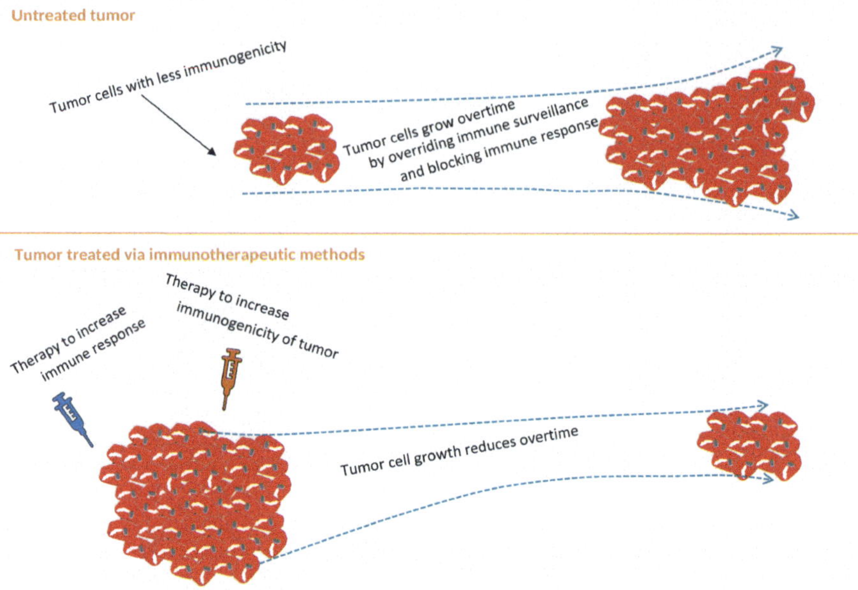

Fig. 4.4 Simplified illustration of immunotherapy. In an untreated scenario, the tumor cells with less immunogenicity remain unrecognized by the immune system. These tumor cells grow overtime by overriding the immune surveillance. However, when treated with immunotherapeutic drugs, the tumor growth is either arrested (dormant) or reduced overtime. The two therapeutic targets are marked in the figure: (1) Therapy that increases the immunogenicity of the tumor and (2) therapy that enhances the immune response (cytotoxicity) of the immune cells

Apart from the classification shown in Fig. 4.3, there is another set of cytokines called as lymphokines. All the cytokines secreted by the lymphocytes (e.g. T cells) are collectively called as lymphokines. For instance, interleukins and interferons secreted by the lymphocytes such as IL2 to IL6, granulocyte-macrophage colony-stimulating factor (GM-CSF), and IFN-γ are lymphokines.

Types of immunotherapeutic strategies: From Fig. 4.2, it is apparent that increasing the immunogenicity of the tumor cells and restricting the immune evasion activities by tumor cells are two important methods to revert the tumor progression. Hence, most of the immunotherapeutic methods make use of the knowledge of tumorigenesis and immune evasion to tailor appropriate counter mechanism to eliminate cancer. Antigenicity of a tumor is another related term that refers to the ability of a tumor to be identified by the antibodies. While antigenicity triggers specific immune fighters, immunogenicity accounts for any trigger that causes an immune response in general. The terms immunogenicity and antigenicity are used interchangeably as well. As identified in [24], there are mainly two categories of immunotherapeutic agents such as

1. Drugs that hinder the immune evasion related activities of tumor cells, and
2. Drugs that are capable of stimulating immunogenic pathways.

As shown in Figs. 4.2 and 4.4, tumor cells with less immunogenicity are more likely to grow uncontrollably by overriding the immune surveillance and immune response. This uncontrolled growth can be restricted by using therapeutic agents that improve immunogenicity of cancer or immune response to cancer. As discussed in the following part of this section, there are several such immunotherapeutic targets and treatment approaches that are currently in use. This is a very novel and dynamic area of cancer research and more pathways are being identified every now and then [22, 37]. However, this chapter presents the following therapeutic approaches for which corresponding mathematical models are also reported:

1. Targeting immune tolerance via co-inhibitory checkpoints.
   (a) Whenever the T cells are activated by the peptide processing mechanism, they start to proliferate and multiply in number (Fig. 4.1). These activated T cells also express the co-inhibitory receptor namely PD-1. The expression of this co-inhibitory receptors is mediated by the signaling proteins such as cytokines (e.g. IL-2, IL-7, IL-15, IL-21). It is known that when the co-inhibitory receptor such as PD-1 that is present on the activated T cells binds with ligands such as PD-L1 and PD-L2, these cells cease to proliferate. This binding of the co-inhibitory receptor (PD-1) and ligands (PD-L1, PD-L2) is an immune system checkpoint to avoid autoimmunity. Several studies point out that the tumor cells are capable of expressing checkpoint ligands such as PD-L1 to stop the proliferation and eventually cause the apoptosis of T cells [24]. Altering this immune evasion pathway using anti-PD-1 or anti-PD-L1 inhibitors and mAbs are important therapeutic targets.
   (b) Similar to PD-1, CTLA-4 is a co-inhibitory receptor protein. The CTLA-4 receptor binds with CD80 (B7-1) or CD86 (B7-2) to send a co-inhibitory signal to the immune system [38]. The CTLA-4 receptor is expressed on immune cells such as T and B cells [39], whereas CD80 (B7-1) and CD86 (B7-2) are expressed on the antigen-presenting cells such as dendritic cells, on activated B cells, and monocytes [38]. The CTLA-4 receptor is called as a co-inhibitory protein since the binding of the CTLA-4 receptor on the T cells with B7-1/B7-2 protein on the antigen-presenting cells switches off the activated T cells and thus downregulates the immune response. Similarly, the CTLA-4 receptors on T regulator cells can also inhibit the immune response. Note that this pathway comes under the category of tolerogenic mechanism depicted in Fig. 4.2. Recent evidence suggests that blocking CTLA-4 mediated immune inhibition to overcome the cancer cell tolerance of the immune system is a very useful approach to improve cancer treatment [40]. Hence, therapeutic anti-CTLA-4 antibodies are used to induce the reduction of T regulator cells or interfere with the co-inhibitory signaling.
   (c) Similarly, T cell immunoglobulin, immunoreceptor tyrosine-based inhibitory motif (ITIM), lymphocyte activation gene-3 (LAG-3), etc are other co-inhibitory receptors. Altering these co-inhibitory receptors can provide a positive outcome to enhance the immune response to tumor.

2. Enhancing anti-tumor responses via co-stimulatory pathways or by increasing the immunogenecity of tumor cells.
    (a) Adoptive transfer of activated T cells or adoptive cell transfer (ACT) is a immune system boosting method in which T cells are cultured *in vitro* and are administrated to the patients. In some cases, the efficacy of these *in vitro* cultured T cells are enhanced by lymphokine activation or gene alteration. ACT is further divided into (a) chimeric antigen receptor (CAR) T-cell therapy, and (b) tumor-infiltrating lymphocyte therapy. Another name for ACT is adoptive cellular immunotherapy (ACI) [41]. Apart from T cells, adoptive cell transfer also uses IL-2 activated natural killer cells [42].
    (b) Monoclonal antibodies (mAbs) are proteins which can be designed to bind to other specific proteins (antigens) to increase immunogenicity or antigenicity of tumor cells. Some mAbs are used to block abnormal proteins on the tumor cells, or to induce cell-cycle arrest leading to cell death. MAb-based immunotherapy utilizes the tumor cell targeting or tumor cell guiding property of monoclonal antibodies. These proteins roam around the body until they identify foreign cells or substance and bind to the antigens present on the surface of the invaders. This antigen-antibody pair acts as a flag that brings the invaders under the notice of the immune system. By figuring out the nature of the antigen present on the cancer cells, appropriate mAbs can be developed to target cancer cells [43, 44].
    (c) The CD-28 receptor is a co-stimulatory protein that binds with CD80 (B7-1) and CD86 (B7-2) to send a co-stimulatory signal to complete the immune response [38]. The CD28 receptor is expressed on immune cells such as T cells [39], whereas CD80 (B7-1) and CD86 (B7-2) are expressed on the antigen-presenting cells such as dendritic cells, on activated B cells, and monocytes [38]. The CD-28 receptor is called as co-stimulatory protein since along with other stimuli that activate the T cells (e.g. TCR signaling), a co-stimulatory signal via CD28 is required to complete the immune response. In the absence of the co-stimulatory signal, the activated T cells either turn unresponsive to immunogenic stimuli or become actively tolerant of tumor-specific antigens [38]. Hence, therapeutic anti-CD-28 antibodies are used to induce the reduction of T regulator cells or interfere with the co-stimulation of T cells by CD28.
    (d) Immunization or vaccination treatment via dendritic cells are also used to stimulate the immune response. As the underlying mechanism involved in the vaccination therapy method is to stimulate the immune system and thus facilitate the tumor regression, vaccination therapy is often considered as a subdivision of immunotherapy [45]. Unlike antiviral vaccines, vaccine therapy for cancer is not a preventive measure against cancer but it promotes cancer regression and prevents relapse of the disease. The therapeutic agents that are used for this treatment method are either derived from patients tumor or developed using other methods [44].

(e) Nonspecific immune stimulation that activates the immune response via activating natural killer cells, or administration of immunostimulatory cytokines is also used [16, 46].

(f) Oncolytic viruses are also used to increase the immunogenicity of tumor cells. Genetically modified viruses can be used to specifically target cancer cells. These oncolytic viruses can get into cancer cells and multiply uncontrollably leading to cancer cell lysis. Such cancer cells that die due to virus overburden, release specific antigens that further increase the immunogenicity of the tumor micro-environment and trigger the immune response [47, 48].

Out of the above listed immunotherapeutic strategies, mathematical models pertaining to adoptive T cell transfer, administration of cytokines, dendritic cell vaccine, and immune checkpoint inhibitors are discussed in this chapter [1, 9–11, 24]. Other methods such as oncolytic virotherapy and monoclonal antibody-based targeted therapy are discussed in Chap. 8 under the heading of miscellaneous therapies. Various researches are carried out in the field of immunotherapy with the help of mathematical models to foster various therapeutic options, for promoting optimal protocol for treatment scheduling and vaccine administration. In the case of immunotherapy, mathematical models are used to analyze tumor-immune interactions when external adjuvants are administrated. It is apparent that the cell types, cell signaling molecules, and mechanisms involved in the tumor-immune interaction are highly complex and yet to be understood clearly. Mathematical models are formulated by accounting for some of the known and significant mechanisms in cancer dynamics. Specifically, the dynamics of the naive or mature form of immune cells such as helper T cells, memory T cells, T regulator cells, cytotoxic T cells, dendritic cells, and influence of anti-tumor cytokines (IL-2), pro-tumor cytokines (TGF-β, IL-10) are presented [2, 49]. In the next sections of this chapter, the following five mathematical models of immunotherapy are presented:

1. Model that involves adoptive cellular therapy and cytokine injection,
2. Model with DC vaccination,
3. Model that involves immune checkpoint inhibition,
4. Model with DC vaccination that accounts for time delay, and
5. An elaborate model on tumor-immune interaction.

Tables 4.1 and 4.2 summarize the notations used in this chapter.

4.1 Immunotherapy Model that Involves Adoptive Cellular Therapy and Cytokine Injection

In this section, the Kirschner-Panetta model [50] is discussed which is one of the most widely used models of immunotherapy [49, 51–54]. This non-spatial dynamical model encompasses the interactions among tumor cells, effector cells, and IL-2 cytokine. In this model, the term "effector cells" represents all the activated immune

Table 4.1 Parameter notations in immunotherapy

Param.	Description	Param.	Description
g	Steepness coefficient	b	Reciprocal carrying capacity
c	Competition rate	d	Death rate or depletion rate
r	Growth rate	m	Mutation (cell transition) rate
a	Fractional cell-kill rate due to therapy	d_{U}	Depletion (elimination) rate of therapeutic agent from tumor site
s	Immune cell influx rate	μ	Half-saturation constant
ρ	Immune response rate or maximum proliferation rate	ψ_{pp}	Inhibition of T cell proliferation due to PD-1-PD-L1 binding
α_{50}	Half-saturation constant	α_{a}	Antigenicity of tumor
C^{50}	Half-saturation constant related to cytokine	ψ_1	Inhibition or inactivation of NK cells by T regulator cells
E_C^{50}	Concentration of the cytokine related to half-saturation of T cell proliferation	E_R^{50}	Number of T regulator cells related to half normal value of DC maturization
λ_{a}	Licensing rate of dendritic cells by helper T cells	d_{U}	Depletion (elimination) rate of therapeutic agent
κ	Fraction of tumor cells that leads to production of mature DCs	p	Smoothness of transition
τ	Time delay or time taken for one cell division		

cells that can kill tumor cells. The next element of this model is the cytokine IL-2. As mentioned in the introduction of this chapter, there are different varieties of interleukins. These cytokines are involved in inflammatory reactions, inhibition of the synthesis of other cytokines, hematopoiesis, and stimulation of the cellular immune response. Among the various types of interleukins identified till now, IL-2 plays a significant role in mediating the expression of co-inhibiting receptors such as PD-1 which regulates the growth and differentiation of immune cells (T and B cells). In [50], it is assumed that as the dose of IL-2 increases, there will be corresponding increase in the number of effector cells.

Regression of tumor when two continuous treatment schemes of immunotherapy namely, the adoptive cellular immunotherapy and cytokine injection is discussed in [50] and the model is given by ([55]):

$$\frac{\mathrm{d}E(t)}{\mathrm{d}t} = \alpha_{\mathrm{a}} A(t) - d_1 E(t) + a_1 u_1(t) + \frac{\rho_1 E(t) C(t)}{\alpha_{50_1} + C(t)}, \tag{4.1}$$

$$\frac{\mathrm{d}A(t)}{\mathrm{d}t} = r_1 A(t)(1 - bA(t)) - \frac{c_1 E(t) A(t)}{\alpha_{50_2} + A(t)}, \tag{4.2}$$

$$\frac{\mathrm{d}C(t)}{\mathrm{d}t} = a_2 u_2(t) + \frac{\rho_2 E(t) A(t)}{\alpha_{50_3} + A(t)} - d_{\mathrm{U}} C(t), \tag{4.3}$$

Table 4.2 Different types of cells and biochemicals in immunotherapy

Var.	Description	Var.	Description
$A(t)$	Tumor cells	$C(t)$	Cytokine concentration
$E_{\rm NC}(t)$	Naive T cells	$E_{\rm NK}(t)$	Natural killer cells
$E_{\rm UD}(t)$	Unlicensed dendritic cells	$E_{\rm D}(t)$	Dendritic cells
$E_{\rm H}(t)$	Helper T cells	$E_{\rm NH}(t)$	Naive helper T cells
$E_{\rm MH}(t)$	Memory helper T cells	$E_{\rm PH}(t)$	Helper T cells in proliferation stage
$E_{\rm 1H}(t)$	Type 1 helper T cells	$E_{\rm MC}(t)$	Memory cytotoxic T cells
$E(t)$	Active or mature cytotoxic T cells, or general effector cells	$E_{\rm PC}(t)$	Cytotoxic T cells in proliferation stage
$E_{\rm R}(t)$	T regulator cells	$E_{\rm PR}(t)$	T regulator cells in proliferation stage
$E_{\rm MR}(t)$	Memory T regulator cells	$u(t)$	Therapeutic input
$U_{\rm AP}(t)$	Concentration of anti-PD-1 inhibitor	$U_{\rm PP}(t)$	Concentration of PD-1-PD-L1 receptor-ligand pair

where $E(t)$, $A(t)$, and $C(t)$ denote the volume of effector cells, cancer cells, and concentration of IL-2, respectively, $u_1(t)$ represents the control input corresponding to any type of ACT such as the lymphokine-activated killer (LAK) cell therapy or tumor-infiltrating lymphocyte (TIL) therapy, and $u_2(t)$ is the second input that accounts for administration of IL-2 injection as an immune-boosting adjuvant [55]. It is easier to explain the tumor-immune interaction terms used in (4.1)–(4.3) using the general model (1.1) and (1.2) discussed in Chap. 1. It can be seen that similar to the general model in (1.1) and (1.2), here there are terms that correspond to cell growth ($\mathscr{G}(\cdot)$), apoptosis ($\mathscr{A}(\cdot)$), competition ($\mathscr{C}(\cdot)$), and the infusion of external adjuvants ($\mathscr{D}(\cdot)$).

First, whenever the immunosurveillance mechanism detects the tumor, it initiates the proliferation of effector cells. This increase in the effector cell population is modeled in (4.1) using the term $\alpha_a A(t)$, where α_a is the parameter modeling antigenicity of the tumor which represents the extent to which tumor cells express their antigens. Recall that the antigens expressed on tumor cells help the immune system to recognize tumor cells as abnormal cells [56]. The apoptosis of effector cells is expressed using $\mathscr{A}(\cdot) = d_1 E(t)$, where d_1 is the death rate of effector cells. The terms $\mathscr{D}(\cdot) = a_1 u_1(t)$ and $\mathscr{D}(\cdot) = a_2 u_2(t)$ in (4.1) and (4.3) model the application of external adjuvants to facilitate immunotherapy, where a_1 and a_2 are the treatment factors that enhance the effector cell populations and IL-2 concentration, respectively, where a dose dependent increase in $E(t)$ and $C(t)$ is assumed [51].

The nonlinear immune boosting facilitated by $u_1(t)$ and $u_2(t)$ is modeled in (4.1) and (4.3) using the terms $\frac{\rho_1 E(t)C(t)}{\alpha_{50_1}+C(t)}$ and $\frac{\rho_2 E(t)A(t)}{\alpha_{50_3}+A(t)}$, where ρ_1 and ρ_2 are immune response rates, and α_{50_1} and α_{50_3} are the half-saturation constants. These terms model the growth of effector cells due to IL-2 and an increase in the production rate of IL-2 due to effector-tumor interaction in Michaelis-Menten form [51]. Note that, the activated T cells produce IL-2 which promotes differentiation of naive T cells to hunting T and memory T cells (Fig. 4.1).

The first term in (4.2) models the tumor growth in logistic form. The increase in tumor growth and restriction in growth due to limitation in carrying capacity is modeled using the terms $\mathscr{G}(\cdot) = r_1 A(t)$ and $\mathscr{K}(\cdot) = br_1 A^2(t)$, respectively, where r_1 is the growth rate and b is the inverse carrying capacity. The second term in (4.2) such as $\mathscr{C}(\cdot) = \frac{c_1 E(t)A(t)}{\alpha_{50_2}+A(t)}$ accounts for tumor cell-lysis that occurs as a result of competition between tumor cells and effector cells, where c_1 is the competition rate and α_{50_2} is the half-saturation constant. Note that, the function $\mathscr{C}(A(t), E(t))$ accommodates the drug effect as well, that is the influence of the immune boosting injection $u_1(t)$ and $u_2(t)$ on increasing $E(t)$ and thus decreasing $A(t)$.

In (4.3), the first and second terms account for the cytokine injection and the recruitment of immune cells to the tumor micro-environment due to the injection of immunotherapeutic agents. The natural reduction or depletion in the IL-2 proteins is expressed using $\mathscr{D}_{\mathrm{c}}(\cdot) = d_{\mathrm{U}} C(t)$, where d_{U} represents the depletion rate of cytokine [55, 57, 58].

In some studies, different treatment methods of adoptive cellular immunotherapy namely, lymphokine-activated killer cell therapy and tumor-infiltrating lymphocyte therapy are used either in combination or separately [55]. A modified version of Kirschner-Panetta model is proposed in [59] which accounts for the time delay between IL-2 production by the antigen-stimulated T cells and stimulation of effector cells through IL-2 treatment as given by:

$$\frac{\mathrm{d}E(t)}{\mathrm{d}t} = \alpha_{\mathrm{a}} A(t) + \frac{\rho_1 E(t-\tau)C(t-\tau)}{\alpha_{50_1} + C(t-\tau)} - d_1 E(t) + a_1 u_1(t). \tag{4.4}$$

Compared to (4.1), in (4.4), a time delay is added to the immune-recruitment term [50, 55, 59].

Recalling the chemotherapy model discussed in Sect. 3.1 of Chap. 3, it can be seen that the apoptosis terms are modeled as $d_1 E(t)$ in both (3.1) and in (4.1). However, the influx rate s in (3.1) that corresponds to the increase in effector cells in the tumor micro-environment is modeled in (4.1) as $\alpha_a A(t)$. This is to account for the significance of antigenicity or immunogenicity (α_a) of the tumor cells when immunotherapeutic agents are used to enhance cancer management. Also notice that, in (3.1), when the immune cell number is reduced by a factor of $a_1 \left(1 - e^{-U(t)}\right) E(t)$ due to the undesired effect of chemotherapeutic drug, in (4.1) the drug input $u_1(t)$ boosts the number of effector cells. Similarly, comparing (3.2) and (4.2), the growth of tumor cells in case of chemotherapy and immunotherapy are modeled using a logistic term. However, when the competition between the tumor cells and immune

Table 4.3 Parameter values of the immunotherapy model (4.1)–(4.3) [50, 55]

Parameter	Value (unit)	Parameter	Value (unit)
α_a	0-0.05 (days^{-1})	ρ_1	0.1245 (days^{-1})
α_{50_1}	2×10^7 (unit of volume)	d_1	0.03 (days^{-1})
a_1	500	r_1	0.18 (days^{-1})
b	1×10^{-9} (unit of volume)	c_1	1 (days^{-1})
α_{50_2}	1×10^5 (unit of volume)	ρ_2	5 (days^{-1})
α_{50_3}	1×10^3 (unit of volume)	d_U	10 (days^{-1})
a_2	7×10^7		

cells are modeled in (3.2) as $c_1E(t)A(t)$, a nonlinear reduction of tumor cells is modeled in (4.2) using the term $\frac{c_1E(t)A(t)}{\alpha_{50_2}+A(t)}$ as the tumor cell-kill is expected to increase in a nonlinear fashion due to the injection of activated T cells.

Table 4.3 summarizes the parameter values of the immunotherapy model (4.1)–(4.3) [50, 55]. The unit of $E(t)$, $A(t)$, and $C(t)$ is volume and $u_i(t)$, $i = 1, 2$ is volume day^{-1}. The initial conditions for the variables in the model (4.1)–(4.3) are $E(0) = A(0) = C(0) = 1$.

4.2 Model with DC Vaccination

Vaccination is a well known immunotherapeutic strategy that is used to boost our body's efficacy to fight pathogen-specific diseases. Typically, vaccine therapy involves the administration of weakened pathogens or pathogen-derived proteins to the body. These exogenously induced substances are capable of invoking adaptive immunity by stimulating the immune response and facilitating the pathogen-specific immune editing. Even though most of the cancer types do not stem from pathogens, very few pathogens or pathogen-derivatives such as human papillomavirus (HPV), helicobacter pylori (bacteria), and aflatoxin (toxin from a fungus) are identified for initiating cancer [60, 61]. Consequently, few prevention vaccines have also developed. Apart from prevention vaccines, some treatment vaccines are also developed recently which can boost the immune activity against cancer via the antigen-presenting mechanism that can mediate the adaptive immune system activities. Due to this reason, cancer treatment via therapeutic vaccines comes under the broad heading of immunotherapy [24]. Treatment approaches include modifying immune cells derived from a patient's body by adding appropriate substances or cells called as adjuvants to target antigen-presenting mechanism and then injecting them back to the bloodstream.

As shown in Fig. 4.1, dendritic cells are one type of antigen-presenting cell, which can induce regression of emerging tumors and can also become antigen-experienced memory cells. These cells are derived as immature dendritic cells from the bone marrow. When these cells encounter presentable antigens of pathogens/cancer cells, they get mature and migrate to the lymph node. Upon maturation, these cells present the antigen fragments of encountered pathogens at the cell surface using major histocompatibility complex (MHC) molecules. The helper and killer T cells detect these antigens and get activated, thereby boosting the immune response [62].

Dendritic cell vaccine (DCV) therapy is a vaccine-based immunotherapy that makes use of the ability of dendritic cells to efficiently deliver loaded antigen molecules to destination [52]. The dendritic cells extracted from the patient are cultured along with tumor-associated antigens (TAA). Then this TAA loaded dendritic cells are injected back to the patient so that the killer cells recognize these antigens and help in boosting the immune response against those antigens.

A model describing the enhancement of immune response using dendritic cell transfection is given in [52]. This model accounts for the dynamics of only those immune cells, which are able to recognize the tumor-associated antigen. The tumor mass is assumed to be at a range where the effects of vascularization, immunosuppression, and immune evasion are negligible. The model of tumor-immune interaction under DC vaccination is given by ([52, 63]):

$$\frac{\mathrm{d}E_{\mathrm{H}}(t)}{\mathrm{d}t} = s_1 + \rho_1 E_{\mathrm{D}}(t)\Big(r_1 E_{\mathrm{H}}(t)\big(1 - b_1 E_{\mathrm{H}}(t)\big)\Big) - d_1 E_{\mathrm{H}}(t), \tag{4.5}$$

$$\frac{\mathrm{d}E(t)}{\mathrm{d}t} = s_2 + \rho_2 C(t)\big(A(t) + E_{\mathrm{D}}(t)\big)\Big(r_2 E(t)\big(1 - b_2 E(t)\big)\Big) - d_2 E(t), \tag{4.6}$$

$$\frac{\mathrm{d}A(t)}{\mathrm{d}t} = r_3 A(t)\big(1 - b_3 A(t)\big) - c_1 A(t)E(t), \tag{4.7}$$

$$\frac{\mathrm{d}E_{\mathrm{D}}(t)}{\mathrm{d}t} = -c_2 E(t)E_{\mathrm{D}}(t) + u(t), \tag{4.8}$$

$$\frac{\mathrm{d}C(t)}{\mathrm{d}t} = r_4 E_{\mathrm{H}}(t)E_{\mathrm{D}}(t) - c_3 E(t)C(t) - d_3 C(t), \tag{4.9}$$

where $E_{\mathrm{H}}(t)$ and $E(t)$ denote the helper T cells ($\mathrm{CD4}^+$) and tumor-specific cytotoxic T cells ($\mathrm{CD8}^+$), $A(t)$ and $E_{\mathrm{D}}(t)$ denote the tumor cells and TAA loaded mature dendritic cells, respectively, $C(t)$ is the concentration of the cytokine IL-2 which is secreted by helper T cells, and $u(t)$ is the input which represents the administration of TAA loaded dendritic cells prepared in vitro [63].

The terms s_1 and s_2 in (4.5) and (4.6), model the normal birth rate as well as the rate of inflow of helper T cells and killer T cells into the region of tumor localization, respectively. Upon recognizing the tumor-specific antigen presented by dendritic cells, the helper T cells and cytotoxic T cells start proliferating. This non-linear clonal expansion of $E_{\mathrm{H}}(t)$ and $E(t)$ is captured using the terms $\mathscr{G}(\cdot) = \rho_1 E_{\mathrm{D}}(t)\Big(r_1 E_{\mathrm{H}}(t)\big(1 - b_1 E_{\mathrm{H}}(t)\big)\Big)$ and $\mathscr{G}(\cdot) = \rho_2 C(t)\big(A(t) + E_{\mathrm{D}}(t)\big)\Big(r_2 E(t)\big(1 - b_2 E(t)\big)\Big)$ in (4.5) and (4.6), respectively, where, ρ_1 and ρ_2 are the maximum prolif-

Table 4.4 Parameter values of the immunotherapy model (4.5)–(4.9) [52, 63]

Parameter	Value (unit)	Parameter	Value (unit)
s_1	10^{-4} (cells $h^{-1}mm^{-3}$)	ρ_1	10, ρ_2 is a parameter and 10 ($pg^{-}1\ mm^3$) is value(unit)
r_1	10^{-2} ($cells^{-1}h^{-1}mm^3$)	b_1, b_2, b_3	1 ($cells^{-1}mm^3$)
d_1, d_2	0.005 (h^{-1})	s_2	10^{-4} (cells $h^{-1}mm^{-3}$)
r_2	10^{-2} ($cells^{-1}h^{-1}mm^3$) r_4 is a parameter 10^{-2} (pg $cells^{-2}$ $h^{-1}mm^3$) is value (unit)	r_3	0.02 (h^{-1})
c_1, c_2	0.1 ($cells^{-1}h^{-1}mm^3$)	d_3	10^{-2} (h^{-1})
c_3	10^{-7} ($cells^{-1}$ $h^{-1}mm^3$)		

eration constants of the helper and cytotoxic T cells, and b_1 and b_2 are their inverse carrying capacities. The term $E_D(t)$ is included to capture the increase in T cell population proportional to the number of dendritic cells. Hence, these growth terms also accommodate the effect of dendritic cell injection. The last terms in (4.5) and (4.6) model the apoptosis or natural death of helper T cells and effector cells as $\mathscr{A}(\cdot) = d_1 E_H(t)$ and $\mathscr{A}(\cdot) = d_2 E(t)$, where d_1 and d_2 are death rates of these cells.

The logistic growth of tumor cells is modeled in (4.7) as $\mathscr{G}(\cdot) = r_3 A(t)\big(1 - b_3 A(t)\big)$ and the decrease in cell population due to their encounter with the cytotoxic T cells is accounted for using the term $c_1 A(t)E(t)$, where c_1 quantifies the increased cell-cell interaction between tumor cells and killer T cells. Note that, here the increase in the cell-cell interaction is mainly due to the immunotherapeutic drug, that is the DC vaccine. Hence, instead of the competition term $c_1 A(t)E(t)$ in (4.7), one can use a drug effect term such as $\mathscr{D}(\cdot) = aA(t)E(t)$, where a quantifies the drug induced cell-kill rate. In [52], it is assumed that the dendritic cells are also killed at a rate of c_2 by the cytotoxic T cells as they expose tumor peptides. This is modeled in (4.8) using the term $c_2 E_D(t)E(t)$.

Equation (4.9) models the dynamics associated with IL-2 due to the dendritic cell vaccine injection. Upon recognition of antigen experienced dendritic cells by helper T cells, they secrete IL-2 which is modeled as $\mathscr{G}(\cdot) = r_4 E_H(t)E_D(t)$, where r_4 denotes the rate of increase in IL-2 concentration. The second term of this equation accounts for the decrease in IL-2 concentration as it is consumed by cytotoxic T cells for its clonal expansion. Similar to (4.7), in (4.9), the interaction between $E(t)$ and $C(t)$ which leads to the reduction in IL-2 is indirectly due to the influence of dendritic cell vaccine, so instead of the competition term $c_2 E(t)C(t)$ in (4.9), one can also use a drug effect term such as $aE(t)C(t)$. The free interleukin-2 also undergoes degradation at a rate d_3. It can be seen that, the dendritic cell dynamics depicted in (4.8) is similar to (3.4) which models the dynamics of chemotherapeutic agent. Compared to the general equation for drug dynamics provided in (1.2), the difference in (4.8) is that the drug elimination term d_U in (1.2) is replaced by the term $c_2 E(t)$ in (4.8) to accommodate the influence of effector cell interaction rate on the depletion of dendritic cells. Table 4.4 summarizes the parameter values of the immunotherapy model (4.5)–(4.9) [52, 63]. In the model (4.5)–(4.9), the unit of $E_{\mathrm{H}}(t)$, $E(t)$, $A(t)$, and $E_{\mathrm{D}}(t)$ is cell mm^{-3}. The unit of IL-2 secreted by helper T cells, $C(t)$, is pg mm^{-3}. Based on the scaled reciprocal carrying capacity ($b_i = 1$, i=1,2,3, cells^{-1} mm^3), all the state variables in this model vary between 0 and 1 where 0 means no cells or no IL-2 secretion and 1 is the upper bound of all cells or IL-2 secretion.

4.3 Model that Involves Immune Checkpoint Inhibition

As explained earlier, tumor cells use the PD-1-PD-L1 binding to hack the immune response mechanisms and thus evade the cytotoxic actions of T cells. An anti-PD-1 drug can be used to hinder PD-1-PD-L1 binding and thereby making tumor cells prone to immune attack. In this section, a mathematical model that accounts for the effect of an immune checkpoint inhibitor in tumor-immune interactions is discussed. In [64], a complex 13 equations PDE model is used to illustrate the combined effect of dendritic cell vaccine and anti-PD-1 drug on tumor-immune interactions. In [65], the PDE model in [64] is used to derive a simplified ODE model when an anti-PD-1 drug is used. The tumor-immune interactions when an anti-PD-1 drug is used to enhance the immune response is given by ([65]):

$$\frac{\mathrm{d}E(t)}{\mathrm{d}t} = \left(r_1 E_{\mathrm{NC}}(t)\frac{C_1(t)}{C_1^{50} + C_1(t)} + r_2 E(t)\frac{C_2(t)}{C_2^{50} + C_2(t)}\right)\left(\frac{1}{1 + \frac{U_{\mathrm{PP}}(t)}{\psi_{\mathrm{pp}}}}\right) - d_1 E(t), \tag{4.10}$$

$$\frac{\mathrm{d}A(t)}{\mathrm{d}t} = r_3 A(t)\Big(1 - bA(t)\Big) - a_\rho A(t)E(t), \tag{4.11}$$

$$\frac{\mathrm{d}U_{\mathrm{AP}}(t)}{\mathrm{d}t} = u_{\mathrm{AP}}(t) - a_{\mathrm{r1}}U_{\mathrm{FP1}}(t)U_{\mathrm{AP}}(t) - d_{\mathrm{U}_2}U_{\mathrm{AP}}(t), \tag{4.12}$$

where $E(t)$, $E_{\mathrm{NC}}(t)$, and $A(t)$ denote the number of activated T cells, naive cytotoxic T cells, and cancer cells, $C_1(t)$ and $C_2(t)$ denote the concentration of IL-12 and IL-2, respectively, $U_{\mathrm{PP}}(t)$ denotes the concentration of PD-1-PD-L1 complex, $U_{\mathrm{AP}}(t)$ denotes the concentration of anti-PD-1 drug, $u_{\mathrm{AP}}(t)$ denotes the infusion rate of anti-PD-1 drug, and $U_{\mathrm{FP1}}(t)$ denotes the level of free PD-1 concentration. The first growth term in (4.10) models the increase in the number of naive T cells due to IL-12, and the second growth term accounts for the increase in proliferation of the activated T cells due to the stimulation by IL-2, where r_1 is the growth rate of T cells due to the activation by the cytokine (IL-12), r_2 is the growth rate of T cells due to the stimulation by the cytokine (IL-2), and d_1 is the death rate of effector T cells. Note that these two growth terms also account for the saturation effect of the immune response using the Michaelis-Menten form and the parameters C_1^{50} and C_2^{50} denote half-saturation values pertaining to the concentration of IL-12 and IL-2, and its effect on the growth of $E_{\mathrm{NC}}(t)$ and $E(t)$, respectively.

In (4.10), the binding of PD-1 receptor with its ligand PD-L1 which leads to the inhibition of T cell activation is modeled using the term $\frac{1}{1+\frac{U_{\mathrm{PP}}(t)}{\psi_{\mathrm{pp}}}}$, where ψ_{pp} denotes

Table 4.5 Parameter values of the immunotherapy model (4.10)–(4.12) [65]

Parameter	Value (unit)	Parameter	Value (unit)
r_1	8.81 (days^{-1})	C_1^{50}	1.5 $\times 10^{-10}$ (g cm^{-3})
r_2	0.5 (days^{-1})	C_2^{50}	2.37 $\times$ 10^{-11} (g cm^{-3})
ψ_{PP}	1.365$\times 10^{-18}$ (g cm^{-3})	d_1	0.05 (days^{-1})
r_3	0.18-0.67 (days^{-1})	$1/b$	0.8-0.945 (g cm^{-3})
a_ρ	57.5 ($\text{days}^{-1}\text{cm}^3\text{g}^{-1}$)	a_{rl}	4.9085$\times 10^6$–2.07 $\times$ 10^8 (days^{-1} cm^3g^{-1})
ρ_{r}	3.19$\times 10^{-7}$ – 8.49 $\times$ 10^{-7}	d_{U_1}	10 (cm^3g^{-1})
d_{U_2}	3.3$\times 10^{-2}$ – 1.39 (days^{-1})	$C_{1\text{ss}}$	1.5$\times 10^{-10}$ (g cm^{-3})
ϵ_{C}	1–100	$C_{2\text{ss}}$	2.37$\times 10^{-11}$ (g cm^{-3})
σ_{L}	3.56$\times 10^{-7}$–1.967$\times 10^{-6}$		

the rate of inhibition. If the concentration of PD-1-PD-L1 binding is much larger than the inhibition rate, this term reduces the growth rate of activated T cells, and quantifies the immune evasion by cancer cells via the PD-1-PD-L1 co-inhibitory pathway (Fig. 4.2). For simplicity, in [65], the cytokine concentrations $C_1(t)$ and $C_2(t)$ are assumed to change within a tight range and they are replaced by their respective steady-state values such as $C_{1\text{ss}}$ and $C_{2\text{ss}}$, respectively.

In (4.11), the first term models the tumor growth using a logistic form, where r_3 is the growth rate of cancer cells and b is the reciprocal carrying capacity. The second term accounts for the tumor regression due to immunotherapy. The parameter a_ρ models the efficacy of the immunotherapeutic drug (anti-PD-1) in restricting immune evasion by tumor cells and activating the T cells to mediate the tumor regression. It can be seen from (4.11) that, the effect of the anti-PD-1 drug on the growth of tumor cells is modeled as $\left(r_3 - a_\rho E(t)\right) A(t)$, which shows that as the number of cytotoxic T cells ($E(t)$) increases, the growth rate of tumor cells will decrease proportionately.

In (4.12), the drug dynamics of the immune checkpoint inhibitor (anti-PD-1) is modeled. The first term $u_{\text{AP}}(t)$ accounts for the effective level of drug in the tumor micro-environment according to the rate of drug infusion. The second term in (4.12) accounts for the depletion of the anti-PD-1 drug concentration due to usage (blocking by PD-1), where a_{rl} is the blocking rate of the receptor PD-1 by the anti-PD-1 drug. The level of free PD-1 is given by $U_{\text{FP1}}(t) = \left(\rho_{\text{r}} - d_{\text{U}_1} U_{\text{AP}}(t)\right) E(t)$, where ρ_{r} denotes the expression level of the PD-1 on T cells, and d_{U_1} is the depletion of PD-1 by anti-PD-1. The last term $d_{\text{U}_2} U_{\text{AP}}(t)$ accounts for the natural depletion of the drug, where d_{U_2} is the drug degradation rate. In [65], the association and dissociation of PD-L1-PD-1 is assumed to be fast and is given by $U_{\text{PP}}(t) = \sigma U_{\text{FP1}}(t) U_{\text{FL1}}(t)$, where $\sigma = \frac{\delta_{\text{a}}}{\delta_{\text{d}}}$, δ_{a} quantifies the association of PD-1 with PD-L1 and δ_{d} quantifies the dissociation of PD-1-PD-L1 complex, $U_{\text{FL1}}(t)$ denotes the level of free PD-L1 and is given by $U_{\text{FL1}}(t) = \sigma_{\text{L}}\left(E(t) + \epsilon_{\text{C}} A(t)\right)$, where σ_{L} is the level of expression of PD-L1 on the activated T cells and ϵ_{C} is the expression of PD-L1 in tumor cells versus T cells. In this model, the anti-PD-1 drug is assumed to be administrated to a patient as continuous intravenous or intradermal injection at the rate of $u_{\mathrm{AP}}(t) = 10^{-10}\mathrm{days}^{-1}\mathrm{cm}^3\mathrm{g}^{-1}$.

Table 4.5 summarizes the parameter values of the immunotherapy model (4.10)–(4.12) [65]. The initial conditions for the variables in (4.10)–(4.12) are $E(0) = 6 \times 10^{-3}$ (g cm^{-3}), $A(0) = 0.3968$ (g cm^{-3}), and $U_{\mathrm{AP}}(0) = 0$ (g cm^{-3}).

4.4 Model with DC Vaccination that Accounts for Time Delay

Compared to the models discussed in Sects. 4.1 and 4.3, additional immune cell populations and time delay involved in their differentiation are taken into consideration in the model discussed in this section. Specifically, a mathematical model is presented which incorporates the tumor-immune interactions pertaining to helper T cells (both naive and mature), dendritic cells, natural killer cells (NK), cytotoxic T cells (naive and mature), interleukin-2, and regulator T cells [66]. Figure 4.5 shows the main mechanisms that are taken into consideration for model development. Once an abnormal cell type or growth is detected by the immune system, both the non-specific and specific fighters of the immune system start counteracting to annihilate the abnormality. Note that the dendritic cell vaccine injection can contribute to the growth of non-specific immune fighters such as natural killer cells by mediating the secretion of the cytokine interleukin-2. Hence, in [66], the involvement of natural killer cells is considered in the model of tumor-immune interaction. Dendritic cell vaccines can also boost the immune response via the adaptive immune system. This is mainly done by presenting the tumor-associated antigen (TAA) to naive cytotoxic T cells (naive $\mathrm{CD8^+}$ T cells) and thus enhancing its proliferation and maturization to form active cytotoxic T cells ($\mathrm{CD8^+}$ T cells).

As shown in Fig. 4.5, antigen presentation by DC cells activates helper T cells and cytotoxic T cells. The activated helper T cells differentiate into type 1 helper cells which secrete IL-2. The cytokine IL-2 activates T regulator cells which can suppress the activation of NK cells. The T regulator cells can also suppress the type 1 helper cells and cytotoxic T cells. This model also accounts for the production of IL-2 by mature $\mathrm{CD8^+}$ cells as well. Another important factor considered in the model discussed in this section is the immunosuppression facilitated by the tumor cells via the secretion of TGF-β.

Several mathematical models discuss the time-delay involved in tumor-immune interaction such as the delay involved in the activation of helper T cells and effector cells, delay involved in differentiation of cells, or the delay in cell migration or cell development [59, 67–70]. Here, the model proposed in [66] is presented as:

$$\frac{\mathrm{d}A(t)}{\mathrm{dt}} = r_1 A(t)\log\left(\frac{b}{A(t)}\right) - \left(a_1 \frac{\frac{\log(E(t))^5}{\log(A(t))^5}}{\frac{\log(E(t))^5}{\log(A(t))^5} + g_1}\right)A(t) - a_2 E_{\mathrm{NK}}(t)A(t), \tag{4.13}$$

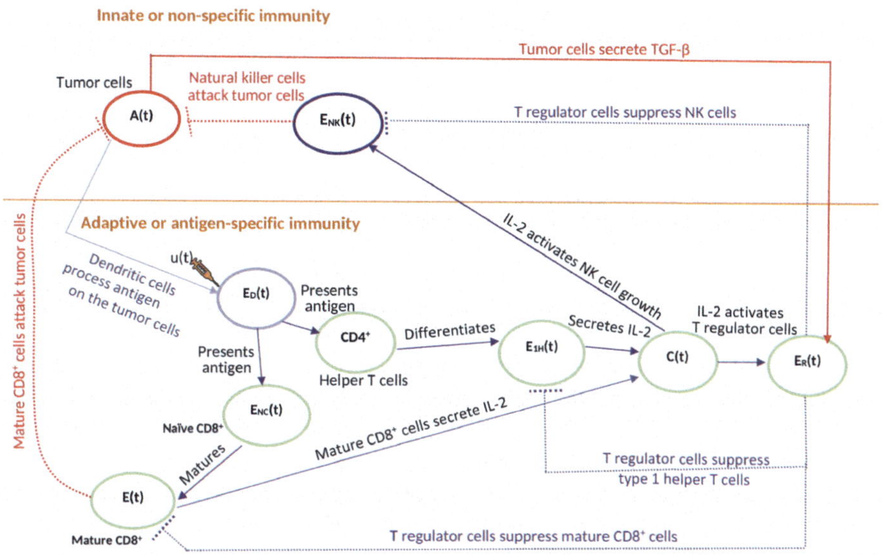

Fig. 4.5 A simplified illustration of the effect of DC vaccination on innate and adaptive immune systems [66]. Natural killer cells who are a member of the innate immune system directly attack cancer cells. However, a member of the adaptive immune system such as DC cells first identifies the type of antigen on the cancer cells and then facilitates the cancer lysis. Once dendritic cells present antigen, naive T cells and helper T cells get activated. Mature T cells attack tumor cells and also secrete IL-2. The type 1 helper T cells also secrete IL-2, which triggers a regulatory action by T regulator cells. Tumor cells are also capable of regulating the immune response by secreting TGF-β. Here, the therapeutic target is DC vaccination and is indicated in the figure as $u(t)$

$$\frac{dE_{NK}(t)}{dt} = s_1 - d_1 E_{NK}(t) + \frac{\rho_1 E_{NK}(t-\tau_1) C(t-\tau_1)}{g_2 + C(t-\tau_1)} - \psi_1 E_{NK}(t) E_R(t), \tag{4.14}$$

$$\frac{dE_{NC}(t)}{dt} = s_2 - d_2 E_{NC}(t) - \rho_2 \frac{E_D(t) E_{NC}(t)}{g_3 + E_D(t)}, \tag{4.15}$$

$$\frac{dE(t)}{dt} = -d_3 E(t) + \frac{\rho_3 E_{NC}(t-7\tau_2) E_D(t-7\tau_2)}{g_3 + E_D(t-7\tau_2)} + m_1 E_D(t-\tau_2) E(t-\tau_2) + \frac{\rho_4 E(t-\tau_2) C^2(t-\tau_2)}{g_4 + C^2(t-\tau_2)} - \psi_2 E(t) E_R(t), \tag{4.16}$$

$$\frac{dE_D(t)}{dt} = -d_4 E_D(t) + \kappa_1 \frac{A(t)}{g_5 + A(t)} + u(t), \tag{4.17}$$

$$\frac{dC(t)}{dt} = \left(s_3 - d_5 C(t) + \rho_5 \frac{E^2(t) C(t)}{g_6 + E^2(t)} + \rho_6 \frac{E_{1H}(t) C(t)}{g_7 + E_{1H}(t)} \right), \tag{4.18}$$

$$\frac{\mathrm{d}E_{\mathrm{R}}(t)}{\mathrm{d}t} = s_4 - d_6 E_{\mathrm{R}}(t) + \rho_7 \frac{E_{\mathrm{R}}(t-\tau_3) A^2 (t-\tau_3)}{g_8 + A^2(t-\tau_3)} + \rho_8 \frac{E_{\mathrm{R}}(t-\tau_3) C(t-\tau_3)}{g_9 + C(t-\tau_3)}, \tag{4.19}$$

$$\frac{\mathrm{d}E_{\mathrm{NH}}(t)}{\mathrm{d}t} = s_5 - d_7 E_{\mathrm{NH}}(t) - \rho_9 \frac{E_{\mathrm{D}}(t) E_{\mathrm{NH}}(t)}{g_3 + E_{\mathrm{D}}(t)}, \tag{4.20}$$

$$\begin{aligned}\frac{\mathrm{d}E_{1\mathrm{H}}(t)}{\mathrm{d}t} = {} & -d_8 E_{1\mathrm{H}}(t) + \frac{m_2 E_{\mathrm{D}}(t-2\tau_3) E_{\mathrm{NH}}(t-2\tau_3)}{g_3 + E_{\mathrm{D}}(t-2\tau_3)} - \psi_3 E_{\mathrm{R}}(t) E_{1\mathrm{H}}(t) \\ & + \frac{\rho_{10} E_{\mathrm{D}}(t-\tau_3) E(t-\tau_3)}{g_3 + E_{\mathrm{D}}(t-\tau_3)},\end{aligned} \tag{4.21}$$

where $A(t)$ and $E_{\mathrm{NK}}(t)$ denote tumor and natural killer cells, $E_{\mathrm{NC}}(t)$ and $E(t)$ denote naive CD8$^+$ and mature CD8$^+$ cells, $E_{\mathrm{D}}(t)$ and $C(t)$ denote dendritic cells and cytokine interleukin-2 (IL-2), $E_{\mathrm{R}}(t)$ and $E_{\mathrm{NH}}(t)$ denote T regulator and naive helper T cells, respectively, and $E_{1\mathrm{H}}(t)$ denotes type 1 helper T cells.

In (4.13), the parameters r_1 and b denote the growth rate and carrying capacity of the tumor cells, a_1 quantifies the saturation level of tumor cell-kill rate influenced by mature CD8$^+$ T cells ($E(t)$), and g_1 is the steepness coefficient related to the interaction (tumor lysis) between $E(t)$ and $A(t)$. The third term $a_2 E_{\mathrm{NK}}(t) A(t)$ accounts for the tumor lysis facilitated by natural killer cells, where a_2 denotes fractional cell-kill rate. It can be see from Fig. 4.5 that the dendritic cell vaccine can facilitate tumor lysis by activating the CD8$^+$ cells and natural killer cells. Hence, these effects are segregated as drug effects and labeled as a_1 and a_2.

In (4.14), the parameters s_1 and d_1 denote the constant influx rate (or production rate) of the natural killer (NK) cells to the tumor micro-environment and their death rate, respectively. In the third term of (4.14), ρ_1 models the maximum production rate of NK cells due to the influence of IL-2 cytokine, g_2 is the steepness coefficient associated with the interaction between NK cells and IL-2. The fourth term given by $\psi_1 E_{\mathrm{NK}}(t) E_{\mathrm{R}}(t)$ quantifies the inhibition or inactivation of NK cells by T regulator cells, where ψ_1 denotes the rate of inhibition.

In (4.15), the parameters s_2 and d_2 denote the constant influx rate and death rate of naive CD8$^+$ cells, respectively, ρ_2 denotes the maximum value of decay rate of naive CD8$^+$ cells with the influence of dendritic cells, and g_3 models the steepness coefficient associated with the decay rate of naive CD8$^+$ cells due to the influence of dendritic cells.

In (4.16), d_3 denotes the death rate of matured CD8$^+$ cells, ρ_3 denotes the maximum production rate of CD8$^+$ cells under the influence of dendritic cells, m_1 is the cell transition rate of naive CD8$^+$ cells to mature CD8$^+$ cells, g_4 is the steepness coefficient of CD8$^+$ cells with respect to the concentration of IL-2 cytokine, and ψ_2 denotes the inhibition or inactivation rate of mature CD8$^+$ by T regulator cells. Here, ρ_4 is the production rate of $E(t)$ under the influence of IL-2. Note that the contribution of DC and IL-2 in increasing the number of mature CD8$^+$ cells is modeled using the two growth terms $m_1 E_{\mathrm{D}}(t-\tau_2) E(t-\tau_2)$ and $\frac{\rho_4 E(t-\tau_2) C^2(t-\tau_2)}{g_4 + C^2(t-\tau_2)}$, respectively.

In (4.17), d_4 denotes the death rate of dendritic cells, κ_1 denotes the fraction of tumor cells that leads to the production of mature dendritic cells (via processing of tumor-associated antigen), g_5 denotes the steepness coefficient associated with the nonlinear production of dendritic cells, and $u(t)$ is the input which is the dendritic cell injection.

In (4.18), s_3 and d_5 denote the influx rate and decay rate of the IL-2 cytokine, ρ_5 and ρ_6 are the maximum value of the IL-2 secretion by the CD8$^+$ cells and type 1 helper T cells, and g_6 and g_7 are the steepness coefficient associated with the secretion of IL-2 cytokine by the CD8$^+$ cells and helper T cells, respectively.

In (4.19), s_4 and d_6 denote the influx rate and death rate of regulator T cells, ρ_7 and ρ_8 are the maximum production rate of T regulator cells due to the influence of tumor cells (via TGF-β secretion) and IL-2, and g_8 and g_9 are the steepness coefficient associated with the production of T regulator cells due to the influence of tumor cells and IL-2, respectively.

In (4.20), s_5 and d_7 denote the influx rate and death rate of naive helper T cells, and ρ_9 is the maximum decay rate or cell transition rate of naive helper T cells as influenced by the dendritic cells. Finally, in (4.21), $\frac{m_2 E_{\mathrm{D}}(t-2\tau_3)E_{\mathrm{NH}}(t-2\tau_3)}{g_3+D(t-2\tau_3)}$ models the cell transition, where m_2 denotes the fraction of naive helper T cells that matures to type 1 helper T cells. Other parameters such as d_8 denotes the death rate of type 1 helper T cells, ψ_3 is rate of cell inhibition or inactivation of type 1 helper T cells by the T regulator cells, and ρ_{10} is the maximum helper T cell production rate facilitated by the dendritic cells.

In (4.14)–(4.20), the parameters $\tau_i, i = 1, 2, 3$, represent the time delay involved in one cell division of NK cells, CD8$^+$ cells, and helper T cells, respectively. These time delays are modeled for one cell division and in some instances several cell division are required for maturization or activation of cells. For instance, in (4.16), the CD8$^+$ cells require 7 cell divisions to complete development. This delay involved in cell transition of naive T cells to active T cells is modeled as $E_{\mathrm{NC}}(t-7\tau_2)$. Similarly, in (4.20), $E_{\mathrm{NH}}(t-2\tau_3)$ models the delay (two cell division of helper cells) involved in the transition of naive helper T cells to type 1 helper T cells. Table 4.6 summarizes the parameter values of the immunotherapy model (4.13)–(4.21) [66]. The initial conditions for the variables in model (4.13)–(4.21) are $A(0) = 5\times10^5$ (cells), $E_{\mathrm{NK}}(0) = 4.4\times10^4$ (cells), $E_{\mathrm{NC}}(0) = 1.2\times10^5$ (cells), $E(0) = 10$ (cells), $E_{\mathrm{D}}(0) = 10$ (cells), $C(0) = 48$ (IU L^{-1}), $E_{\mathrm{R}}(0) = 1.1\times10^6$ (cells), $E_{\mathrm{NH}}(0) = 1.26\times10^5$ (cells), and $E_{\mathrm{IH}}(0) = 10$ (cells).

4.5 An Elaborate Model on Tumor-Immune Interaction

In this section, an elaborate mathematical model is presented that depicts many important interactions in the tumor micro-environment using twelve components. Note that, no specific immunotherapy administration method is incorporated in this model. However, this model accounts for many of the important mechanisms in the tumor-immune interaction. As shown in Fig. 4.2, the immune mechanism involves both immunostimulatory and immunosuppressive mechanisms. The models discussed in Sects. 4.1–4.3 do not account for the immunosuppressive effects. In

Table 4.6 Parameter values of the immunotherapy model (4.13)–(4.21) [66]

Parameter	Value (unit)	Parameter	Value (unit)
r_1	0.16 (days^{-1})	b	5×10^9 (cells)
a_1	6.9 (days^{-1})	g_1	3.5
a_2	7.13×10^{-10} ($\text{cells}^{-1}\text{days}^{-1}$)	s_1	1.32×10^4 (cells days^{-1})
d_1	4.12×10^{-2} (days^{-1})	ρ_1	6.68×10^{-2} (day^{-1})
g_2	2.5×10^4 (cells)	τ_1	1.26 (days)
ψ_1	1×10^{-7}(cells days^{-1})	s_2	5×10^5 (cells days^{-1})
d_2	0.03 (days^{-1})	ρ_2	1.2 (days^{-1})
g_3	$1\times 10^{5.4}$ (cells)	d_3	0.4 (days^{-1})
ρ_3	8.98×10^{-7} (days^{-1})	τ_2	0.45 (days)
m_1	0.38 ($\text{cells}^{-1}\text{days}^{-1}$)	ρ_4	0.19 (days^{-1})
g_4	6.25×10^6 (IU^2L^{-2})	ψ_2	4.3×10^{-7} ($\text{days}^{-1}\text{cells}^{-1}$)
d_4	0.237 (days^{-1})	κ_1	2.438×10^4 (cells days^{-1})
g_5, g_7	10^5 (cells)	s_3	2.805×10^2 ($\text{IUL}^{-1}\text{days}^{-1}$)
d_5	5.5 (days^{-1})	ρ_5	1.1 (days^{-1})
g_6	10^{11} (cells^2)	ρ_6	4.99 (days^{-1})
s_4	3.212×10^5 (cells days^{-1})	d_6	0.3 (days^{-1})
ρ_7	0.26 (days^{-1})	g_8	4.5×10^{17} (cells^2)
τ_3	0.47 (days)	ρ_8	0.399 (days^{-1})
g_9	$10^{4.4}$ (IUL^{-1})	s_5	5.5×10^5 (cells days^{-1})
d_7	0.03 (days^{-1})	ρ_9	1.05 (days^{-1})
ρ_{10}	1.4 (days^{-1})	d_8	0.44 (days^{-1})
m_2	0.45 (days^{-1})	ψ_3	8×10^{-7} ($\text{cells}^{-1}\text{days}^{-1}$)

Sect. 4.4, immunosuppressive effect of TGF-β is modeled in (4.19). In this section, a model that investigates the effect of multiple immunosupression mechanisms on T cell response is presented [2]. Immunosuppression is an important mechanism that has to be considered while modeling tumor-immune interactions since it is mentioned to be the main cause of the immunotherapy failure [66].

Figure 4.6 is a simplified illustration of the mathematical model presented in [2]. The T cell precursors shown in Fig. 4.6 are the antigen-experienced memory immune cells. Upon activation, each T cell precursors (cytotoxic, helper, and regulator) transit to a temporary proliferating stage before it matures to the fully functional stage. The cytotoxic T cells, helper T cells, and T regulator cells are differentiated from each other by evaluating the biomarkers present on them. For instance, the T regulator cells express CD4, CD25, or FOXP3 proteins as biomarkers. Helper T cells express

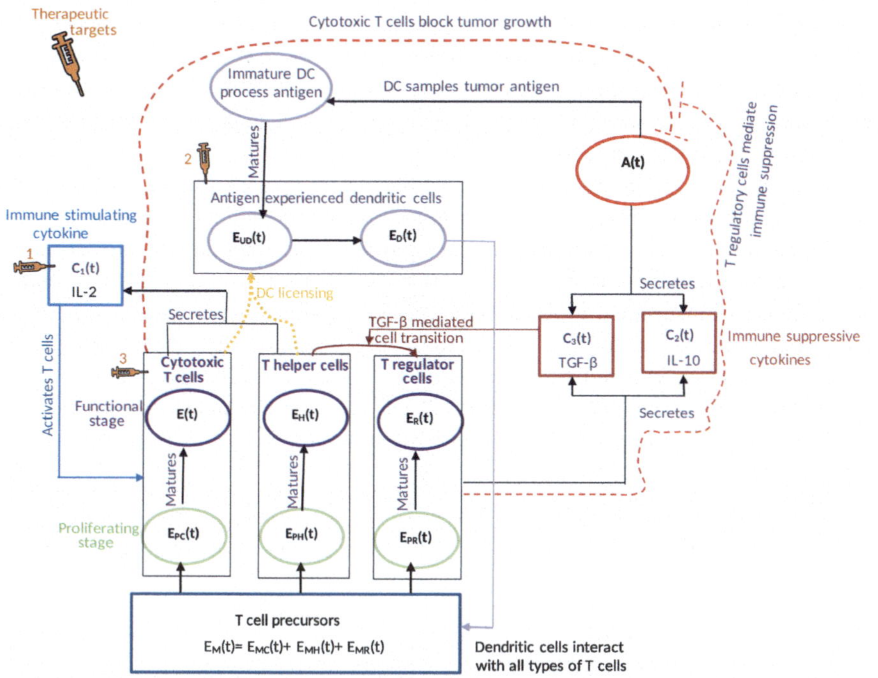

Fig. 4.6 Tumor-immune interaction model [2]. Upon experiencing antigen, the immature DC cells matures. However, licensing of antigen experienced DC cells is completed by the collective action of cytotoxic T cells and helper T cells. Immune stimulating cytokines mediate maturization of proliferating T cells to the respective functional stage. T regulator cells and tumor cells secrete immune regulator cytokines to block the immune response. TGF-β can mediate cell transition of helper T cells to T regulator cells. Three possible therapeutic targets such as immune stimulating cytokine (IL-2) injection, DC vaccination, and activated T cell injection are also marked in the figure

CD4 protein and are called CD4$^+$ cells. Similarly, cytotoxic T cells express CD8 protein and are called as CD8$^+$ cells [2].

As discussed earlier, the immune cell activation involves several co-stimulatory and co-inhibitory signaling to facilitate the desired immune response and to restrict autoimmunity. One such mechanism is the dendritic cell licensing which requires several hand shaking signals from helper T cells and T cells. Dendritic cell licensing is required for these cells to activate more T cell precursors. As shown in Fig. 4.6, when DC cells experience antigen they mature to unlicensed DC cells, and the DC licensing process is completed only with the interaction of helper T cells. The licensed DC cells trigger the proliferation and maturization of more immune cells from T cell precursor pool.

The two main immunosuppressive cytokines such as TGF-β and IL-10 which are secreted by T regulator cells or tumor cells play a role in blocking the immune response facilitated by the cytotoxic T cells. Evidences also suggest that the immunosuppressive cytokine such as TGF-β can mediate the cell transition of helper T cells to T regulator cells which are the main immunoregulators. As modeled in (4.1), (4.6), (4.10), and (4.16), the immune stimulatory cytokine such as IL-2 can contribute to the activation of cytotoxic T cells. Moreover, cytotoxic T cells and helper cells are believed to secrete IL-2 as well.

The tumor-immune interaction model provided in [2] does not dedicate an input term to account for the infusion of an immunotherapeutic agent. This model is still included in this chapter as it involves many significant variables and the model can be used for various therapeutic interventions that makes use of immune system related targets. As only the tumor-immune interaction is considered here without an external agent, then as per the definition of functions in the general model (1.1)–(1.2), the drug effect terms a_i will not be in this model. However, the notation a_i is used to indicate drug effects if (1) IL-2 injection, (2) DC vaccination, and (3) adoptive T cell transfer are used. See Fig. 4.6. The aforementioned model is given as below:

$$\frac{\mathrm{d}A(t)}{\mathrm{d}t} = \frac{A(t)}{\left(\left(\frac{1}{r_1}\right)^p + \left(\frac{A^{1-n}(t)}{r_2}\right)^p\right)^{1/p}} - \frac{a_1 A^*(t)}{\left(1 + g_1 \frac{A^*(t)}{E(t)}\right)} \frac{1}{\left(1 + g_2 \frac{E_{\mathrm{R}}(t)}{E(t)}\right)\left(1 + \frac{C_3(t)}{C_3^{50}}\right)}, \tag{4.22}$$

$$\frac{\mathrm{d}E_{\mathrm{UD}}(t)}{\mathrm{d}t} = \frac{\alpha_{\mathrm{a}} A^*(t)}{\left(1 + \frac{C_2(t)}{C_2^{50}}\right)\left(1 + \frac{E_{\mathrm{R}}(t)}{E_{\mathrm{R}}^{50}}\right)} - \frac{\lambda_{\mathrm{a}} E_{\mathrm{UD}}(t)}{1 + \frac{E_{\mathrm{UD}}(t)}{E_{\mathrm{MH}}(t)}} - d_1 E_{\mathrm{UD}}(t), \tag{4.23}$$

$$\frac{\mathrm{d}E_{\mathrm{D}}(t)}{\mathrm{d}t} = \frac{\lambda_{\mathrm{a}} E_{\mathrm{UD}}(t)}{1 + \frac{E_{\mathrm{UD}}(t)}{E_{\mathrm{MH}}(t)}} - d_2 E_{\mathrm{D}}(t), \tag{4.24}$$

$$\frac{\mathrm{d}E_{\mathrm{PC}}(t)}{\mathrm{d}t} = \frac{a_2 E_{\mathrm{MC}}(t)}{1 + g_4 \frac{E_{\mathrm{M}}(t)}{E_{\mathrm{D}}(t)}} - d_3 E_{\mathrm{PC}}(t), \tag{4.25}$$

$$\frac{\mathrm{d}E(t)}{\mathrm{d}t} = \frac{a_3 E_{\mathrm{PC}}(t) C_1(t)}{\left(1 + \frac{C_3(t)}{E_{C_3}^{50}}\right)\left(E_{\mathrm{C}_1}^{50} + C_1(t)\right)} - d_4 E(t), \tag{4.26}$$

$$\frac{\mathrm{d}E_{\mathrm{PH}}(t)}{\mathrm{d}t} = \frac{a_4 E_{\mathrm{MH}}(t)}{1 + g_4 \frac{E_{\mathrm{M}}(t)}{E_{\mathrm{UD}}(t) + E_{\mathrm{D}}(t)}} - d_5 E_{\mathrm{PH}}(t), \tag{4.27}$$

$$\frac{\mathrm{d}E_{\mathrm{H}}(t)}{\mathrm{d}t} = \frac{a_5 E_{\mathrm{PH}}(t) C_1(t)}{\left(1 + \frac{C_3(t)}{E_{C_3}^{50}}\right)\left(E_{\mathrm{C}_1}^{50} + C_1(t)\right)} - \frac{a_6 E_{\mathrm{H}}(t) C_3(t)}{g_5 + C_3(t)} - d_6 E_{\mathrm{H}}(t), \tag{4.28}$$

$$\frac{\mathrm{d}E_{\mathrm{PR}}(t)}{\mathrm{d}t} = \frac{a_7 E_{\mathrm{MR}}(t)}{1 + g_4 \frac{E_{\mathrm{M}}(t)}{E_{\mathrm{D}}(t)}} - d_7 E_{\mathrm{PR}}(t), \tag{4.29}$$

$$\frac{\mathrm{d}E_{\mathrm{R}}(t)}{\mathrm{d}t} = \frac{a_8 E_{\mathrm{PR}}(t) C_1(t)}{\left(E_{\mathrm{C}_1}^{50} + C_1(t)\right)} + \frac{a_6 E_{\mathrm{H}}(t) C_3(t)}{g_5 + C_3(t)} - d_8 E_{\mathrm{R}}(t), \tag{4.30}$$

$$\frac{\mathrm{d}C_1(t)}{\mathrm{d}t} = \frac{a_9 E_{\mathrm{PH}}(t)}{\left(1 + \frac{C_3(t)}{C_{C_3}^{50}}\right)\left(1 + \frac{C_2(t)}{C_{C_2}^{50}}\right)} - \frac{C_1(t)}{\tau_1}, \tag{4.31}$$

$$\frac{dC_2(t)}{dt} = r_3 E_R(t) + r_4 A(t) - \frac{C_2(t)}{\tau_2}, \tag{4.32}$$

$$\frac{dC_3(t)}{dt} = r_5 E_R(t) + r_6 A(t) - \frac{C_3(t)}{\tau_3}, \tag{4.33}$$

where $A(t)$ denotes tumor cells, $E_{UD}(t)$ and $E_D(t)$ are unlicensed and licensed dendritic cells, $E_{PC}(t)$ and $E(t)$ are cytotoxic T cells in the proliferating stage and active or fully functional cytotoxic T cells, $E_{PH}(t)$ and $E_H(t)$ are helper T cells in the proliferating stage and active helper T cells, and $E_{PR}(t)$ and $E_R(t)$ are T regulator cells in the proliferating stage and active T regulator cells, respectively, and $C_1(t)$, $C_2(t)$, and $C_3(t)$ denote the concentration of the cytokines interleukin-2 (IL-2), interleukin-10 (IL-10), and transforming growth factor-β (TGF-β), respectively. Note that all the antigen-experienced T cells are called as memory T cells and their sum is given by $E_M(t) = E_{MC}(t) + E_{MH}(t) + E_{MR}(t)$, where $E_{MC}(t)$, $E_{MH}(t)$, and $E_{MR}(t)$ are the memory T, memory T helper, and memory T regulator cells, respectively. The antigen-experienced memory T cells goes through a short lived proliferation stage $(E_{PC}(t), E_{PH}(t), E_{PR}(t))$ before turning to respective active or fully function cells $(E(t), E_H(t), E_R(t))$.

In (4.22), a combined exponential-power growth law is used for depicting the growth of cancer cells. It is known that small and large tumors have different growth rates and the volume doubling time of a tumor scales with the size of the tumor [71]. Consequently, studies report an initial exponential growth and then a transition to power growth law. This transition is modeled in (4.22), where p is used to quantify the smoothness of this transition, and r_1 and r_2 are used to model the growth coefficients for exponential and power growth, respectively and $r_1 = r_2(A_1)^{n-1}$, where A_1 is the transition size of tumor, and n is power-law exponent. Another important feature of this model is that, the cell-kill rate of cytotoxic T cells is included in the tumor cell dynamics by accounting for the possible extent of accessibility of the tumor cells by the killer cells. Specifically, $A^*(t)$ represents the fraction of tumor cells accessible to the immune system. This limited accessibility may be due to spatial constraints or poor vascularization. Wherever, this spatial constraint is relevant, the term $A^*(t)$ is used instead of $A(t)$, where $A^*(t) = \frac{A(t)}{\left(1+\left(\frac{A^{1-q}(t)}{g_3}\right)^p\right)^{1/p}}$. The second term in (4.22) quantifies the tumor regression due to the immune response where g_1 is the steepness coefficients associated with the interaction curve of tumor cells with cytotoxic T cells and g_2 is the T regulator cells with cytotoxic T cells. Here, C_3^{50} is the concentration of TGF-β that causes 50% tumor cell-kill effect.

In (4.23), the parameter α_a denotes the antigenicity of the tumor, C_2^{50} and E_R^{50} are the concentration of IL-10 and the number of T regulator cells at which the dendritic cell maturization markers are at half normal levels. As shown in Fig. 4.6, helper T cells are involved in licensing the dendritic cells and thus the ratio of unlicensed dendritic cells to helper T cells modeled by λ_a determines the rate of licensing. It can be seen that for abundant helper T cells and few unlicensed dendritic cells

$(E_{\mathrm{UD}}(t) << E_{\mathrm{MH}}(t))$, the term $\frac{\lambda_a E_{\mathrm{UD}}(t)}{1+\frac{E_{\mathrm{UD}}(t)}{E_{\mathrm{MH}}(t)}}$ reduces to $\lambda_a E_{\mathrm{UD}}(t)$, and for $E_{\mathrm{UD}}(t) >> E_{\mathrm{MH}}(t)$ the licensing rate is limited by the availability of helper T cells $(\lambda_a E_{\mathrm{MH}}(t))$. The third term accounts for the cell death or inactivation of unlicensed dendritic cells using the parameter d_1.

In (4.24), the first term accounts for the growth of dendritic cells as contributed by the licensing of $E_{\mathrm{UD}}(t)$ denoted in (4.23). The second term of this equation models the death of licensed dendritic cells or expiration of the antigen presentation by using the term d_2.

In (4.25), a_2 is the growth rate or recruiting rate of $E_{\mathrm{PC}}(t)$, d_3 denotes the death rate or inactivation rate of cytotoxic T cells in the short living proliferating stage, g_4 is the steepness coefficient associated with the interaction curve that depicts the transition of T cell precursors $(E_{\mathrm{M}}(t))$ to proliferative T cells $(E_{\mathrm{PC}}(t))$ by the action of matured dendritic cells $(E_{\mathrm{D}}(t))$.

In (4.26), a_3 denotes the growth rate or maturization rate of E_{PC} to $E(t)$, d_4 is the death rate or inactivation rate of $E(t)$, $E_{\mathrm{C}_1}^{50}$ and $E_{\mathrm{C}_3}^{50}$ account for the concentration of IL-2 and TGF-β that control the saturation of T cell proliferation, and $E_{\mathrm{C}_1}^{50}$ and $E_{\mathrm{C}_3}^{50}$ denote the concentrations that result in 50% T cell proliferation. As shown in Fig. 4.6, TGF-β and IL-2 have opposing functions, TGF-β inhibits T cell proliferation while IL-2 enhances T cell proliferation.

In (4.27), a_4 is the growth rate or recruiting rate of $E_{\mathrm{PH}}(t)$, d_5 denotes the death rate or inactivation rate of proliferating helper T cells, and g_4 is the steepness coefficient associated with the interaction curve that depicts the transition of T cell precursors $(E_{\mathrm{M}}(t))$ to proliferative helper T cells $(E_{\mathrm{PH}}(t))$ by the action of dendritic cells $(E_{\mathrm{UD}}(t)$ and $E_{\mathrm{D}}(t))$.

In (4.28), a_5 denotes the growth rate or maturization rate of $E_{\mathrm{PH}}(t)$ to $E_{\mathrm{H}}(t)$, and d_6 is the death rate or inactivation rate of $E_{\mathrm{H}}(t)$. As shown in Fig. 4.6, TGF-β facilitates the immune suppression by mediating the conversion of helper T cells to T regulator cells. As the value of $c_1(t)$ (concentration of TGF-β) increases, this cell transition saturates to $a_6 E_{\mathrm{H}}(t)$.

Similar to (4.25), in (4.29), a_7 is the growth rate or recruiting rate of $E_{\mathrm{PR}}(t)$, and d_7 denotes the death rate or inactivation rate of the same. The conversion of helper T cells to T regulator cells is modeled using the term $\frac{a_6 E_{\mathrm{H}}(t) C_3(t)}{g_5+C_3(t)}$ in (4.28) and (4.30). The parameters a_8 and d_8 denote the growth and decay of $E_{\mathrm{R}}(t)$, respectively.

In (4.31), a_9 and τ_1 are the production rate of IL-2 cytokine by helper T cells and their removal rate from the system. As shown in Fig. 4.6, the immune-suppressive cytokines can inhibit the production of IL-2. This is modeled in the first term of (4.31), where $C_{\mathrm{C}_2}^{50}$ and $C_{\mathrm{C}_3}^{50}$ denote the concentration of IL-10 and TGF-β, respectively, that can cause 50% suppression of IL-2 cytokine.

As shown in Fig. 4.6, the cytokine IL-10 and TGF-β are produced by the regulator T cells and tumor cells. This is modeled in (4.32) and (4.33) using the parameters r_i, $i = 3, \ldots, 6$ which indicate the production rates and τ_i, $i = 1, 2$ which indicate the removal of the cytokines from the system (4.31).

Table 4.7 summarizes the parameter values of the immunotherapy model (4.22)–(4.32) [2]. The initial conditions for the variables in model (4.22)–(4.33) are $A(0) = 1$

Table 4.7 Parameter values of the immunotherapy model (4.22)–(4.32) [2]

Parameter	Value (unit)	Parameter	Value (unit)
r_2	333 (days^{-1})	p	3
r_1	100-1000 ($\text{cells}^{1-r_2}\text{days}^{-1}$)	n	$\frac{1}{2}$
a_1	0.9 (days^{-1})	g_1	1.2
g_2	11	C_3^{50}	3.5 (ng ml^{-1})
g_3	100 (cells^{1-q})	q	$\frac{2}{3}$
C_2^{50}	0.4 (ng ml^{-1})	α_{a}	$10^{-5} - 10^5$ (days^{-1})
E_{R}^{50}	2×10^7 (cells)	λ_{a}	0.5 (days^{-1})
d_1	0.14 (days^{-1})	d_2	0.5 (days^{-1})
a_2	23 (days^{-1})	g_4	0.33
d_3, d_5, d_7	0.2 (days^{-1})	a_3	16 (days^{-1})
$E_{C_3}^{50}$	2.9 (ng ml^{-1})	$E_{C_1}^{50}$	0.3 (ng ml^{-1})
d_4	1 (days^{-1})	r_5	1.8×10^{-8} ($\text{ng ml}^{-1}\text{days}^{-1}\text{cells}^{-1}$)
a_4	9.9 (days^{-1})	a_5	1.9 (days^{-1})
a_6	0.022 (days^{-1})	g_5	1.7 (ng ml^{-1})
d_6, d_8	0.1 (days^{-1})	a_7	5.1 (days^{-1})
a_8	2.1 (days^{-1})	a_9	1.7×10^{-5}($\text{ng ml}^{-1}\text{cells}^{-1}\text{days}^{-1}$)
$C_{C_3}^{50}$	0.9 (ng ml^{-1})	$C_{C_2}^{50}$	0.75 (ng ml^{-1})
τ_1	0.08 (days)	r_3	1.4×10^{-8} ($\text{ng ml}^{-1}\text{days}^{-1}\text{cells}^{-1}$)
τ_2	0.05 (days)	r_4	1.3×10^{-10} ($\text{ng ml}^{-1}\text{days}^{-1}\text{cells}^{-1}$)
τ_3	0.07 (days)	r_6	1.1×10^{-7} ($\text{ng ml}^{-1}\text{days}^{-1}\text{cells}^{-1}$)

(cell) and $C_1(0) = C_2(0) = C_3(0) = 0\,(\text{ng ml}^{-1})$. Initial values of all other variables are set to either zero or a very small value 10^{-5} to avoid singularity.

4.6 Summary

One of the advantages of immunotherapy, compared to other anti-tumor treatments, is that immunotherapy is very specific in targeting the tumor cells alone while leaving the healthy cells unaffected [72]. Hence, as shown in all of the 5 models discussed in this chapter, the dynamics of the normal cell population are ignored while discussing tumor-immune interactions. The main disadvantage of the immunotherapy method lies in the fact that, since most tumor cells are proficient in tricking the immune system by immune editing and suppressing immunogenic clones, immunotherapy methods such as DC vaccination, IL-2 injection, LAK or TIL injections do not give positive outcomes in some of the patients [24]. Immune checkpoint inhibitors are the immunotherapeutic agents that restrict such immune evasions. However, immune-related adverse events are not rare with the use of immune checkpoint inhibitors [73].

As explained earlier, the immune response to tumor cells has a significant correlation to the antigenicity of tumor cells. The basic understanding is that, as the antigenicity of tumor cells increases, they are more detectable to the immunosurveillance team of the immune system leading to a corresponding increase in the immune response. However, the analysis in [2] suggests that there exists an optimal antigenicity of the tumor for which the immune response is maximum. The results of [2] suggests that if the antigenicity of a fast-growing tumor is minimal, then the immune response is low. However, if the antigenicity is higher, a high immunosuppressive response is triggered by regulator T cells and TGF-β, besides the large immune response. Incorporating such details while modeling tumor-immune interaction is desirable.

In general, as the tumor grows, there is a proportional increase in immune cell-mediated cell-kill of the tumor cells. In (3.2), (4.7), and (4.11) the reduction in tumor cells due to the immune response is modeled using the term $-cE(t)A(t)$ and it varies according to the value of c ($c = 0.5$ in (3.2) and $c = 0.1$ in (4.7)). In (4.11), the immunotherapy drug restricts immune evasion and more cancer cells are visible to the immune system and hence $c = 57.5$ is used to account for the significant increase in immune cell-mediated cell-kill. In Sects. 4.2–4.5 that include DC vaccination and immune checkpoint evasion models, attacking cells or immune cells are not injected directly, instead, immunogenicity (that is the likelihood of being seen and recognized by the immune system) of the tumor cells is increased by using drugs. Hence, as $A(t)$ increases there will be a proportional increase in attack and thus tumor cells decrease proportionally. However, in Sect. 4.1, the nonlinear increase in $E(t)$ due to the direct injection of externally cultured immune cells (LAK injection) is modeled. Hence, the reduction in $A(t)$ is modeled using the term $-\frac{A(t)E(t)}{A(t)+\alpha_{50}}$, where for a small value of $A(t)$, there will be a proportional increase in cell-kill and LAK injection is enough to achieve a tumor-free state. Thus, when the tumor is small complete eradication can be achieved using LAK injection. But with an increase in $A(t)$, the overall cell-kill effect will not increase but saturates. Moreover, in large tumors, not all tumor cells have similar antigenicity (due to tumor cell heterogeneity). In the case of large tumors, as immunotherapy in form of LAK injection alone is insufficient to completely eradicate the tumor, combined therapy to increase antigenicity of the tumor (eg. DC vaccination or immune checkpoint inhibition) along with LAK injection is recommended for better treatment response. In essence, when we use immunotherapy to increase $E(t)$, a proportional increase in immune-mediated cell-kill can happen only if all the tumor cells are immunogenic/antigenic so that the avalanche of immune cells generated as a result of immunotherapy can identify all tumor cells. If all the tumor cells are immunogenic, the proportional cell-kill model is appropriate to model immune cell-mediated cell-kill, otherwise, a saturation model needs to be used.

The model discussed in Sect. 4.1 describes the main interactions in tumor microenvironment. However, the effect of dendritic cells, helper T cells and regulator T cells, in stimulating the immune response and the immunosuppressive effects are ignored [50, 52]. The dynamics of some of these cell population and effect of immunosuppression are accounted for in models discussed in later sections. However, each mathematical model focuses on certain aspects and assumes that the influence of others are negligible. Hence, an overall model that includes normal cells, components of innate and adaptive immune system, immunosuppression, and multiple inputs is desirable.

References

1. F.D. Barber, Recent developments in oncology immunotherapy, adverse effects Part 2. J. Nurse Pract. **14**(4), 259–266 (2018)
2. M. Robertson Tessi, A. El Kareh, A. Goriely, A mathematical model of tumor-immune interactions. J. Theor. Biol. **294**, 56–73 (2012)
3. K.E. Hellström, I. Hellström, Lymphocyte-mediated cytotoxicity and blocking serum activity to tumor antigens, in *Advances in Immunology*, vol. 18 (Elsevier, Amsterdam, 1974), pp. 209–277
4. C.D. Wimmer, M. Rentsch, A. Crispin, W.D. Illner, H. Arbogast, C. Graeb, K.W. Jauch, M. Guba, The janus face of immunosuppression-de novo malignancy after renal transplantation: the experience of the transplantation center Munich. Kidney Int. **71**(12), 1271–1278 (2007)
5. T. Boon, J.C. Cerottini, B. Van den Eynde, P. Van der Bruggen, A. Van Pel, Tumor antigens recognized by T lymphocytes. Annu. Rev. Immunol. **12**(1), 337–365 (1994)
6. G.P. Dunn, C.M. Koebel, R.D. Schreiber, Interferons, immunity and cancer immunoediting. Nat. Rev. Immunol. **6**(11), 836–848 (2006)
7. S.A. Rosenberg, Decade in review-cancer immunotherapy: entering the mainstream of cancer treatment. Nat. Rev. Clin. Oncol. **11**(11), 630 (2014)
8. C.A. Pennell, K. Ellis, Demystifying cancer immunotherapy for lay audiences. Front. Immunol. **10**, 2488 (2019)
9. A. Cappuccio, M. Elishmereni, Z. Agur, Cancer immunotherapy by interleukin-21: potential treatment strategies evaluated in a mathematical model. Cancer Res. **66**(14), 7293–7300 (2006)
10. A. Ghaffari, N. Naserifar, Optimal therapeutic protocols in cancer immunotherapy. Comput. Biol. Med. **40**(3), 261–270 (2010)
11. B. Piccoli, F. Castiglione, Optimal vaccine scheduling in cancer immunotherapy. Phys. A **370**(2), 672–680 (2006)
12. B. Alberts, A. Johnson, J. Lewis, M. Raff, K. Roberts, P. Walter, Helper T cells and lymphocyte activation, in *Molecular Biology of the Cell*, 4th edn. (Garland Science, 2002)
13. A.M. Brandsma, S. Bondza, M. Evers, R. Koutstaal, M. Nederend, J. Jansen, T. Rösner, T. Valerius, J.H. Leusen, T. Ten Broeke, Potent Fc receptor signaling by Iga leads to superior killing of cancer cells by neutrophils compared to IgG. Front. Immunol. **10**, 704 (2019)
14. K.R. Chaudhari, M. Ukawala, A.S. Manjappa, A. Kumar, P.K. Mundada, A.K. Mishra, R. Mathur, J. Mönkkönen, R.S.R. Murthy, Opsonization, biodistribution, cellular uptake and apoptosis study of PEGylated PBCA nanoparticle as potential drug delivery carrier. Pharm. Res. **29**(1), 53–68 (2012)
15. P.G. Sasikumar, M. Ramachandra, Small-molecule immune checkpoint inhibitors targeting PD-1/PD-L1 and other emerging checkpoint pathways. BioDrugs **32**(5), 481–497 (2018)
16. E.P. Juliá, A. Amante, M.B. Pampena, J. Mordoh, E.M. Levy, Avelumab, an IgG1 anti-PD-L1 immune checkpoint inhibitor, triggers NK cell-mediated cytotoxicity and cytokine production against triple negative breast cancer cells. Front. Immunol. **9**, 2140 (2018)
17. T.F. Chen, K.K. Li, E.F. Zhu, C.F. Opel, M.J. Kauke, H. Kim, E. Atolia, K.D. Wittrup, Artificial anti-tumor opsonizing proteins with fibronectin scaffolds engineered for specificity to each of the murine FcγR types. J. Mol. Biol. **430**(12), 1786–1798 (2018)
18. I. Faiena, A.L. Cummings, A.M. Crosetti, A.J. Pantuck, K. Chamie, A. Drakaki, Durvalumab: an investigational anti-PD-L1 monoclonal antibody for the treatment of urothelial carcinoma. Drug Des., Dev. Ther. **12**, 209 (2018)

19. L. Chen, Co-inhibitory molecules of the B7-CD28 family in the control of T-cell immunity. Nat. Rev. Immunol. **4**(5), 336–347 (2004)
20. K. Peggs, S. Quezada, J.P. Allison, Cancer immunotherapy: co-stimulatory agonists and co-inhibitory antagonists. Clin. Exp. Immunol. **157**(1), 9–19 (2009)
21. E. Contardi, G.L. Palmisano, P.L. Tazzari, A.M. Martelli, F. Fala, M. Fabbi, T. Kato, E. Lucarelli, D. Donati, L. Polito et al., CTLA-4 is constitutively expressed on tumor cells and can trigger apoptosis upon ligand interaction. Int. J. Cancer **117**(4), 538–550 (2005)
22. R. Padmanabhan, H.S. Kheraldine, N. Meskin, S. Vranic, A.E. Al Moustafa, Crosstalk between HER2 and PD-1/PD-L1 in breast cancer: from clinical applications to mathematical models. Cancers **12**, no. 3, 636 (2020)
23. Y. Wang, H. Wang, H. Yao, C. Li, J.Y. Fang, J. Xu, Regulation of PD-L1: emerging routes for targeting tumor immune evasion. Front. Pharmacol. **9**, 536 (2018)
24. V. Velcheti, K. Schalper, Basic overview of current immunotherapy approaches in cancer. Am. Soc. Clin. Oncol. Educ. Book **36**, 298–308 (2016)
25. N. Jorgensen, G. Persson, T.V.F. Hviid, The tolerogenic function of regulatory T cells in pregnancy and cancer. Front. Immunol. **10**, 911 (2019)
26. F. Salamanna, V. Borsari, D. Contartese, V. Costa, G. Giavaresi, M. Fini, What is the role of interleukins in breast cancer bone metastases? A systematic review of preclinical and clinical evidence. Cancers **11**(12), 2018 (2019)
27. B.E. Lippitz, R.A. Harris, Cytokine patterns in cancer patients: a review of the correlation between interleukin 6 and prognosis. OncoImmunology **5**, no. 5 (2016)
28. J.A. Bridge, J.C. Lee, A. Daud, J.W. Wells, J.A. Bluestone, Cytokines, chemokines, and other biomarkers of response for checkpoint inhibitor therapy in skin cancer. Front. Med. **5**, 351 (2018)
29. N. Nagarsheth, M. Wicha, W. Zou, Chemokines in the cancer microenvironment and their relevance in cancer immunotherapy. Nat. Rev. Immunol. **17**, 05 (2017)
30. A.E. Vilgelm, A. Richmond, Chemokines modulate immune surveillance in tumorigenesis, metastasis and response to immunotherapy. Front. Immunol. **10**, 333 (2019)
31. A. Zlotnik, Chemokines and cancer. Int. J. Cancer **119**(9), 2026–2029 (2006)
32. H. Zhao, N. Dong, T. Liu, P. Zhang, Y. Zheng, L. Yang, X. Ren, Clinical significance of serum Type III interferons in patients with gastric cancer. J. Interf. Cytokine Res. **39**(3), 155–163 (2019)
33. A.K. Knuth, S. Rösler, B. Schenk, L. Kowald, S.J. van Wijk, S. Fulda, Interferons transcriptionally up-regulate MLKL expression in cancer cells. Neoplasia **21**(1), 74–81 (2019)
34. J.J. Huang, G.C. Blobe, Dichotomous roles of TGF-β in human cancer. Biochem. Soc. Trans. **44**(5), 1441–1454 (2016)
35. C.M. Filippi, A.E. Juedes, J.E. Oldham, E. Ling, L. Togher, Y. Peng, R.A. Flavell, M.G. von Herrath, Transforming growth factor-β suppresses the activation of CD8+ T-cells when naive but promotes their survival and function once antigen experienced: A two-faced impact on autoimmunity. Diabetes **57**(10), 2684–2692 (2008)
36. A. Dahmani, J.S. Delisle, TGF-β in T cell biology: implications for cancer immunotherapy. Cancers **10**(6), 194 (2018)
37. M.J. Gorbet, A. Ranjan, Cancer immunotherapy with immunoadjuvants, nanoparticles, and checkpoint inhibitors: recent progress and challenges in treatment and tracking response to immunotherapy. Pharmacol. Ther. **207**, 107456 (2020)
38. D. Sansom, CD28, CTLA-4 and their ligands: who does what and to whom? Immunology **101**(2), 169 (2000)
39. P.T. Sage, A.M. Paterson, S.B. Lovitch, A.H. Sharpe, The coinhibitory receptor CTLA-4 controls B cell responses by modulating T follicular helper, T follicular regulatory, and T regulatory cells. Immunity **41**(6), 1026–1039 (2014)
40. R.K. Vaddepally, P. Kharel, R. Pandey, R. Garje, A.B. Chandra, Review of indications of FDA-approved immune checkpoint inhibitors per NCCN guidelines with the level of evidence. Cancers **12**(3), 738 (2020)

41. M.W. Rohaan, S. Wilgenhof, J.B. Haanen, Adoptive cellular therapies: the current landscape. Virchows Arch. **474**(4), 449–461 (2019)
42. D.A. Lee, Cellular therapy: adoptive immunotherapy with expanded natural killer cells. Immunol. Rev. **290**(1), 85–99 (2019)
43. L.G. de Pillis, W. Gu, A.E. Radunskaya, Mixed immunotherapy and chemotherapy of tumors: modeling, applications and biological interpretations. J. Theor. Biol. **238**(4), 841–862 (2006)
44. C.J. Wheeler, A. Das, G. Liu, J.S. Yu, K.L. Black, Clinical responsiveness of glioblastoma multiforme to chemotherapy after vaccination. Clin. Cancer Res. **10**(16), 5316–5326 (2004)
45. A.G. Dalgleish, Vaccines versus immunotherapy: overview of approaches in deciding between options. Hum. Vaccines Immunother. **10**(11), 3369–3374 (2014)
46. A. Diefenbach, E.R. Jensen, A. Jamieson, D.H. Raulet, Rae1 and H60 ligands of the NKG2D receptor stimulate tumor immunity. Nature **413**, 165–71 (2001)
47. A.S. Novozhilov, F.S. Berezovskaya, E.V. Koonin, G.P. Karev, Mathematical modeling of tumor therapy with oncolytic viruses: regimes with complete tumor elimination within the framework of deterministic models. Biol. Direct **1**, 6 (2006)
48. A.L. Jenner, A.C.F. Coster, P.S. Kim, F. Frascoli, Treating cancerous cells with viruses: insights from a minimal model for oncolytic virotherapy. Lett. Biomath. **5**(sup1), S117–S136 (2018)
49. R. Eftimie, J.L. Bramson, D.J.D. Earn, Interactions between the immune system and cancer: a brief review of non-spatial mathematical models. Bull. Math. Biol. **73**(1), 2–32 (2011)
50. D. Kirschner, J.C. Panetta, Modeling immunotherapy of the tumor-immune interaction. J. Math. Biol. **37**(3), 235–252 (1998)
51. A. Rivaz, M. Azizian, M. Soltani, Various mathematical models of tumor growth with reference to cancer stem cells: a review. Iran. J. Sci. Technol., Trans. A: Sci. **43**(2), 687–700 (2019)
52. F. Castiglione, B. Piccoli, Optimal control in a model of dendritic cell transfection cancer immunotherapy. Bull. Math. Biol. **68**(2), 255–274 (2006)
53. A. Tsygvintsev, S. Marino, D.E Kirschner, A mathematical model of gene therapy for the treatment of cancer. Math. Methods Model. Biomed., 01 (2013)
54. J. Arciero, T. Jackson, D. Kirschner, A mathematical model of tumor-immune evasion and siRNA treatment. Discret. Contin. Dyn. Syst.-B **4**, 39 (2004)
55. K.R. Fister, J.H. Donnelly, Immunotherapy: an optimal control theory approach. Math. Biosci. Eng. **2**(3), 499–510 (2005)
56. A. Konstorum, A.T. Vella, A.J. Adler, R.C. Laubenbacher, Addressing current challenges in cancer immunotherapy with mathematical and computational modelling. J. R. Soc. Interface **14**(131), 20170150 (2017)
57. V.A. Kuznetsov, I.A. Makalkin, M.A. Taylor, A.S. Perelson, Nonlinear dynamics of immunogenic tumors: parameter estimation and global bifurcation analysis. Bull. Math. Biol. **56**(2), 295–321 (1994)
58. R. De Boer, P. Hogeweg, H. Dullens, R.A. De Weger, W. Den Otter, Macrophage T lymphocyte interactions in the anti-tumor immune response: a mathematical model. J. Immunol. **134**(4), 2748–2758 (1985)
59. S. Banerjee, Immunotherapy with interleukin-2: a study based on mathematical modeling. Int. J. Appl. Math. Comput. Sci. **18**(3), 389–398 (2008)
60. F.S. Cyprian, H.F. Al Farsi, S. Vranic, S. Akhtar, A.E. Al Moustafa, Epstein–Barr virus and human papillomaviruses interactions and their roles in the initiation of epithelial-mesenchymal transition and cancer progression. Front. Oncol. **8**, 111 (2018)
61. H. Al Thawadi, L. Ghabreau, T. Aboulkassim, A. Yasmeen, S. Vranic, G. Batist, A.E. Al Moustafa, Co-incidence of epstein–Barr virus and high-risk human papillomaviruses in cervical cancer of Syrian women. Front. Oncol. **8**, 250 (2018)
62. A. Radunskaya, L. de Pillis, A. Gallegos, A model of dendritic cell therapy for melanoma. Front. Oncol. **3**, 56 (2013)
63. A. Minelli, F. Topputo, F. Bernelli Zazzera, Controlled drug delivery in cancer immunotherapy: stability, optimization, and Monte Carlo analysis. SIAM J. Appl. Math. **71**, no. 6, 2229–2245 (2011)

64. X. Lai, A. Friedman, Combination therapy of cancer with cancer vaccine and immune checkpoint inhibitors: a mathematical model. PloS One **12**, no. 5 (2017)
65. E. Nikolopoulou, L.R. Johnson, D. Harris, J.D. Nagy, E.C. Stites, Y. Kuang, Tumour-immune dynamics with an immune checkpoint inhibitor. Lett. Biomath. **5**(sup1), S137–S159 (2018)
66. M. Qomlaqi, F. Bahrami, M. Ajami, J. Hajati, An extended mathematical model of tumor growth and its interaction with the immune system, to be used for developing an optimized immunotherapy treatment protocol. Math. Biosci. **292**, 1–9 (2017)
67. S. Banerjee, R.R. Sarkar, Delay-induced model for tumor-immune interaction and control of malignant tumor growth. Biosystems **91**(1), 268–288 (2008)
68. M. Mackey, Unified hypothesis for the origin of aplastic anemia and periodic hematopoiesis. Blood **51**(5), 941–956 (1978)
69. Y. Dong, G. Huang, R. Miyazaki, Y. Takeuchi, Dynamics in a tumor immune system with time delays. Appl. Math. Comput. **252**, 99–113 (2015)
70. C.K. Osborne, D.H. Boldt, G.M. Clark, J.M. Trent, Effects of tamoxifen on human breast cancer cell cycle kinetics: accumulation of cells in early G1 Phase. Cancer Res. **43**(8), 3583–3585 (1983)
71. H.E. Skipper, Kinetics of mammary tumor cell growth and implications for therapy. Cancer **28**(6), 1479–1499 (1971)
72. B. Joshi, X. Wang, S. Banerjee, H. Tian, A. Matzavinos, M.A. Chaplain, On immunotherapies and cancer vaccination protocols: a mathematical modelling approach. J. Theor. Biol. **259**(4), 820–827 (2009)
73. M.A. Postow, R. Sidlow, M.D. Hellmann, Immune-related adverse events associated with immune checkpoint blockade. N. Engl. J. Med. **378**(2), 158–168 (2018)

Chapter 5
Anti-angiogenic Therapy Models

Anti-angiogenic therapy is used to interrupt the development of blood vessels towards and into the tumors from the existing blood vessels that surround the tumor micro-environment [1]. The two main processes that are involved in the formation and maintenance of the vascular network in our body are vasculogenesis and angiogenesis. Vasculogenesis is the formation of new blood vessels in our body. Even though vasculogenesis is most prevalent during the embryonic stage, it also ensues when new vessels are required to bypass blocked vessels, or during the formation of new vessels after injury. Angiogenesis refers to the development of existing vasculature by means of vessel sprouting and splitting. In healthy tissues, this process is regulated by the balanced action of pro-angiogenic and anti-angiogenic factors [2, 3].

Tumor cells are also capable of initiating angiogenesis in the tumor micro-environment for their existence [4]. Tumor cells facilitate angiogenesis primarily by altering the balance that exists between pro-angiogenic and anti-angiogenic factors in a healthy condition. This is referred to as an angiogenesis switch [4]. In contrast to the selectively permeable blood vessels in the host tissues, the newly formed vascular networks in the tumor micro-environment are often malformed, highly permeable, and leaky. These abnormally formed vascular networks favor metastasis by letting the cancer cells to get into the bloodstream [1]. In short, angiogenesis is a milestone in the tumor progression which allows the transition of a benign tumor to a malignant one. Inhibiting the process of angiogenesis in tumors will curtail the supply of nutrients and oxygen to tumors and hence their growth beyond a few millimeters [5]. Moreover, since malformed and leaky blood vessels favor tumor metastasis, restricting angiogenesis in tumors can considerably improve the overall longterm outcome of the patients. The scope of anti-angiogenesis in cancer treatment was pointed out in the early 1970s itself [6]. Currently, there are many approved inhibitors and monoclonal antibodies (mabs) that can facilitate anti-angiogenesis.

Compared to chemotherapy, one of the main advantages associated with the anti-angiogenic therapy method is that since the target here is the normal (non-mutated)

R. Padmanabhan et al., *Mathematical Models of Cancer and Different Therapies*, Series in BioEngineering, https://doi.org/10.1007/978-981-15-8640-8_5

endothelial cells which are genetically stable there is a less probability of encountering two hits of mutation which leads to the development of drug (angiogenesis inhibitor) resistance. In simple words, compared to chemotherapy, the development of drug resistance is less evident with this therapy mode. Moreover, angiogenesis inhibitors have mild-toxicity and exhibit fewer side effects [7]. Anti-angiogenic therapy is proved to be effective in slowing down tumor growth and preventing metastasis. However, the main limitation of this therapy is that it cannot eradicate cancer, but can only limit the growth of the tumor. In addition to that, research suggests the necessity for a life long treatment to eliminate the chance of dormant cancer cells being active again in the absence of therapy. Hence, angiogenesis inhibitors are often used along with other (adjuvant therapy) mainstay therapeutic agents that are used for cancer management [8]. Despite the fact that the anti-angiogenic therapy methods are inadequate to eradicate cancer, the acceptance of this mode of therapy along with other therapy methods (combination therapy) is due to its potential to block metastasis which is the leading cause of cancer-induced mortality.

As mentioned earlier, the cell populations involved in a mathematical model vary according to the focus of interest of the model. In the case of anti-angiogenic therapy, one of the main cell populations that comes into the picture is the endothelial cells which are a specialized form of epithelial cells. Epithelial cells are the cells which line the outer surface and inner cavities of many organs, they form glands, and play an important role in protection, sensation, absorption, and filtration. The endothelial cells are the cells which line blood vessels and are involved in the development and extension of existing blood vessels by means of cell proliferation, migration, and differentiation. These cells regulate vascular contraction, vascular relaxation, blood clotting, immune function, and platelet adhesion [1].

As mentioned earlier, a balance between the pro-angiogenic and anti-angiogenic factors plays an important role in the development and maintenance of the life-supporting vascular network in our body. Angiogenesis occurs only when the pro-angiogenic factors are activated and are important for the normal growth and development of our body as well as during pregnancy and wound healing. Typically, abnormal vasculogenesis and angiogenesis are observed in case of disease conditions such as arthritis, neovascularization in choroid and iris of the eye, duodenal ulcers, and cancer. Angiogenesis in tumors involves the secretion of a number of tumor chemicals which are together referred to as tumor angiogenic factors (TAFs). These chemicals are produced by the cancer cells to initiate capillary sprouting from the nearby normal tissues towards the location of the tumor and thus facilitate extensive angiogenesis in the tumors. The TAFs include both stimulatory (pro-angiogenic) and inhibitory (anti-angiogenic) agents.

Figure 5.1 shows various stages in angiogenesis. As shown in this figure, when small avascular tumors (<2 mm) experience hypoxia, they generate TAFs. These angiogenic factors move around and bind with the receptors on the endothelial cells of the nearby blood vessels. As mentioned earlier, in a normal condition, a balance is maintained between the pro-angiogenic and anti-angiogenic inhibitors. However, TAFs disrupt this balance and mediate several mechanisms, which enhance the action of angiogenesis promoters and thereby initiate angiogenesis towards the tumor. This

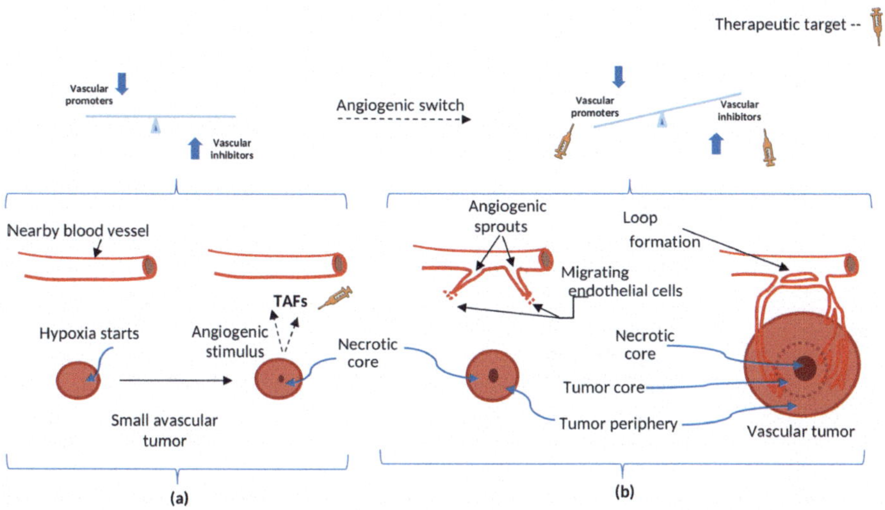

Fig. 5.1 Illustrative diagram showing the transition of an avascular tumor to a vascular tumor: **a** shows that when a tumor grows beyond few millimeters, the cells in the center experience hypoxia. Hypoxia is an angiogenic stimulus that can induce the secretion of many TAFs (tumor angiogenic factors), which disrupts the balance between vascular promoters and inhibitors and thus toggles the angiogenic switch, and **b** shows that once vascular promoters overweigh the vascular inhibitors angiogenesis is induced, which is marked by the migration of endothelial cells and the development of angiogenic sprouts. Joining of two such growing sprouts can result in a loop formation. Repeated sprouting, looping, and splitting of vessels inside the tumor facilitates angiogenesis in tumors. Therapeutic targets such as inhibition of the action of TAFs, inhibition of vascular promoters, and enhancing the production and action of vascular inhibitors are also marked in this figure

is indicated as an angiogenic switch in Fig. 5.1. Basically, the process of angiogenesis involves endothelial cell migration followed by capillary sprout formation and then the extension of these new sprouts occurs by means of cell proliferation. Later on loop formation (anastomosis) ensues to facilitate interconnection between newly formed capillaries (Fig. 5.1).

Research suggests that the expression of vascular endothelial factor (VEGF) serves an important role in initiating angiogenesis and thereby facilitating metastasis of tumors [1]. Along with VEGF, expression of several other biomarkers such as acidic fibroblast growth factor (a-FGF), basic fibroblast growth factor (b-FGF), etc. are identified to be associated with the angiogenesis in tumors. Anti-angiogenic treatment stems from the experimental evidences on the reduction of capillary network formation by using anti-angiogenic agents [9]. In order to prevent angiogenesis in tumors, several endogenous (angiogenin, endostatin, etc.) and exogenous inhibitors are used currently. Drugs such as aflibercept, bevacizumab, ranibizumab, and TNP-470 are exogenous angiogenesis inhibitors. Mechanism of action of anti-angiogenic agents includes inhibition of vascular endothelial growth factor (VEGF), inhibition of proliferation and migration of endothelial cells, stimulating the production of

Table 5.1 Different types of cells and biochemicals in anti-angiogenic therapy

Param.	Description	Param.	Description
$A_r(t)$	Radius of the tumor	$A_c(t)$	Number of live cells in the core of the tumor
$A_p(t)$	Number of live cells in the periphery of the tumor	$A_n(t)$	Number of dead (necrotized) cells in the core of the tumor
$V_b(t)$	Volume of the vascular network in the tumor	$V_{bc}(t)$	Volume of the vascular network in the core of the tumor
$V_{bp}(t)$	Volume of the vascular network in the periphery of the tumor	$U_{NP}(t)$	Nutrient concentration in the periphery of the tumor
$U_{NC}(t)$	Nutrient concentration in the core of the tumor	$U_{A_p}(t)$	Density of the tumor cells in the periphery

endogenous angiogenesis inhibitors, and inhibition of binding of angiogenic stimulators, to name some.

In [9], many spatiotemporal models of angiogenesis are discussed using PDEs which account for the main defining characteristics of angiogenesis such as the mean sprout density, sprout branching, expansion rate of the capillary network, structure and shape of the capillary network and also the influence of the extracellular component namely fibronectin in facilitating cell adhesion, migration and guiding of sprouting tip cells during angiogenesis. However, the main focus of this book is on ODE models.

Anti-angiogenic therapy models primarily involved the dynamics of tumor cells, endothelial cells, angiogenesis inhibitory agents, and angiogenesis stimulatory agents. Interactions between these cells and agents involve many common dynamics similar to that explained in the general model given by (1.1) and (1.2) in Chap. 1. Even though there exist several models with slight modifications that represent anti-angiogenic therapy [8–12], the following two main models are considered in this chapter, namely:

1. Model that accounts for the dynamics of the tumor cells and endothelial cells under anti-angiogenic therapy, and
2. Model that involves the dynamics of the vasculature in the core and periphery of the tumor under anti-angiogenic therapy.

Tables 5.1 and 5.2 summarize the notations used in this chapter.

Table 5.2 Parameter notations used in anti-angiogenic therapy

Var.	Description	Var.	Description
m	Mutation (cell transition) rate	r	Growth rate
a	Fractional cell-kill rate due to therapy	d_U	Depletion (elimination) rate of therapeutic agent from tumor site
V_c	Volume of the core of the tumor	V_x	Density of the external vasculature
V_p	Volume of periphery of the tumor	υ_{11}	Factor of decreasing tumor volume
ΔV_c	Increment in volume of core of the tumor	ΔV_p	Increment in volume of periphery of the tumor
U_{A_p}	Tumor expansion in terms of the density of the tumor cells in the periphery of the tumor	κ	Parameter associated with tumor growth or necrosis
υ_{12}	Spontaneous loss of functional vasculature	ξ_S	Angiogenic stimulatory effect of tumor
ξ_I	Angiogenic inhibition due to endothelial cell death	ξ_E	Efficiency of the anti-angiogenic agent

5.1 Dynamics of Tumor Cells and Endothelial Cells Under Anti-angiogenic Therapy

Among the available mathematical models of anti-angiogenic therapy, the most widely accepted model is the one that portrays the dynamics of tumor cells and endothelial cells given in [10]. This model is developed by using the experimental results from mice with Lewis lung carcinoma reported in [10] itself. In general, experiments and clinical trials suggest that, the factors that can influence the volume of the vascular network are the intrinsic loss rate, stimulatory/inhibitory influences from the tumor, and inhibition via externally administered inhibitors [8, 10–12]. Hence, in [10], two compartments are used where the first one models the dynamics in the tumor volume and the second one accommodates the changes in the volume of the vascular network. In [13, 14], the basic model given in [10] is modified by adding an integral term to quantify the dynamics of the administrated inhibitor. The modified model is given by:

$$\frac{\mathrm{d}A(t)}{\mathrm{d}t} = -\upsilon_{11} A(t) \ln\left(\frac{A(t)}{V_{\mathrm{b}}(t)}\right), \tag{5.1}$$

$$\frac{\mathrm{d}V_{\mathrm{b}}(t)}{\mathrm{d}t} = -\upsilon_{12} V_{\mathrm{b}}(t) + \xi_S A(t) - \xi_I V_{\mathrm{b}}(t) A^{\frac{2}{3}}(t) - a V_{\mathrm{b}}(t) U(t), \tag{5.2}$$

$$U(t) = \int_0^t u(t') \mathrm{e}^{(-d_{\mathrm{U}}(t-t'))} \mathrm{d}t', \tag{5.3}$$

where $A(t)$ is the tumor volume, $V_{\mathrm{b}}(t)$ is the volume of the vascular network (endothelial volume), $U(t)$ is the concentration of the exogenous inhibitor administrated, $u(t)$ is the drug (angiogenic inhibitor) infusion rate, $d_{\mathrm{U}}(t)$ denotes the drug clearance rate, r denotes the tumor growth rate, υ_s denotes the spontaneous loss of functionality of the vascular network, ξ_S denotes the stimulatory effect of the tumor via secretion of growth factors such as VEGF, ξ_I denotes the inhibition effect of the tumor, and a accounts for the drug-dependent reduction.

As mentioned earlier, the bidirectional control mediated by the TAFs decides how well angiogenesis ensues in tumors and this tumor-induced angiogenesis, in turn, controls how fast the tumor grows. In terms of the angiogenesis, this bidirectional effect makes the carrying capacity of the tumor a time-varying parameter. Hence, unlike the constant reciprocal carrying capacity b used in chemotherapy and immunotherapy, in the case of anti-angiogenic therapy, the volume of the vascular network, which is denoted as $V_{\mathrm{b}}(t)$, represents the carrying capacity of the tumor. Note that the term $V_{\mathrm{b}}(t)$ indicates the influence of the volume of the vascular network on the carrying capacity of the tumor. Hence, the variable $k(t)$ defined in (1.1) in Chap. 1 can be alternatively used in place of $V_{\mathrm{b}}(t)$.

Even though the type of therapy used differs, the underlying mechanisms involved in the progression and regression of cancer share many common factors. Analyzing these therapy-specific mathematical models with respect to the general model given by (1.1)–(1.2) in Chap. 1 throws light on the important mechanisms addressed and the assumptions involved in specific models.

In (5.1), the growth of the tumor cells given by $\mathscr{G}(\cdot)$ is modeled by using a Gompertzian growth pattern which accounts for the slowing down of tumor growth with respect to the carrying capacity $V_{\mathrm{b}}(t)$ with the parameter υ_{11} denoting the decreasing factor of tumor volume. In (5.2), the first term models the spontaneous loss of functional vasculature in terms of υ_{12} and the second term models the inherent angiogenic stimulation in terms of ξ_S. The term $\mathscr{A}(\cdot) = -\xi_I V_{\mathrm{b}}(t)^{\frac{2}{3}} A(t)$ represents the apoptosis of the endothelial cells, where ξ_I denotes the reduction in the carrying capacity of the vascular network due to the death or disaggregation of endothelial cells. The effect of anti-angiogenic agent is modeled using the term $a V_{\mathrm{b}}(t) U(t)$.

Using the fact that the concentration of the angiogenic inhibitor in the tumor site is proportional to the rate of infusion of the angiogenic inhibitor [13, 15, 16], the drug dynamics given by (5.3), is rewritten as:

$$\frac{\mathrm{d}U(t)}{\mathrm{d}t} = -d_{\mathrm{U}} U(t) + u(t), \tag{5.4}$$

Table 5.3 Parameter values of the anti-angiogenic therapy model (5.1)–(5.3) [10, 13, 14, 16]

Parameter	Value (unit)	Parameter	Value (unit)
ν_{11}	0.192 (days^{-1})	ν_{12}	0 (days^{-1})
ξ_S	5.85 (days^{-1})	ξ_I	0.00873 (days^{-1}mm^{-2})
d_U	1.3 (days^{-1})	a	0.66 (kg days^{-1}mg^{-1})

where d_U is the elimination (clearance) rate of the inhibitor, $U(t)$ is the concentration of the inhibitor, and $u(t)$ is the rate of infusion of the inhibitor. In [10], a quantitative analysis using the anti-angiogenic agents such as endostatin, angiostatin, and TNP-470 is also provided. The original model presented in [10] has been extensively studied [8, 17, 18]. In [8], a slight modification by adding spatial aspects of the diffusion of anti-angiogenic agents are also incorporated along with the dynamics of tumor cells and vasculature. Table 5.3 summarizes the parameter values of the anti-angiogenic therapy model (5.1)–(5.3) [10, 13, 14]. The initial conditions for the variables in model (5.1)–(5.3) are $A(0) = V_b(0) = 17347$ (mm^3) and $U(0) = 0$ (mg kg^{-1}).

5.2 Dynamics of Vasculature in Core and Periphery of Tumor Under Anti-angiogenic Therapy

In this subsection, a mathematical model given in [19] is discussed which incorporates more details regarding the geometry and diffusion of the vasculature in order to investigate the effect of an anti-angiogenic agent on the tumor dynamics. This model is validated using experimental mice data of colorectal carcinoma [20]. The model accounts for the dynamics of the vasculature in the core and periphery of the tumor and is given by:

$$\frac{dA_r(t)}{dt} = r_1 g(U_{A_p}(t)), \tag{5.5}$$

$$\frac{dA_c(t)}{dt} = \frac{\Delta V_c}{V_p} A_p(t) - m\left(\frac{1}{1+e^{\frac{p_3-U_{NC}(t)}{\kappa_3}}}\right)^{\theta_1} A_c(t), \tag{5.6}$$

$$\frac{dA_p(t)}{dt} = -\frac{\Delta V_c}{V_p} A_P(t) + r_2\left(\frac{1}{1+e^{\frac{p_1-U_{NP}(t)}{\kappa_1}}}\frac{1}{1+e^{\frac{p_2-U_{A_p}(t)}{\kappa_2}}}\right) A_p(t), \tag{5.7}$$

$$\frac{dA_n(t)}{dt} = m\left(\frac{1}{1+e^{\frac{p_3-U_{NC}(t)}{\kappa_3}}}\right)^{\theta_1} A_c(t), \tag{5.8}$$

$$\frac{dV_{bc}(t)}{dt} = r_3 A_r^{\beta}(t)\frac{\Delta V_c}{V_p} V_{bp}(t) + \left(a_1 e^{-U(t)\xi_E}\right)\left(\frac{1}{1+e^{\frac{p_4-U_{NC}(t)}{\kappa_4}}}\right)^{\theta_2} V_{bp}(t), \tag{5.9}$$

$$\frac{\mathrm{d}V_{\mathrm{bp}}(t)}{\mathrm{d}t} = \Delta V_{\mathrm{t}} V_{\mathrm{x}} - r_3 A_{\mathrm{r}}^{\beta}(t) \frac{\Delta V_{\mathrm{c}}}{V_{\mathrm{p}}} V_{\mathrm{bp}}(t) + \left(a_1 e^{-U(t)\xi_{\mathrm{E}}}\right) \left(\frac{1}{1 + e^{\frac{p_4 - U_{\mathrm{NC}}(t)}{\kappa_4}}}\right)^{\theta_2} V_{\mathrm{bp}}(t), \tag{5.10}$$

$$\frac{\mathrm{d}U(t)}{\mathrm{d}t} = -d_{\mathrm{U}} U(t) + u(t), \tag{5.11}$$

where $A_{\mathrm{r}}(t)$ denotes the radius of the tumor, $A_{\mathrm{c}}(t)$ is the number of live cells in the core of the tumor, $A_{\mathrm{p}}(t)$ is the number of live cells in the periphery of the tumor, $A_{\mathrm{n}}(t)$ is the number of dead (necrotized) cells in the core of the tumor, $V_{\mathrm{bc}}(t)$ denotes the volume of the vascular network in the core of the tumor, $V_{\mathrm{bp}}(t)$ is the volume of the vascular network in the periphery of the tumor, $U_{A_{\mathrm{p}}}(t)$ denotes the density of tumor cells in the periphery, $U_{\mathrm{NP}}(t)$ is the nutrient concentration in the periphery of the tumor, $U_{\mathrm{NC}}(t)$ is the nutrient concentration in the core of the tumor, $U(t)$ is the concentration of the anti-angiogenic agent, and $u(t)$ is the rate of infusion of the anti-angiogenic agent. The function $g(U_{A_{\mathrm{p}}}(t))$ in (5.5) models the tumor expansion in terms of the density of tumor cells in the periphery and is given by $g(U_{A_{\mathrm{p}}}(t)) = \frac{1}{1+e^{\frac{p_{\mathrm{g}} - U_{A_{\mathrm{p}}}(t)}{\kappa_{\mathrm{g}}}}}$, where p_{g} and κ_{g} are parameters associated with the tumor growth.

In (5.5), the increase in the radius of the tumor in terms of density of tumor cells in the periphery is modeled, where r_1 is the growth rate. Note that, as the tumor grows in size, the cells which are earlier considered as part of the periphery move inside the tumor and become part of the core (Fig. 5.1). This transition of the cells from the periphery of the tumor to the core of the tumor is modeled using the term $\frac{\Delta V_{\mathrm{c}}}{V_p} A_{\mathrm{P}}(t)$ in (5.6) and (5.7). Next, the term $m\left(\frac{1}{1+e^{\frac{p_3 - U_{\mathrm{NC}}(t)}{\kappa_3}}}\right)^{\theta_1}$ in (5.6) represents the reduction of tumor cells due to necrosis, where m denotes the per capita depletion rate of the live tumor cells in the core. It is apparent that as necrosis increases, the number of necrotized tumor cells in the core increases, hence the same term is used in (5.8). Cells removed from the necrotic core by phagocytosis is assumed to be negligible.

In (5.7), the term $r_2\left(\frac{1}{1+e^{\frac{p_1 - U_{\mathrm{NP}}(t)}{\kappa_1}}} \frac{1}{1+e^{\frac{p_2 - U_{A_{\mathrm{p}}}(t)}{\kappa_2}}}\right) A_{\mathrm{p}}(t)$ models the increase in the cancer cell population in the periphery of the tumor via proliferation. This term is analogous to the growth function $\mathscr{G}(\cdot)$ in (1.1), where the tumor growth is modeled with respect to the concentration of the nutrient supply and density of the cells in the periphery of the tumor in which r_2, p_1, p_2, κ_1 and κ_2 are parameters associated with proliferation of the tumor cells. This model accounts for the fact that the rate of cell proliferation is limited when $U_{A_{\mathrm{p}}}(t)$ is too high and $U_{\mathrm{NP}}(t)$ is low. The rate at which cells in the core undergo necrosis is modeled in (5.8), where m is the cell transition from the core to necrotic core (see (5.6) and Fig. 5.1). The parameters V_{c}, V_{p}, ΔV_{c}, and ΔV_{t} are given by [19]:

$$V_c = \frac{4}{3}(d_c A_r)^3 \pi, \tag{5.12}$$

$$V_p = \frac{4}{3}(A_r)^3 \pi - V_c, \tag{5.13}$$

$$\Delta V_c = \frac{4}{3}(d_c(A_r + \Delta A_r))^3 \pi - V_c, \tag{5.14}$$

$$\Delta V_t = \frac{4}{3}\pi(A_r + \Delta A_r)^3 - \frac{4}{3}\pi A_r^3, \tag{5.15}$$

where V_c and V_p are the volumes of the core and periphery of the tumor, ΔV_c is the increment in volume of the core, ΔV_t is the increment in volume of the tumor, d_c is the core-periphery ratio which quantifies whether the cells are closer to the center or periphery of the tumor, and ΔA_r is the increment in the radius of the tumor. The core-periphery ratio of the tumor is modeled in terms of the radius and is given by $d_c(A_r) = \left(\frac{1}{1+e^{\frac{0.5-A_r}{0.333}}}\right)^{2.2} - 0.15$. Nutrition concentration in the core ($U_{NC}(t)$) and periphery ($U_{NP}(t)$) are calculated using:

$$U_{NC}(t) = \frac{r_c}{r_v^{ref}}, \quad r_c = \frac{V_{bc}(t)}{V_c}, \tag{5.16}$$

$$U_{NP}(t) = \frac{r_p}{r_v^{ref}}, \quad r_p = \frac{V_{bp}(t)}{V_p}, \tag{5.17}$$

where r_v^{ref} is the reference vasculature ratio that denotes the necessary percentage of vasculature in a unit volume of tissue that is sufficient to support tumor cells, and $U_{NC}(t)$ and $U_{NP}(t)$ are normalized using r_v^{ref} and hence dimensionless.

In (5.9) and (5.10), the term $\left(\frac{1}{1+e^{\frac{p_4-U_{NC}(t)}{\kappa_4}}}\right)^{\theta_2}$ models the effect of the production of tumor angiogenic factor (TAF) on the volume of vasculature in the core and periphery, respectively. This term accounts for the fact that the tumor cells initiate production of TAF when the nutrition supply goes to a very low value. The term $a_1 e^{-U(t)\xi_E}$ in (5.9) and (5.10) accounts for the effect of anti-angiogenic therapy in terms of parameter a_1 that quantifies drug effect and drug concentration. It can be seen from (5.9) that the term $r_3 A_r^{\beta}(t)\frac{\Delta V_c}{V_P} V_{bp}(t)$ models the increase of the volume of the vascular network inside the core ($V_{bc}(t)$). The term V_x in (5.10) is the density of the external vasculature and ξ_E denotes the efficiency of the anti-angiogenic agent. As the tumor grows, the volume of the vascular network in the periphery is more and more internalized and becomes a part of the core. Hence, the value of $V_{bc}(t)$ increases in line with the increase in $V_{bp}(t)$ and $A_r(t)$. Note that the same increment of tumor radius (ΔA_r) contributes to a much larger volume increase when the radius is large compared to a small value of radius. This is captured by the term A_r^{β}, where $\beta > 1$

Table 5.4 Parameter values of the anti-angiotherapy model (5.5)–(5.11) [19]

Parameter	Value (unit)	Parameter	Value (unit)
r_1	1.2 (mm days^{-1})	m	1 ($\text{mm}^3\text{days}^{-1}$)
p_1	1	κ_2	–45000 (mm^{-3})
θ_1, θ_2	0.3	r_2	12 (days^{-1})
p_2	4×10^5 (mm^{-3})	κ_3	–0.04
κ_1	0.17	p_3	0.2
r_3	0.06	β	1.2
a_1	1 (kg mg^{-1} day^{-1})	ξ_{E}	0.8
p_4	0.45	κ_4	–0.06
d_{U}	$\frac{\log(2)}{3.9}$ (days^{-1})	$r_{\text{v}}^{\text{ref}}$	0.005
κ_{g}	55000 (mm^{-3})	p_{g}	4×10^5 (mm^{-3})

is a constant. Finally, (5.11) models the drug dynamics, where d_{U} is the elimination (clearance) rate of the anti-angiogenic agent.

Table 5.4 summarizes the parameter values of the anti-angiotherapy model (5.5)–(5.11) [19]. The initial conditions for the variables in model (5.5)–(5.11) are $A_{\text{r}}(0) = 13$ (mm), $A_{\text{c}}(0) = 3$, $A_{\text{p}}(0) = 495$, $A_{\text{n}}(0) = 0$, $V_{\text{bc}}(0) = 0$ (mm^3), $V_{\text{bp}}(0) = 0$ (mm^3), and $U(0) = 0$ (mg kg^{-1}).

5.3 Summary

The main difference between the two models discussed in this chapter and the models discussed in earlier chapters is the use of a time-varying parameter $V_{\text{b}}(t)$ for modeling the carrying capacity. Note that, in both the angiotherapy models discussed in this chapter, the effect of the immune system on tumor dynamics and the effect of normal cells on tumor cells are ignored.

Angiogenesis is a complex process that involves the collective action of several cytokines, pro-angiogenic factors, and anti-angiogenic factors. Apart from endothelial cells, other cells such as immune cells, mural cells, and bone marrow pericytes are involved in angiogenesis. For instance, immune cells secrete pro-angiogenic factors as a part of the inflammatory response, which can mediate neovascularisation [3]. Developing mathematical models that elucidate the contribution of immune cells, bone marrow pericyte, mural cells, etc., in the orchestration of angiogenesis is imperative to analyze cancer dynamics [2]. Similarly, several stimuli induce angiogenesis. For instance, hypoxia induces the dimerization of hypoxia-inducible factors (HIF-α and HIF-β), which in turn initiates the transcription of several growth factors and cytokines (e.g. VEGF, erythropoietin, angiopoietin, interleukins, and chemokines). All these growth factors and cytokines collectively mediate angiogenesis through various signal transduction pathways. Consequently, these pathways opened up many therapeutic targets. However, mathematical models that particularly depict the mechanism of action of all these growth factors, cytokines, and respective therapeutic targets related to angiogenesis are yet to be devised.

References

1. J. Folkman, Role of angiogenesis in tumor growth and metastasis. Semin. Oncol. **29**(6), Sup16, 15–18 (2002)
2. G. Mangialardi, A. Cordaro, P. Madeddu, The bone marrow pericyte: an orchestrator of vascular niche. Regen. Med. **11**(8), 883–895 (2016)
3. W. Liang, N. Ferrara, The complex role of neutrophils in tumor angiogenesis and metastasis. Cancer Immunol. Res. **4**(2), 83–91 (2016)
4. H. Rieger, M. Welter, Integrative models of vascular remodeling during tumor growth. Wiley Interdiscip. Rev. Syst. Biol. Med. **7**(3), 113–129 (2015)
5. B. Al Husein, M. Abdalla, M. Trepte, D.L. DeRemer, P.R. Somanath, Antiangiogenic therapy for cancer: an update. Pharmacother.: J. Hum. Pharmacol. Drug Ther. **32**(12), 1095–1111 (2012)
6. J. Folkman, Tumor angiogenesis: therapeutic implications. N. Engl. J. Med. **285**(21), 1182–1186 (1971)
7. R.S. Kerbel, A cancer therapy resistant to resistance. Nature **390**(6658), 335 (1997)
8. A. Ergun, K. Camphausen, L.M. Wein, Optimal scheduling of radiotherapy and angiogenic inhibitors. Bull. Math. Biol. **65**(3), 407–424 (2003)
9. A. Anderson, M. Chaplain, Continuous and discrete mathematical models of tumor-induced angiogenesis. Bull. Math. Biol. **60**(5), 857–899 (1998)
10. P. Hahnfeldt, D. Panigrahy, J. Folkman, L. Hlatky, Tumor development under angiogenic signaling: a dynamical theory of tumor growth, treatment response, and postvascular dormancy. Cancer Res. **59**(19), 4770–4775 (1999)
11. C.J.W. Breward, H.M. Byrne, C.E. Lewis, A multiphase model describing vascular tumour growth. Bull. Math. Biol. **65**, 609–640 (2003)
12. A. d'Onofrio, U. Ledzewicz, H. Maurer, H. Schättler, On optimal delivery of combination therapy for tumors. Math. Biosci. **222**(1), 13–26 (2009)
13. J. Sápi, D.A. Drexler, I. Harmati, Z. Sápi, L. Kovács, Linear state-feedback control synthesis of tumor growth control in antiangiogenic therapy, in *10th International Symposium on Applied Machine Intelligence and Informatics (SAMI)* (2012), pp. 143–148
14. U. Ledzewicz, H. Schättler, A synthesis of optimal controls for a model of tumor growth under angiogenic inhibitors, in *Proceedings of the 44th IEEE Conference on Decision and Control* (2005), pp. 934–939
15. D.A. Drexler, L. Kovács, J. Sápi, I. Harmati, Z. Benyó, Model-based analysis and synthesis of tumor growth under angiogenic inhibition: a case study. IFAC Proc. Vol. **44**(1), 3753–3758 (2011)
16. P. Yazdjerdi, N. Meskin, M. Al Naemi, A.E. Al Moustafa, L. Kovács, Reinforcement learning-based control of tumor growth under anti-angiogenic therapy. Comput. Methods Programs Biomed. **173**, 15–26 (2019)
17. J. Sápi, D.A. Drexler, L. Kovács, Comparison of mathematical tumor growth models, in *2015 IEEE 13th International Symposium on Intelligent Systems and Informatics (SISY)* (2015), pp. 323–328
18. D.A. Drexler, L. Kovács, J. Sápi, I. Harmati, Z. Benyó, Model-based analysis and synthesis of tumor growth under angiogenic inhibition: a case study. IFAC Proc. **44**(1), 3753–3758 (2011). 18th IFAC World Congress

19. D. Csercsik, J. Sápi, T. Gönczy, L. Kovács, Bi-compartmental modelling of tumor and supporting vasculature growth dynamics for cancer treatment optimization purpose, in *2017 IEEE 56th Annual Conference on Decision and Control (CDC)* (2017), pp. 4698–4702
20. J. Sápi, L. Kovács, D.A. Drexler, P. Kocsis, D. Gajári, Z. Sápi, Tumor volume estimation and quasi-continuous administration for most effective bevacizumab therapy. PLoS One **10**(11), e0142190 (2015)

Chapter 6
Radiotherapy Models

Using radiation for the diagnosis and treatment of cancer has a history of more than 100 years [1, 2]. The external beam therapy for cancer treatment uses high energy beams of photons (X-rays), protons, and neutrons to bring about detrimental changes in the irradiated cells. These ionizing radiations primarily cause damage to the DNA of the cells and thereby impair the cell mitosis which eventually leads to cell death [3]. The definition of cell death is different for different types of cells. For differentiated cells that do not proliferate further (e.g., muscle, nerve), loss of cell function is considered to be cell death [3]. However, for a proliferating cell like a hematopoietic cell or intestinal epithelial cells, loss of capability to proliferate is considered as cell death. There is another type of death that happens when the cells try to divide due to abnormal or damaged chromosome and is called as mitotic cell death. Mitotic cell death (mitotic catastrophe) is the common form of death that occurs due to radiation [3].

Figure 6.1 shows various types of DNA damage that occur due to irradiation and its effect on cell survival. Radiation can mediate cell death either by causing direct damage to the DNA or can induce the cell death indirectly by facilitating the release of free radicals. As shown in Fig. 6.1, the damage caused to the single strand or double strand of DNA can have different effects on the fate of the irradiated cells. Even though the cell-kill effect of ionizing radiation is useful for annihilating cancer cells, the fact that radiation is carcinogenic emphasizes the need for the use of the optimal radiation dose particularly targeting the cancer cells while sparing normal cells [4].

As illustrated in Fig. 6.2, if the target of radiotherapy is a tumor tissue in an internal organ, then the intense energy beams can damage the normal tissues from the body surface to the target and beyond the target. Note that the strength of the beam reduces exponentially as it goes towards the target. Hence, it can cause more harm during initial penetration than post tumor, or beyond the tumor. Due to this initial high dose impact, appropriate targeting mechanism and dose optimization algorithms are used to fine-tune the dose delivery [5–7].

R. Padmanabhan et al., *Mathematical Models of Cancer and Different Therapies*, Series in BioEngineering, https://doi.org/10.1007/978-981-15-8640-8_6

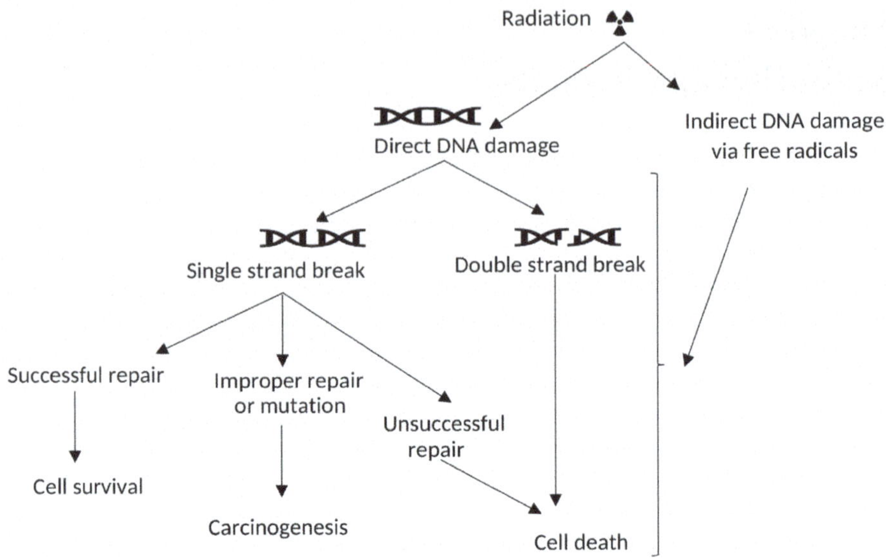

Fig. 6.1 Illustrative diagram showing the direct and indirect effect of ionizing radiation on the cells. Direct DNA damage may be either single strand break or double strand break. Double strand break can lead to cell death. Successful repair of single strand break leads to survival of cells and improper repair can lead to carcinogenesis or cell death. Cell death is also facilitated in an indirect manner via the free radicals released due to the effect of ionizing radiation

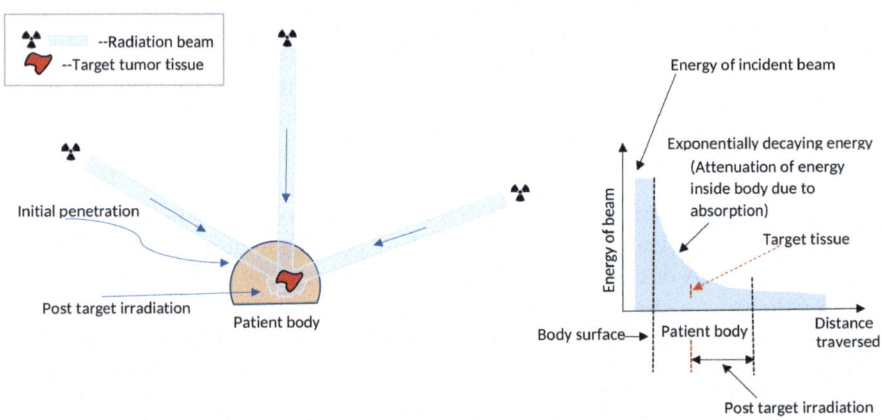

Fig. 6.2 Targeting specific tumor tissue in an internal organ using photon beams. Initial penetration and post target irradiation on a patient's body and respective energy profile is shown in the figure

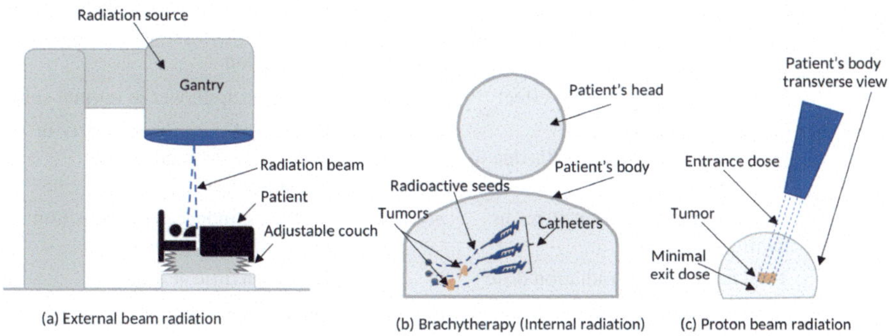

Fig. 6.3 Illustrative diagram showing **(a)** external beam radiotherapy, **(b)** internal beam radiotherapy, and **(c)** proton therapy. **(a)** In the case of external beam therapy, the radiation source is housed in a gantry and an adjustable patient couch is used to position the patient appropriately. **(b)** In the case of internal beam therapy or brachytherapy for breast cancer, internal radiation is facilitated by using radioactive seeds and radiation catheters. **(c)** In the case of proton beam therapy, the proton beam can be controlled to irradiate the target tumor tissue to limit the minimal exit dose

Over the years, several methods have been developed to deliver radiation (photon or proton) precisely to the target tumor tissue and thus minimize cell damage in the surrounding areas of the tumor. External beam radiotherapy and internal beam radiotherapy (brachytherapy) are two main methods that uses X-rays (photons) for tumor regression (Fig. 6.3). As shown in Fig. 6.2, the photon beam-based therapy can result in post target irradiation and hence often computer controlled algorithms are used to facilitate precision radiotherapy. In the case of brachytherapy, radioactive material is added to the site (target) by implantation or injection. Compared to photon beam-based therapy, in the case of the proton therapy, since the delivery of protons are related to its mass and density, it can be programmed/targeted to reach a specific distance by adjusting its initial dose. Hence, the proton beam delivers limited radiation to the healthy tissues beyond the site of the tumor. The concept of post target irradiation and minimal exit dose are illustrated in Figs. 6.2 and 6.3, respectively.

Dose conformity is a commonly used term in the radiation therapy to assess the treatment plan in terms of the percentage radiation dose that will be delivered to the target [8]. Some methods that are currently in used include the three dimensional conformal radiation therapy (3D CRT), intensity modulated therapy (IMRT), volumetric modulated arc therapy (VMAT), stereotactic radiation therapy (SRT), adaptive radiation therapy (ART), and image-guided radiation therapy (IGRT) [1]. These methods have many advantages that make them specifically suitable for treating certain types of cancer. For instance, image-guided radiation therapy is particularly used for treating moving tumors such as that in the lungs. Even though intensity modulated therapy and volumetric modulated arc therapy have good dose conformity, latter one has a better time of delivery [5–7]. The radiosensitivity of different cell types is different, and typically radiations from a moderate dose to high dose are used to kill cancer cells. Experiments and clinical trials suggest that the radiosensitivity of the cells in the

Table 6.1 Parameter notations used in radiotherapy

Param.	Description	Param.	Description
a	Dose dependent radiation effect	ϵ	Radiation spill over to normal cells
a_γ	Degree of inhibition of growth/proliferation of cells due to radiation	a_u	Potency of the radiosensitizer in enhancing accumulation of radiation dose
a_p	Potency of the radiosensitizer in facilitating cell-kill	m_a	Radiation induced cell transition rate of the dying cells
u_{tot}	Total accumulated radiation dose	u_t	Radiation dose at time t
α	Linear parameter	β	Quadratic parameter

Table 6.2 Different types of cells and biochemicals in radiotherapy

Var.	Description	Var.	Description
$A(t)$	Cancer cells	$A_i(t), i = 1, \ldots, 6$	Cancer cells with different degrees of damage due to irradiation
$N(t)$	Normal cells	$U_s(t)$	Plasma concentration of radiosensitizer
$u(t)$	Radiation dose		

G_2 and mitotic phases of the cell-cycle are higher than those cells in S-phase (DNA synthesis). Note that many types of radiosensitizers are also used during radiotherapy to enhance the accumulation of radiation dose in the target [5–7].

As mentioned earlier, the cell populations involved in a mathematical model varies according to the focus of interest of the model. In case of mathematical models developed for radiotherapy, the cell populations involved are categorized based on whether they are healthy, diseased, lethally irradiated, or according to the phase of the cell-cycle they are in. In this chapter, the following special cases of the general model (1.1)–(1.2) are discussed that account for the dynamics of different cell populations with respect to radiotherapy, namely:

1. Two cell-based competition model of tumor dynamics under radiotherapy,
2. Linear-quadratic cell survival model of tumor dynamics due to radiotherapy.

Tables 6.1 and 6.2 summarize the notations that are used in this chapter.

6.1 Two Cell-Based Competition Model

Based on the discussions pertaining to chemotherapy, immunotherapy, and anti-angiogenic therapy, it is apparent that the competition between different cell populations plays a key role in deciding the overall tumor dynamics. Similarly, here the

Lotka-Volterra competition model of tumor dynamics with respect to radiotherapy is considered as ([9]):

$$\frac{dN(t)}{dt} = r_1 N(t)\left(1 - b_1 N(t)\right) - c_1 N(t)A(t), \quad N(0) \geq 0, \tag{6.1}$$

$$\frac{dA(t)}{dt} = r_2 A(t)\left(1 - b_2 A(t)\right) - c_2 N(t)A(t) - \mathscr{D}\left(a, N(t), A(t)\right), \quad A(0) \geq 0, \tag{6.2}$$

where $N(t)$ denotes the concentration of normal cells, $A(t)$ denotes the concentration of abnormal (tumor) cells, $\mathscr{D}(a, N(t), A(t))$ is the radiation control term, where a is the radiation dose-dependent cell-kill rate, r_i and c_i, $i = 1, 2$, are the growth rates and competition rates used to model $\mathscr{G}(r, N(t))$ and $\mathscr{C}(N(t), A(t), c)$, respectively. The drug effect term $\mathscr{D}(a, N(t), A(t))$ can be modeled to account for a constant dose, a dose proportional to the tumor size, or proportional to the ratio of the cancer cells to the normal cells as $\mathscr{D}(a, N(t), A(t)) = a$, $aA(t)$, or $a\frac{A(t)}{N(t)}$, respectively. From (6.2), it can be seen that, these terms can model the reduction in tumor growth rate as $r_2 A(t) - a$, $(r_2 - a)A(t)$, or $\left(r_2 - \frac{a}{N(t)}\right) A(t)$, for various radiation doses.

The model given in [9] is then extended by additionally accounting for the *spill-over* of radiation to healthy cells by using the term $\mathscr{D}_1(a, N(t), A(t))$ and is given by:

$$\frac{dN(t)}{dt} = r_1 N(t)\left(1 - b_1 N(t)\right) - c_1 N(t)A(t) - \mathscr{D}_1\left(a, N(t), A(t)\right), \quad N(0) \geq 0, \tag{6.3}$$

$$\frac{dA(t)}{dt} = r_2 A(t)\left(1 - b_2 A(t)\right) - c_2 N(t)A(t) - \mathscr{D}_2\left(a, N(t), A(t)\right), \quad A(0) \geq 0, \tag{6.4}$$

where the radiation control term modeled using the function $\mathscr{D}_i(a, N(t), A(t))$, $i = 1, 2$ can be in the form (1) $\mathscr{D}_1(\cdot) = a_1$ and $\mathscr{D}_2(\cdot) = a_2$ which account for the irradiation of tumor site with a constant amount of radiation, (2) $\mathscr{D}_1(\cdot) = a_1 A(t)$ and $\mathscr{D}_2(\cdot) = a_2 A(t)$ wherein the irradiation is linearly dependent on the instantaneous value of the concentration of the cancer cells, (3) $\mathscr{D}_1(\cdot) = a_1 \frac{A(t)}{N(t)}$ and $\mathscr{D}_2(\cdot) = a_2 \frac{A(t)}{N(t)}$ wherein the irradiation is proportional to the ratio $\frac{A(t)}{N(t)}$, or (4) a periodic irradiation wherein $\mathscr{D}_1(\cdot) = a_1$ and

$$\mathscr{D}_2(\cdot) = \begin{cases} a_2 & nT \leq t < nT + \tau \\ 0 & nT + \tau \leq t < (n+1)T, \quad n = 0, 1, 2, \ldots \end{cases}, \tag{6.5}$$

where T is the period and τ is the duration of administration of radiation in the periodic step function $\mathscr{D}_2(a, N(t), A(t))$ [10]. Clinical trials suggest that typically $\mathscr{D}_1(\cdot) < \mathscr{D}_2(\cdot)$ [11]. Similar to (6.3), in [10], a perturbation term ϵ is considered to account for the possible spill over of the radiation on to the surrounding tissues, i.e. $\mathscr{D}_1(\cdot) =$

Table 6.3 Parameter values of the radiotherapy model (6.1)–(6.5) [9, 10]

Param.	Value	Param.	Value	Param.	Value
$a_i, i = 1, 2$	0.01–0.2	r_1	0.008	c_1	0.01
$b_i, i = 1, 2$	1	r_2	0.4	c_2	0.15
ϵ	0.001				

$\epsilon a N(t)$. Note that (6.1)–(6.4) neglect the change in the cell number due to the natural death (apoptosis) of the cell populations, cell transition (alterations) due to mutation or any other reasons, and dynamics of the therapeutic agent (Fig. 1.4). Table 6.3 summarizes the parameter values of the radiotherapy model (6.1)–(6.5) [10]. The initial conditions for the variables in model (6.1)–(6.4) are $N(0) = 0.5 \leq \frac{1}{b_1}$ and $A(0) = 0.8 \leq \frac{1}{b_2}$.

6.2 Linear-Quadratic Cell Survival Model

Another most widely accepted mathematical model that depicts the effects of radiotherapy is based on the linear-quadratic model of cell survival [12, 13]. As shown in Fig. 6.1, under radiotherapy, the cell death is mediated by a single lethal mutation or by the accumulation of several mutations. Hence, in the following model the effects of mutation and double strand break in DNA is accounted for using a dose protraction parameter. The fraction of surviving cells is denoted by σ_{T} whose dynamics depends on the radiation dose and time interval of irradiation as given by:

$$\ln \sigma_{\mathrm{T}} = -\alpha u_{\mathrm{tot}} - \beta G_{\mathrm{T}} u_{\mathrm{tot}}^2, \tag{6.6}$$

where α and β are the linear and quadratic parameters associated with the linear-quadratic model of radiology, and u_{tot} is the cumulative radiation dose during an irradiation interval of T. In particular, α and β represent the lethal damage to DNA caused by one-track action and two-track action, respectively. Here, G_{T} denotes the Lea-Catcheside dose-protraction factor given by ([13]):

$$G_{\mathrm{T}} = 2\int_0^T \frac{u(t)}{u_{\mathrm{tot}}} \mathrm{d}t \int_0^t \frac{u\left(t'\right)}{u_{\mathrm{tot}}} e^{\lambda(t'-t)} \mathrm{d}t', \tag{6.7}$$

where u_{tot} is the total dose of radiation till time T, $u(t)$ is the time varying dose, and λ is the repair time constant. The dose protraction fraction model given by (6.7) accounts for the effects of lethal double-strand break in DNA at time t and its secondary interaction at time t'. The main advantage of the LQ model is that, using the dose protraction fraction G, this model can predict the prolonged effect for each of the four different types of radiation doses $\mathscr{D}_i\ (a, N(t), A(t)), i = 1, 2$ mentioned earlier. The biologically effective dose (BED) or extrapolated response dose (ERD) associated with the radiation therapy is calculated in terms of the fraction of the surviving cells and is given by:

$$\mathrm{BED} = -\frac{\ln(\sigma_\mathrm{T})}{\alpha} = u_{tot}\left(1 + \frac{u_\mathrm{d}}{\alpha/\beta}\right), \tag{6.8}$$

where u_d is the dose per fraction. As mentioned earlier, radiosensitizers are often used to enhance the efficacy of radiation therapy. In [14], the pharmacokinetics of the radiosensitizer using a one-compartment model is given as:

$$\frac{\mathrm{d}U_\mathrm{s}(t)}{\mathrm{d}t} = -d_\mathrm{U}U_\mathrm{s}(t), \quad U_\mathrm{s}(0) = \frac{u_0 B}{V}, \tag{6.9}$$

where $U_\mathrm{s}(t)$ is the plasma concentration of the radiosensitizer used, d_U is the elimination rate of the radiosensitizing agent, V is the distribution volume, u_0 is the dose of the agent administrated at time $t = 0$, and B is the bioavailability.

The mathematical model of the tumor dynamics with respect to radiation and radiosensitizing agent presented in [14] is an extension of the model given in [2]. The extended model given in [14] accounts for both short-term and long-term growth dynamics due to treatment and are validated by pre-clinical trials using mice xenograft models. Several experimental trials support the assumption that the irradiated cells undergo one or multiple cell divisions before dying (mitotic catastrophe) [2, 15]. With radiotherapy, the growth of the surviving cancer cells in the tumor micro-environment is often impeded due to the impaired vascular support of the region and mutations involved. These effects are considered as the secondary effect of radiation. In [14], important effects of the ionizing radiations such as the immediate killing of cells and preventing the capability to proliferate are modeled using six compartments, namely: (1) A_1 models the compartment that includes the proliferating abnormal (cancer) cells, (2) A_i, $i = 2, 3$, and 4 are transit compartments which categorize the dying cancer cells with different degrees of damage, and (3) $A_i, i = 5$ and 6 model the compartments which include the cancer cells which are lethally irradiated. The compartment A_5 is used to include the cells which are capable of one more cell division before apoptosis and A_6 is used include the cells which die without further proliferation. The cell dynamics in the first compartment is given by:

$$\frac{\mathrm{d}A_1(t)}{\mathrm{d}t} = rA_1(t)\mathrm{e}^{-a_\gamma u_\mathrm{tot}} - m_1 A_1(t), \quad t \neq t_i, \tag{6.10}$$

$$A_1\left(t_i^+\right) = A_1\left(t_i^-\right) - \mathscr{M}\left(u(t_i), U_\mathrm{s}(t_i)\right) A_1(t), \quad i = 1, \ldots, n, \tag{6.11}$$

where r is the growth rate, m_1 is the cell transition rate due to radiation, u_tot is the accumulated radiation dose, and a_γ quantifies the degree of inhibition of growth/proliferation of cells. With respect to the general model given by (1.1)–(1.2), here the cell transition function $\mathscr{M}\left(u(t_i), U_\mathrm{s}(t_i)\right)$ models the transition of cells from one compartment to another, where $u(t_i)$ and $U_\mathrm{s}(t_i)$ are the dose of radiation and concentration of the radiosensitizer administrated concurrently at time t_i and is given by:

$$\mathcal{M}\left(u(t_i), U_s(t_i)\right) = 1 - e^{\left(-\left(1+a_p U_s(t_i)\right)\left(\alpha u(t_i)+\beta u^2(t_i)\right)\right)}, \tag{6.12}$$

where a_p is the potency of the radiosensitizer. Note that here $\mathcal{M}(\cdot)$ denotes the fraction cells that are lethally irradiated. The extent of irradiation depends on the dose $u(t_i)$ and exposure to the radiosensitizer $U_s(t_i)$ (6.9). The volume of cells in each compartment is denoted by $A_i(t)$, $i = 2, 3,$ and 4 and the dynamics are given by:

$$\frac{\mathrm{d}A_2(t)}{\mathrm{d}t} = m_1 A_1(t) + m_1 A_5(t) + m_1 A_6(t) - m_1 A_2(t), \tag{6.13}$$

$$\frac{\mathrm{d}A_3(t)}{\mathrm{d}t} = m_1 A_2(t) - m_1 A_3(t), \tag{6.14}$$

$$\frac{\mathrm{d}A_4(t)}{\mathrm{d}t} = m_1 A_3(t) - m_1 A_4(t). \tag{6.15}$$

It can be seen from (6.13)–(6.15) that, due to radiation, m_1 fraction of cells transit between compartments. Any cells from the lethally irradiated compartments such as A_5 and A_6, which survive more than one cell division are added to the compartment A_2. This is modeled by using the term $m_1 A_5(t) + m_1 A_6(t)$ in (6.13). The term $m_1 A_2(t)$ in (6.13) and (6.14) models the transition of dying cells to the next stage represented by the compartment $A_3(t)$. Similar explanation holds for the rest of the terms in (6.13)–(6.15). Finally, the dynamics in A_5 and A_6 are given by:

$$\frac{\mathrm{d}A_5(t)}{\mathrm{d}t} = -r A_5(t) - m_1 A_5(t), \quad t \neq t_i, \tag{6.16}$$

$$A_5\left(t_i^+\right) = A_5\left(t_i^-\right) + \mathcal{M}\left(u(t_i), U_s(t_i)\right) A_1(t), \quad i = 1, \ldots, n, \tag{6.17}$$

$$\frac{\mathrm{d}A_6(t)}{\mathrm{d}t} = 2r A_5(t) - m_1 A_6(t), \tag{6.18}$$

where $A_5\left(t_i^+\right)$ and $A_5\left(t_i^-\right)$ denote the volume of the cells in the compartment A_5 just before and after the time of irradiation t_i. The transition of the fraction of lethally irradiated cells from compartment A_1 to A_5 is modeled using the term $\pm\mathcal{M}\left(u(t_i), U_s(t_i)\right) A_1(t)$ in (6.11) and (6.17). Note, that the cells from compartment A_5 undergoes cell division to form two daughter cells (Fig. 6.4). These daughter cells are categorized into compartment A_6. Hence, even though $r A_5(t)$ cells leave compartment A_5, $2r A_5(t)$ enters the compartment A_6; see equations (6.16) and (6.18).

The action of radiosensitizer has an effect on the total radiation that accumulates in an irradiated site and is given by:

$$u_{\mathrm{tot}}\left(t_i^+\right) = u_{\mathrm{tot}}\left(t_i^-\right) + \left(1 + a_u U_s(t_i)\right) u(t_i), \tag{6.19}$$

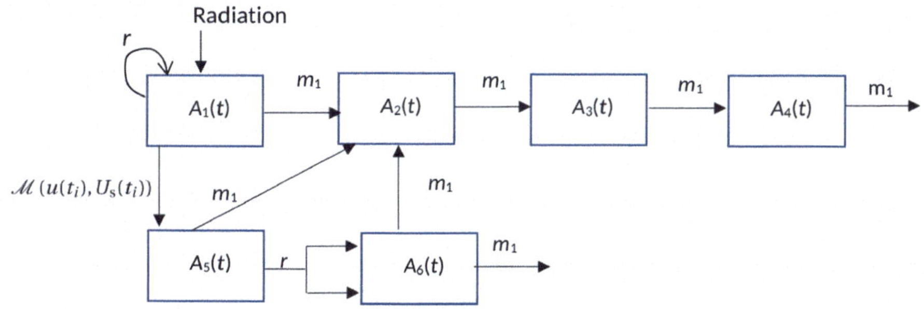

Fig. 6.4 Illustrative diagram showing the cell transition between six compartments defined in model (6.10)–(6.18), where A_1 models the compartment that includes the proliferating cancer cells, A_i, $i = 2, 3$, and 4 are transit compartments which categorize the dying cancer cells with different degrees of damage, and A_i, $i = 5$ and 6 models the compartments which include the cancer cells which are lethally irradiated

where a_u denotes the potency of the radiosensitizer in enhancing accumulation of radiation dose. Note that the initial conditions are given by:

$$A_i(0) = A_0 \left(\frac{m_1}{r}\right)^{i-1}, i = 1, \ldots, 4, \quad A_i(0) = 0, \quad i = 5, 6, \quad u_{tot}(0) = 0. \tag{6.20}$$

In short, the mathematical model of the combined effect of radiation and radiosensitizer given by (6.9)–(6.20) mainly accommodates two effects such as (1) immediate cell-kill effect (short-term effect) and (2) inhibition of proliferation of surviving cells (long-term effect), where the fraction of irradiated cells (6.12) is modeled according to the LQ approach of radiotherapy. This model is able to describe post-treatment events including tumor regrowth and is useful to evaluate parameters such as tumor static concentration (TSC) and tumor static exposure (TSE), which are used to study the cell-kill efficacy, synergy in action, and toxicity in the case of combined administration of radiation and chemicals.

As mentioned earlier, the cell death is triggered when the ionizing radiation induces unrepairable damage to DNA strands in cells [16]. Apart from the loss of cells due to radiotherapy, the PDE-based model presented in [16] also accounts for the net proliferation, cell death, haptotaxis (movement/migration of cells), and effect of random motility in tumor dynamics. Table 6.4 summarizes the parameter values of the radiotherapy model (6.9)–(6.20) [13, 14]. The initial conditions for the variables discussed in this section are given by (6.9) and (6.20), where $U_s(0)$ (mg kg^{-1}) is calculated using $u_0 = [25, 100]$ (mg kg^{-1}) in (6.9) and $A_i(0)$, $i = 1, \ldots, 6$ are calculated using $A_0 = 27$ mm^3 in (6.20).

Table 6.4 Parameter values of the radiotherapy model (6.9)–(6.20) [13, 14]

Parameter	Value (unit)	Parameter	Value (unit)
r	0.04 (days^{-1})	α	54 (kGy^{-1})
m_1	0.26 (days^{-1})	α/β	10 (Gy)
A_0	27 (mm^3)	a_p	0.42 (mL μg^{-1})
a_γ	4.0 (kGy^{-1})	a_u	0.15 (mL μg^{-1})
λ	1 (h)	u_d	1.8–2 (Gy)
d_U	0.231 (h^{-1})		

6.3 Summary

Compared to the models discussed in Chaps. 3 to 5, models discussed in this chapter mainly account for the cell dynamics with respect to the effect of radiation alone. The influence of immune system, presence or absence of tumor vasculature, and cell-cell interactions in the tumor micro-environment are neglected.

The association of circulating lymphocytes and cytokines with the survival of a patient after undergoing radiotherapy is a clear implication of the influence of immune interaction related to this therapy [17]. Many studies report the immuno-suppressive effects of radiotherapy [17, 18]. A few studies, including the preclinical study reported in [19], report reduced efficacy of radiotherapy in immuno-deficient mice [17, 18]. Similarly, the fact that radiation-induced cell-damage is positively correlated with the supply of oxygen highlights the importance of tumor vasculature in deciding the treatment efficacy of radiotherapy [18]. All these studies highlight the importance of further investigating the tumor-immune interaction and tumor vasculature on the radiotherapy [18]. Hence, developing mathematical models that account for both systemic and regional interaction of radiotherapy is imperative.

Apart from these, another area is the post-irradiation toxicity models that make use of the association of biomarkers for predicting the treatment efficacy after radiotherapy. For instance, in [20], such a model is presented that predicts the possibility of radiation-induced pneumonitis in patients who received radiotherapy for lung cancer. Several genetic and nongenetic factors as well as radiation parameters can contribute to such toxicities. The model reported in [20] rely on a single biomarker which is the site-specific probability of radiation pneumonitis obtained from GLM-NET (generalised linear model via elastic net). More specific models that account for the association of multiple parameters to predict the efficacy of radiation therapy and post-irradiation toxicities are desirable.

References

1. W. Wang, J. Lang, Strategies to optimize radiotherapy based on biological responses of tumor and normal tissue. Exp. Ther. Med. **4**(2), 175–180 (2012)
2. T. Cardilin, J. Almquist, M. Jirstrand, A. Zimmermann, S. El Bawab, J. Gabrielsson, Model-based evaluation of radiation and radiosensitizing agents in oncology. CPT: Pharmacomet. Syst. Pharmacol. **7**(1), 51–58 (2018)
3. B. Wouters, Cell death after irradiation: how, when and why cells die. Basic Clin. Radiobiol. 27–40 (2009)
4. J.B. Little, Radiation carcinogenesis. Carcinogenesis **21**(3), 397–404 (2000)
5. D. Pflugfelder, J.J. Wilkens, S. Nill, U. Oelfke, A comparison of three optimization algorithms for intensity modulated radiation therapy. Zeitschrift für Medizinische Physik **18**(2), 111–119 (2008)
6. J.M. Pakela, H.H. Tseng, M.M. Matuszak, R.K. Ten Haken, D.L. McShan, I. El Naqa, Quantum inspired algorithm for radiotherapy planning optimization. Med. Phys. **47**(1), 5–18 (2020)
7. M. Wilson, Optimization of the radiation shielding capabilities of bismuth-borate glasses using the genetic algorithm. Mater. Chem. Phys. **224**, 238–245 (2019)
8. D.L. Holyoake, M. Robinson, D. Grose, D. McIntosh, D. Sebag-Montefiore, G. Radhakrishna, N. Patel, M. Partridge, S. Mukherjee, M.A. Hawkins, Conformity analysis to demonstrate reproducibility of target volumes for margin-intense stereotactic radiotherapy for borderline-resectable pancreatic cancer. Radiother. Oncol. **121**(1), 86–91 (2016)
9. G. Belostotski, H.I. Freedman, A control theory model for cancer treatment by radiotherapy. Int. J. Pure Appl. Math. **25** (2005)
10. Z. Liu, C. Yang, A mathematical model of cancer treatment by radiotherapy. Comput. Math. Methods Med. 1–12 (2014)
11. H.I. Freedman, G. Belostotski, Perturbed models for cancer treatment by radiotherapy. Differ. Equ. Dyn. Syst. **17**, 115–133 (2009). Apr
12. R. Sachs, L. Hlatky, P. Hahnfeldt, Simple ODE models of tumor growth and anti-angiogenic or radiation treatment. Math. Comput. Model. **33**(12), 1297–1305 (2001)
13. S.F.C. O'Rourke, H. McAneney, T. Hillen, Linear quadratic and tumour control probability modelling in external beam radiotherapy. J. Math. Biol. **58**, 799 (2008). Sep
14. T. Cardilin, J. Almquist, M. Jirstrand, A. Zimmermann, F. Lignet, S. El Bawab, J. Gabrielsson, Modeling long-term tumor growth and kill after combinations of radiation and radiosensitizing agents. Cancer Chemother. Pharmacol. **83**(6), 1159–1173 (2019)
15. H.B. Forrester, C.A. Vidair, N. Albright, C.C. Ling, W.C. Dewey, Using computerized video time lapse for quantifying cell death of X-irradiated rat embryo cells transfected with c-myc or c-Ha-ras. Cancer Res. **59**(4), 931–939 (1999)
16. H. Enderling, M.A.J. Chaplain, P. Hahnfeldt, Quantitative modeling of tumor dynamics and radiotherapy. Acta Biotheor. **58**(4), 341–353 (2010)
17. C. Grassberger, S.G. Ellsworth, M.Q. Wilks, F.K. Keane, J.S. Loeffler, Assessing the interactions between radiotherapy and antitumour immunity. Nat. Rev. Clin. Oncol. 1–17 (2019)
18. R.S.A. Goedegebuure, L.K. de Klerk, A.J. Bass, S. Derks, V.L.J.L. Thijssen, Combining radiotherapy with anti-angiogenic therapy and immunotherapy: a therapeutic triad for cancer? Front. Immunol. **9**, 3107 (2019)
19. H.B. Slone, L.J. Peters, L. Milas, Effect of host immune capability on radiocurability and subsequent transplantability of a murine fibrosarcoma. J. Natl. Cancer Inst. **63**(5), 1229–1235 (1979)
20. L. Du, N. Ma, X. Dai, W. Yu, X. Huang, S. Xu, F. Liu, Q. He, Y. Liu, Q. Wang et al., Precise prediction of the radiation pneumonitis in lung cancer: an explorative preliminary mathematical model using genotype information. J. Cancer **11**(8), 2329 (2020)

Chapter 7
Hormone Therapy Models

Hormone therapy or endocrine therapy is used along with other treatment strategies to alleviate different types of human cancers including prostate and breast [1–4]. The idea of using hormone therapy for the regression of cancer stems from the understanding that many hormones play key roles in the progression of certain cancers. Hence, hormone therapy involves treatment methods that use agents that can regulate the production of hormones or influence the mechanism of action of hormones to facilitate cancer cure. Hormone therapy has a history of 80 years which started with the identification of the positive benefits of hormone deprivation in patients with metastatic prostate cancer in 1941 [5]. Note that, as hormone deprivation alone is often insufficient to eradicate cancer, this treatment method is used along with (adjuvant therapy) or prior to (neoadjuvant therapy) chemotherapy or radiation therapy to enhance the overall treatment outcome of the patient. Hormone therapy is facilitated by (1) chemical castration which involves hormone deprivation by using therapeutic agents and/or (2) surgical castration which is the removal of the hormone-secreting gland.

Even though hormone therapy is useful for managing various cancers, it is predominantly used for treating prostate cancer [2, 4]. Testosterone (TST) and estrogen are the primary male and female sex hormones, respectively. While the TST mediated treatments for the prostate cancer are categorized as hormone therapy, most of the estrogen-mediated treatments for the breast cancer are discussed under the heading of targeted therapy in the literature [6]. Hence, in this chapter, the example of hormone-mediated growth of prostate cancer cells and associated therapeutic targets is presented to discuss mathematical models pertaining to hormone therapy.

Androgen is the common name for a group of hormones that is responsible for the masculine characteristics in a human being. TST and androstenedione are principle members of androgens. Hormone therapy for prostate cancer is facilitated by using therapeutic agents that are capable of lowering the production of TST. Evidence suggests that along with testes and adrenal gland, tumor cells can also secrete androgens [7]. Hence, the removal of testes (orchiectomy/surgical castration) alone is often

R. Padmanabhan et al., *Mathematical Models of Cancer and Different Therapies*, Series in BioEngineering, https://doi.org/10.1007/978-981-15-8640-8_7

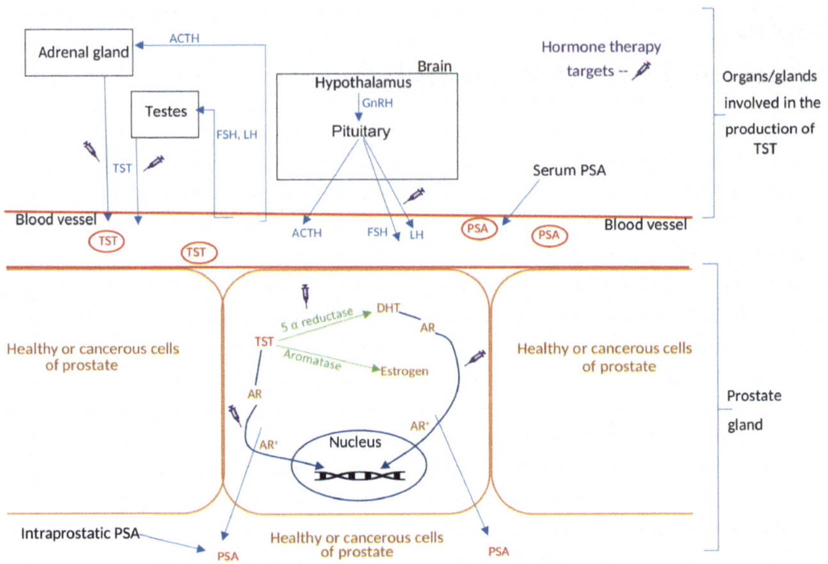

Fig. 7.1 Illustrative diagram showing (1) the brain mediated regulation of the secretion of TST (testosterone) by testes and adrenal gland, (2) enzyme-mediated conversion of TST to DHT, and (3) activated androgen receptor (AR^+) mediated regulation of gene expression that results in the secretion of prostate-specific antigen (PSA) in the epithelial cells of the prostate gland. Hormones of hypothalamus, pituitary, testes, and adrenal gland such as GnRH (gonadotrophin-releasing hormone), ACTH (adrenocorticotropic hormone), FSH (follicle-stimulating hormone), LH (luteinizing hormone), TST (testosterone), and DHT (dihydrotestosterone) are involved in the production of TST and thereby in the secretion of PSA

inadequate for the regression of androgen-dependent cancer cells. Therefore, drugs that can block multiple pathways related to the production and action of TST are also needed to achieve complete chemical castration and to facilitate the annihilation of androgen-dependent (AD) cancer cells.

As shown in Fig. 7.1, GnRH (gonadotrophin-releasing hormone) that is secreted by the hypothalamus regulates the release of FSH (follicle-stimulating hormone), LH (luteinizing hormone), and ACTH (Adrenocorticotropic hormone) by the pituitary gland. These hormones which are released to the circulatory system can control the production of TST in testes and adrenal gland. About 95% of TST in the blood is secreted by the testes and remaining by the adrenal gland. The circulatory system carries TST to the prostate cells wherein the enzyme 5 α reductase mediates the conversion of the majority of TST to more potent derivative dihydrotestosterone (DHT). A small portion of TST is converted to estrogen by the enzyme aromatase. An androgen receptor (AR) is a nuclear receptor in the cytoplasm of the cells which can sense hormones such as TST and DHT in the cell. As shown in Fig. 7.1, upon getting bonded with androgens (hormones), these receptors are activated to AR^+ and get translocated to the nucleus of the cell where they regulate gene expression associated with the cell proliferation, metabolism, in addition to the secretion of prostate-specific antigen (PSA). This TST mediated gene regulation pathway that facilitates proliferation and metabolism of healthy prostate cells is also utilized by most of the prostate cancer cells for their growth and multiplication [3, 4]. Hence, blocking the activation of AR, altering the stability of relevant proteins/hormones, interrupting the production of TST, and regulating the production of GnRH or LH are potential targets for hormone therapy. Several such hormone therapy targets are marked in Fig. 7.1. Commonly used agents that facilitate hormone therapy include GnRH agonists, androgen receptor antagonists (anti-androgens), and steroidogenesis inhibitors.

Another important factor associated with prostate cancer is the significant correlation between the level of androgen in blood and the production of PSA by prostate cells [8, 9]. PSA is a glycoprotein secreted by the prostate gland, urethral lining, and bulbourethral gland. Under normal conditions, very little PSA levels are detected in the blood. However, due to increased glandular size or abnormal nature of the prostate cancer tissues, often an increased level of PSA is released to the circulatory system. Even though higher level of PSA does not necessarily indicate prostate cancer, it is considered as one of the important biomarkers for this disease. As shown in Fig. 7.1, binding of TST with AR results in the activation of AR. In response to activation of AR, epithelial lining (both healthy and cancerous) of the prostate gland secretes PSA. The level of PSA is significantly correlated with the size of the tumor as well [7]. Hence, along with other biomarkers and diagnostics tests, the PSA levels of the patients also are examined for screening for primary as well as metastatic prostate cancer.

Research reveals that, the hormone TST and its derivative DHT promote the growth and reduce the apoptosis of prostate cancer cells [9]. Consequently, reducing the level of such tumor growth-promoting hormones in the body can hinder the progression of cancer. Anti-androgens can deactivate androgens by binding with the androgen receptors and thus blocking signal transduction pertaining to growth and apoptosis. However, it is also identified that a prolonged treatment period can provoke the transition (alteration) of hormone-dependent cells to hormone-independent cells that are resistant to treatment [2, 3, 8, 9]. As shown in Fig. 7.2, during the period of treatment (androgen deprivation), the AD cancer cells may switch to either reversible or irreversible androgen-independent (AI) types. However, during the off-treatment period, reversible AI cancer cells may switch back to AD type. This alteration of cells which results in the development of castration insensitive (castration-resistant) cells explains why often tumor relapse is reported after the hormone deprivation therapy.

This chapter is mainly focused on the mathematical models that represent tumor dynamics under hormone therapy. Specifically, how tumor dynamics are portrayed in the following six mathematical models with respect to the general model given by (1.1)–(1.2) is investigated:

1. Hormone-dependent and -independent tumor dynamics model.
2. Tumor growth model under intermittent hormone therapy.
3. Cell-quota-based model of tumor dynamics for hormone therapy.

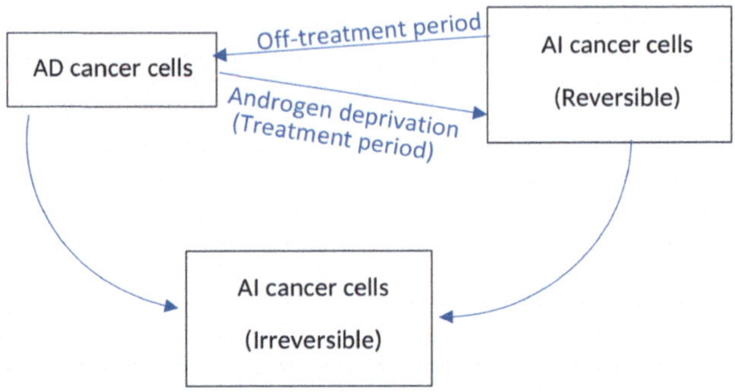

Fig. 7.2 Illustrative diagram showing the cell transition between AD and AI cancer cells with respect to androgen deprivation therapy. Reversible (adapted) AI cells turn back to AD cells in the absence of treatment, i.e. during the off-treatment period. Irreversible (mutated) AI cells remain as such during the on- or off-treatment period

4. Androgen receptor dynamics based model of tumor dynamics for hormone therapy.
5. Piecewise linear tumor growth model under intermittent hormone therapy.
6. Cell-cycle based model of tumor dynamics for hormone therapy.

Models (1)–(5) listed above discuss mathematical models of hormone therapy for prostate cancer and model 6 is a cell-cycle-based model of hormone therapy for the management of breast cancer. Tables 7.1 and 7.2 summarize the notations used in this chapter.

7.1 Hormone-Dependent and Hormone-Independent Tumor Dynamics Model

Androgen deprivation therapy (ADT) is one of the main treatment strategies for prostate cancer which involves either continuous androgen suppression (CAS) or intermittent androgen suppression (IAS) methods. In this section, a model that use CAS for treatment of prostate cancer is presented. As mentioned earlier, the main difference between various mathematical models of cancer therapy lies in the type of the cell populations ($C_{pi}(t)$, $i = 1, 2, \ldots$) that are involved in each case. In the case of prostate cancer, the efficacy of hormone treatment primarily depends on the number of cancer cells that rely on androgen for their progression. Hence, the dynamics pertaining to prostate cancer and hormone therapy is depicted in terms of the cell dynamics of AD and AI cancer cells as given by ([4]):

Table 7.1 Parameter notations in hormone therapy

Param.	Description	Param.	Description
a	Efficacy of CAS	b	Reciprocal carrying capacity
c	Competition rate	d	Death rate or depletion rate
m_{m}	Mutation rate of cells in mitotic phase	m	Mutation (cell transition) rate
m_{x}	Maximum mutation rate	m_{g}	Mutation rate of cells in growth phase
q_{m}	Maximum cell-quota	q	Minimum cell-quota
σ	Independent production rate of PSA	γ_{P}	Leakage rate of PSA into the blood
δ	Binding affinity of drug	s	Influx of circulating lymphocytes
m_{50}	Half-saturation level of mutation	U_0	Normal level of androgen in blood
m_{s}	Mutation rate of cells in DNA synthesis phase	r	Growth rate or hormone production rate
d_{U}	Depletion rate of therapeutic agent/hormone/PSA	r_0	Baseline value of PSA production rate
v_{m}	Maximum value of cell-quota uptake rate	v_{50}	Half-saturation level of cell-quota uptake rate
ρ_{50}	Half-saturation level of PSA production	n	Steepness coefficient associated with cell-quota and mutation rate
θ	Steepness coefficient associated with cell-quota and PSA production	$w_{y,z}^{x}$	Contribution of population z to the net growth of y, during xth period
k_{ij}	Rate of mass transfer from ith to jth compartment	κ	Parameters related to proliferation and apoptosis
K_{P}	PSA leakage parameter		

Table 7.2 Different types of cells and biochemicals in hormone therapy

Var.	Description	Var.	Description
$A(t)$	Cancer cells	$A_{\text{D}}(t)$	Androgen-dependent tumor cells
$A_{\text{I}}(t)$	Androgen-independent tumor cells	$A_{\text{IR}}(t)$	Reversible androgen-independent cancer cells
$A_{\text{II}}(t)$	Irreversible androgen-independent cancer cells	$A_{\text{g}}(t)$	Cancer cells in the growing phase
$A_{\text{s}}(t)$	Cancer cells in the DNA synthesis phase	$A_{\text{m}}(t)$	Cancer cells in the mitotic phase
$u(t)$	Rate of administration of therapeutic agent	$U_{\text{SA}}(t)$	Concentration of serum androgen
$U_{\text{P}}(t)$	Concentration of prostate-specific antigen (PSA) in blood	$C_Q(t)$	Cell-quota of prostate cancer cell
$U_{\text{IP}}(t)$	Intraprostatic PSA concentration	$U_{\text{T}}(t)$	Concentration of AR activated by TST
$U_{\text{D}}(t)$	Concentration of AR activated by DHT	$U_{\text{X}}(t)$	Concentration of tamoxifen
$U_{\text{H}}(t)$	Concentration of 4-hydroxytamoxifen	$X(t)$	Mass of the drug in a compartment
$E_{\text{CL}}(t)$	Circulating lymphocytes		

$$\frac{\mathrm{d}A_{\mathrm{D}}(t)}{\mathrm{d}t} = r_1 U_{\mathrm{SA}}(t)\Big(1 - b\big(A_{\mathrm{D}}(t) + c_1 A_{\mathrm{I}}(t)\big)\Big)A_{\mathrm{D}}(t) - (d_1 + m_1)\left(1 - \frac{U_{\mathrm{SA}}(t)}{U_0}\right)A_{\mathrm{D}}(t), \tag{7.1}$$

$$\frac{\mathrm{d}A_{\mathrm{I}}(t)}{\mathrm{d}t} = r_2\Big(1 - b\big(A_{\mathrm{I}}(t) + c_2 A_{\mathrm{D}}(t)\big)\Big)A_{\mathrm{I}}(t) + m_1\left(1 - \frac{U_{\mathrm{SA}}(t)}{U_0}\right)A_{\mathrm{D}}(t), \tag{7.2}$$

$$\frac{\mathrm{d}U_{\mathrm{SA}}(t)}{\mathrm{d}t} = -d_{\mathrm{U}}\left(U_{\mathrm{SA}}(t) - U_0\right) - U_0 d_{\mathrm{U}} u(t), \tag{7.3}$$

where $A_{\mathrm{D}}(t)$ and $A_{\mathrm{I}}(t)$ are the androgen-dependent and androgen-independent cancer cells, respectively, and $U_{\mathrm{SA}}(t)$ is the concentration of androgen in the blood (serum).

Comparing the general model of cancer dynamics given by (1.1)–(1.2) to the model of tumor dynamics under hormone therapy given by (7.1)–(7.3), one can see that the latter model is a special case of the former general model. Similar to (1.1)–(1.2), in (7.1)–(7.3) the proliferation of AD and AI cells are modeled in terms of growth rate r_i, $i = 1, 2$, d_1 accounts for the apoptosis of AD cells, b is the growth limitation due to carrying capacity, c_i, $i = 1, 2$, is the competition rate of AD and AI cells, respectively, m_1 is the rate of irreversible cell transition of the AD cells to AI cells, d_{U} denotes the elimination rate of androgen, and U_0 represents the normal androgen concentration. The term $r_1 U_{\mathrm{SA}}(t)\Big(1 - b\big(A_{\mathrm{D}}(t) + c_1 A_{\mathrm{I}}(t)\big)\Big)A_{\mathrm{D}}(t)$ in (7.1), models the increase in the number of AD cells with respect to the level of $U_{\mathrm{SA}}(t)$ in the blood and its restriction due to the carrying capacity of tumor micro-environment and competition between AD and AI cells. Similarly, the growth of AI cells is modeled in (7.2) using the same logistic pattern but without the term $U_{\mathrm{SA}}(t)$ as the growth is independent of $U_{\mathrm{SA}}(t)$.

The term $m_1\left(1 - \frac{U_{\mathrm{SA}}(t)}{U_0}\right)A_{\mathrm{D}}(t)$ in (7.1) and (7.2) represents the transition of AD cells to AI cells depending upon the level of androgen relative to the normal level given by U_0. Note that, in the case of CAS or IAS, the administration of therapeutic agents blocks the androgen production and thus the androgen level in the blood falls from the normal level. This is accounted for by using the term $u(t)$ in (7.3). In [4], this input term is selected as $u(t) = a$, where a is a positive constant to quantify the efficacy of the CAS approach in facilitating the androgen suppression. Note that, in (7.3) there is a decrease in the concentration of the serum androgen with an increase in the drug input. As mentioned earlier, when there is no treatment, testosterone homeostasis mediated by the hypothalamus keeps the level of androgen in the blood close to the normal level, i.e. $U_{\mathrm{SA}}(t) \approx U_0$. Hence, the transition of AD cells to AI cells modeled using the term $-m_1 A_{\mathrm{D}}(t) + m_1 \frac{U_{\mathrm{SA}}(t)}{U_0} A_{\mathrm{D}}(t)$ in (7.1) is close to zero as $m_1 A_{\mathrm{D}}(t) \approx m_1 \frac{U_{\mathrm{SA}}(t)}{U_0} A_{\mathrm{D}}(t)$, which represents no cell transition when androgen level is normal. However, as $U_{\mathrm{SA}}(t)$ decreases due to ADT, then $m_1 A_{\mathrm{D}}(t) > m_1 \frac{U_{\mathrm{SA}}(t)}{U_0} A_{\mathrm{D}}(t)$ and the increased transition of AD cells to AI cells in an androgen deprived environment is accordingly modeled.

The model (7.1)–(7.3) assumes that the apoptosis of AI cells, influence of normal epithelial cells of prostate, and the effect of immune response on the AI cells and AD cells are negligible. A detailed equilibrium point analysis of the model (7.1)–(7.3)

Table 7.3 Parameter values of the hormone therapy model (7.1)–(7.3) [4]

Parameter	Value (unit)	Parameter	Value (unit)
r_1	0.025 (days^{-1})	b	0.091×10^{-9} (days^{-1})
c_1	0.9	d_1	0.064 (days^{-1})
m_1	5×10^{-5} (days^{-1})	U_0	20 (ng mL^{-1})
r_2	0.006 (days^{-1})	c_2	0.8
d_{U}	0.08 (days^{-1})		

is given in [4]. Table 7.3 summarizes the parameter values of the hormone therapy model (7.1)–(7.3) [4]. The initial conditions for the variables in model (7.1)–(7.3) are $A_{\mathrm{D}}(0) = [1, 10]$ (cells), $A_{\mathrm{I}}(0) = 0.14$ (cells), $U_{\mathrm{SA}}(0) = 20\,(\mathrm{ng\,ml^{-1}})$, and $u(0) = a$, $0.6 \leq a \leq 0.9$.

7.2 Tumor Growth Model Under Intermittent Hormone Therapy

As mentioned earlier, a prolonged use of hormone therapy via CAS methods is associated with reversible (adapted) or irreversible (mutated) transition of AD cancer cells to AI cancer cells (Fig. 7.2). Such AI cancer cells are responsible for the relapse of the disease after hormone-based treatment. In order to combat with this side effect of CAS, the efficacy of IAS is investigated in [3, 8, 10, 11]. In the case of IAS, a certain predefined threshold value of the PSA level is used as a criterion to decide on the time of commencement and termination of treatment. The model discussed in this section categorizes the prostate cancer cells as two subtypes androgen-dependent and androgen-independent instead of three subtypes shown in Fig. 7.2. The model in the context of IAS therapy is given by ([10]):

$$\begin{aligned}\frac{\mathrm{d}A_{\mathrm{D}}(t)}{\mathrm{d}t} =& r_1\left(\kappa_1 + (1-\kappa_1)\frac{U_{\mathrm{SA}}(t)}{U_{\mathrm{SA}}(t)+\kappa_2}\right)A_{\mathrm{D}}(t) - d_1\left(\kappa_3 + (1-\kappa_3)\frac{U_{\mathrm{SA}}(t)}{U_{\mathrm{SA}}(t)+\kappa_4}\right)A_{\mathrm{D}}(t)\\ &- m_1\left(1-\frac{U_{\mathrm{SA}}(t)}{U_0}\right)A_{\mathrm{D}}(t), \qquad (7.4)\\ \frac{\mathrm{d}A_{\mathrm{I}}(t)}{\mathrm{d}t} =& m_1\left(1-\frac{U_{\mathrm{SA}}(t)}{U_0}\right)A_{\mathrm{D}}(t) + r_2\left(1-\frac{U_{\mathrm{SA}}(t)}{U_0}\right)A_{\mathrm{I}}(t) - d_2A_{\mathrm{I}}(t), \qquad (7.5)\\ \frac{\mathrm{d}U_{\mathrm{SA}}(t)}{\mathrm{d}t} =& -d_{\mathrm{U}}\left(U_{\mathrm{SA}}(t)-U_0\right) - U_0 d_{\mathrm{U}} u(t), \qquad (7.6)\end{aligned}$$

where $A_{\mathrm{D}}(t)$ and $A_{\mathrm{I}}(t)$ are the androgen-dependent and androgen-independent cancer cells, respectively, $U_{\mathrm{SA}}(t)$ is the concentration of androgen in the blood, and $u(t)$ is the drug infusion. The temporal variation of the PSA in blood is assumed to be a linear function as given by $U_{\mathrm{P}}(t) = x_1A_{\mathrm{D}}(t) + x_2A_{\mathrm{I}}(t)$, where $U_{\mathrm{P}}(t)$ is the serum PSA concentration and x_i, $i = 1, 2$, is a constant [10]. Drug infusion in case of IAS therapy is modeled as:

$$u(t) = \begin{cases} 0 \to 1, & \text{when } U_P(t) = h_1 \text{ and } \frac{dU_P(t)}{dt} > 0, \\ 1 \to 0, & \text{when } U_P(t) = h_0 \text{ and } \frac{dU_P(t)}{dt} < 0. \end{cases} \tag{7.7}$$

Here, the drug administration is suspended when the concentration of PSA in the blood (measured) falls below h_0 during on-treatment periods and it is re-instituted when the concentration of PSA in the blood exceeds h_1 during off-treatment periods [10].

In (7.4), the first and second terms model the growth and apoptosis of AD cells and the third term accounts for the mutation of AD cells to AI cells, where r_1, d_1, and m_1 are the growth rate, death rate, and mutation rate, respectively. Proliferation and apoptosis rates of the AD cells depend on the androgen level in the tumor micro-environment. Hence, the terms $\left(\kappa_1 + (1-\kappa_1)\frac{U_{SA}(t)}{U_{SA}(t)+\kappa_2}\right)$ and $\left(\kappa_3 + (1-\kappa_3)\frac{U_{SA}(t)}{U_{SA}(t)+\kappa_4}\right)$ in (7.4) are used to quantify the effect of androgen deprivation therapy on the growth rate and the apoptosis rate of AD cells, where κ_1, κ_2, κ_3, and κ_4 are the model parameters chosen to fit the proliferation and apoptosis versus androgen concentration curve obtained under hormone therapy. Note that it is not straightforward to quantify the number of AD and AI cells in the tumor micro-environment. Hence, an obvious question here is how the model parameters are obtained for such a case. Here the values of the parameters r_1 and d_1 which are associated with the dynamics of AD cells are derived from experimental data from patients who respond to hormonal treatment, whereas that of r_2 and d_2 which are associated with AI cells are obtained from patients who failed to respond to hormonal treatment [10]. Another important parameter of the model discussed in this section is the maximum mutation rate (m_1) which decides the possibility for the relapse of the tumor and the expected duration for a relapse.

In (7.5), the first term accounts for the increase in AI cells due to mutation of AD cells to AI cells, the second term models the growth of AI cells, and third term models the apoptosis. Here, r_2 and d_2 are the growth and death rates, respectively. In (7.6), androgen dynamics in the context of IAS therapy is modeled, where a predefined lower threshold and upper threshold values of PSA level is used to on or off the treatment under IAS therapy.

The influence of the androgen level in the blood and the dynamics of AD cancer cells is apparent. Apart from that, many experimental data suggest that there exists a certain level of dependence between the androgen level and the dynamics of AI cell population as well [12–14]. Based on the experimental data discussed in [15], it is pointed out in [3] that the net growth rate of AI cells can be negative when the androgen level is normal, i.e. when the androgen deprivation therapy is withdrawn (off treatment). It is apparent that there can be an increasing number of AD cells due to the normal supply of androgen in the tumor micro-environment. The reported decrease in (negative) growth rate of AI cells during off-treatment period can be due to the competition of these cells with the actively proliferating AD cells or due to the reversible mutation.

Table 7.4 Parameter values of the hormone therapy model (7.4)–(7.6) [10, 16]

Parameter	Value (unit)	Parameter	Value (unit)
r_1	0.0204 (days^{-1})	κ_1	0
κ_2	2 (nmol L^{-1})	κ_3	8
d_1	0.0076 (days^{-1})	m_1	0.00001-0.00005
r_2	0.0242 (days^{-1})	U_0	8–35 (nmol L^{-1})
d_2	0.0168 (days^{-1})	κ_4	0.5 (nmol L^{-1})
h_0	10 (ng mL^{-1})	h_1	15 (ng mL^{-1})
x_1, x_2	1	d_U	0.08 (days^{-1})

In [3], a review of various mathematical models suggested for IAS therapy is presented. The IAS therapy model given in [3, 16] is an extension of the model (7.4)–(7.6) given in [10]. In the modified one, a competition term given by $\mathcal{C}(\cdot) = -c_1 A_D(t) A_I(t)$, where $c_1 > 0$ is used in (7.4) and (7.5) to account for the reduction in cell populations due to the interaction between AD and AI cells. Table 7.4 summarizes the parameter of the hormone therapy model (7.4)–(7.6) [10, 16]. The initial conditions for the variables in model (7.4)–(7.6) are $A_D(0) = 5$ (cells), $A_I(0) = 0$ (cells), and $U_{SA}(0) = U_0$, $8 \leq U_0 \leq 35$ nmol L^{-1}. Drug administration is switched on or off according the serum PSA concentration $U_P(t)$ measured in ng mL^{-1}.

7.3 Cell-quota-based Model of Tumor Dynamics for Hormone Therapy

In this section, a model that accounts for the dependence between the androgen level and the dynamics of prostate cancer cells using a cell-quota parameter is discussed. The cell-quota-based model is common in ecological stoichiometry and was first used in 1968 to model the growth dynamics (Droop's cell-quota model) of algae in terms of its internal nutrient status [17, 18]. This model is used to quantify the growth rate of microorganism (e.g. phtyoplankton) in terms of the available nutrient (nutrient quota) in an ecosystem. As the internal nutrient concentration increases, the growth rate increases and saturates like a sigmoid curve when there is abundant nutrients. This behavior is modeled as:

$$r(C_Q(t)) = r_\infty \left(1 - \frac{q}{C_Q(t)}\right), \tag{7.8}$$

where $r(C_Q(t))$ is the cell-quota dependent growth rate, $C_Q(t)$ is the internal nutrient quota, r_∞ is the maximum growth rate when $C_Q(t) \to \infty$, and q is the minimum cell-quota, that is the cell-quota when $r(C_Q(t)) = 0$ [19]. The uptake of nutrient can be defined in terms of Michaelis-Menten kinetics as given by:

$$v(R_{\mathrm{Q}}(t)) = v_{\max}\frac{R_{\mathrm{Q}}(t)}{g + R_{\mathrm{Q}}(t)}, \tag{7.9}$$

where $v(R_{\mathrm{Q}}(t))$ is the rate of uptake of external nutrient, $R_{\mathrm{Q}}(t)$ is the concentration of external nutrient, $v_{\max}$ is the maximum uptake rate, and g is the half-saturation constant related to the uptake of external nutrients. Using (7.8) and (7.9), the growth dynamics of the phytoplankton biomass is modeled as:

$$\frac{\mathrm{d}C_{\mathrm{Q}}(t)}{\mathrm{d}t} = v(R_{\mathrm{Q}}(t)) - r(C_{\mathrm{Q}}(t))C_{\mathrm{Q}}(t), \tag{7.10}$$

$$\frac{\mathrm{d}P_{\mathrm{p}}(t)}{\mathrm{d}t} = r(C_{\mathrm{Q}}(t))P_{\mathrm{p}}(t) - dP_{\mathrm{p}}(t), \tag{7.11}$$

where $P_{\mathrm{p}}(t)$ is the phytoplankton biomass and d is the death rate of the phytoplankton.

In [8], a cell-quota-based model that accounts for the influence of androgen on the proliferation and apoptosis of cancer cells owing to its similarity to the ecosystem dynamics is presented. Similar to an ecosystem, a tumor micro-environment involves interaction and competition between its components (producer-gazer/predator-prey) and the overall growth rate of the populations is according to the availability of food. A similar relationship exists between the growth rate of cancer cells and the concentration of androgen present in the tumor micro-environment.

In [8], it is pointed out that the models which assume a constant growth rate of AD cells show poor accuracy when fitted with clinical data. In the context of hormone therapy, the cell-quota model is particularly relevant as the activation of AR and subsequent signal transduction rely on the internal androgen status. Specifically, as the AR-TST and AR-DHT binding (Fig. 7.1) depend on the level of intracellular androgen, Droop's cell-quota model can be used to model the growth dynamics with the intracellular androgen level as cell-quota. The model discussed in [8] is given by:

$$\frac{\mathrm{d}A_{\mathrm{D}}(t)}{\mathrm{d}t} = r_{\mathrm{m}}\left(1 - \frac{q_1}{C_{Q_1}(t)}\right)A_{\mathrm{D}}(t) - d_1A_{\mathrm{D}}(t) - m_1\left(C_{Q_1}(t)\right)A_{\mathrm{D}}(t) + m_2\left(C_{Q_2}(t)\right)A_{\mathrm{I}}(t), \tag{7.12}$$

$$\frac{\mathrm{d}A_{\mathrm{I}}(t)}{\mathrm{d}t} = r_{\mathrm{m}}\left(1 - \frac{q_2}{C_{Q_2}(t)}\right)A_{\mathrm{I}}(t) - d_2A_{\mathrm{I}}(t) + m_1\left(C_{Q_1}(t)\right)A_{\mathrm{D}}(t) - m_2\left(C_{Q_2}(t)\right)A_{\mathrm{I}}(t), \tag{7.13}$$

$$\frac{\mathrm{d}C_{Q_i}(t)}{\mathrm{d}t} = v_{\mathrm{m}}\frac{q_{\mathrm{m}} - C_{Q_i}(t)}{q_{\mathrm{m}} - q_i}\frac{U_{\mathrm{SA}}(t)}{U_{\mathrm{SA}}(t) + v_{50}} - r_{\mathrm{m}}\left(C_{Q_i}(t) - q_i\right) - d_3C_{Q_i}(t),\ i = 1, 2, \tag{7.14}$$

$$\frac{\mathrm{d}U_{\mathrm{P}}(t)}{\mathrm{d}t} = r_0\left(A_{\mathrm{D}}(t) + A_{\mathrm{I}}(t)\right) + r_1A_{\mathrm{D}}(t)\frac{C_{Q_1}^{\theta}(t)}{C_{Q_1}^{\theta}(t) + \left(\rho_{50}^1\right)^{\theta}} + r_2A_{\mathrm{I}}(t)\frac{C_{Q_2}^{\theta}(t)}{C_{Q_2}^{\theta}(t) + \left(\rho_{50}^2\right)^{\theta}} - d_{\mathrm{U}}U_{\mathrm{P}}(t), \tag{7.15}$$

where $A_{\mathrm{D}}(t)$ and $A_{\mathrm{I}}(t)$ are the AD and AI cancer cells, respectively, $C_{Q_i}(t), i = 1, 2$ is the cell-quota, $U_{\mathrm{P}}(t)$ is the concentration of prostate-specific antigen (PSA) in blood, and $U_{\mathrm{SA}}(t)$ denotes the serum androgen measurement. In (7.12) and (7.13), r_{m} quantifies the maximum proliferation rate of AD and AI cells, $q_i, i = 1, 2$ denotes the minimum quota, and d_1 and d_2 denote the death rates of AD and AI cells, respectively. The term $r_{\mathrm{m}}\left(1 - \frac{q_i}{C_{Q_i}(t)}\right), i = 1, 2$ accounts for the androgen dependent proliferation rate of AD and AI cells. As the cell-quota of the ith cell increases, the term

$\left(1 - \frac{q_1}{C_{Q_1}(t)}\right) \to 1$ and the proliferation rate of ith cell approaches the maximum proliferation rate $r_{\rm m}$. The mutation rates or cell transition rates between AD and AI cells are assumed to be a function of respective cell-quotas and are modeled as:

$$m_1(C_{Q_1}(t)) = m_{\rm x_1} \frac{m_{50_1}^n}{C_{Q_1}^n(t) + m_{50_1}^n}, \tag{7.16}$$

$$m_2(C_{Q_2}(t)) = m_{\rm x_2} \frac{C_{Q_2}^n(t)}{C_{Q_2}^n(t) + m_{50_2}^n}, \tag{7.17}$$

respectively, where n is the steepness coefficient associated with the cell-quota and mutation rate, $m_{\rm x_i}$, $i = 1, 2$, denote the maximum mutation rate of AD cells to AI cells and AI cells to AD cells, respectively, and m_{50_i}, $i = 1, 2$, are the half-saturation level of mutation of AD cell to AI cells and AI cells to AD cells, respectively. In (7.16), for normal or higher than normal values of cell-quota ($C_{Q_1}(t)$), the mutation rate ($m_1(C_{Q_1}(t))$) of AD cells to AI cells will be less and for low values of $C_{Q_1}(t)$, the mutation rate of AD cells approaches the maximum mutation rate, i.e. $m_1(C_{Q_1}(t)) \to m_{\rm x_1}$. Thus, the low mutation rate in the presence of abundant androgen and high mutation rate in the context of androgen deprivation (treatment) is accounted for in (7.16). In contrast to this, in (7.17), for high value of $C_{Q_2}(t)$, $m_2(C_{Q_2}(t)) \to m_{\rm x_2}$ and a low value of $C_{Q_2}(t)$ results in a low mutation rate $m_2(C_{Q_2}(t))$. This implies that there will not be reversible switching (AI to AD) in an androgen deprived environment (See Fig. 7.2).

In (7.14), $v_{\rm m}$ is the maximum value of cell-quota uptake rate of AD and AI cells, $q_{\rm m}$ is the maximum cell-quota of AD and AI cells, v_{50} is the half-saturation level of cell-quota uptake, and d_3 is the cell-quota degradation rate. It is assumed that, as the serum androgen level ($U_{\rm SA}(t)$) increases, the uptake of androgen into the cells approaches its maximum value $v_{\rm m}$. This is modeled in the first term of (7.14). Serum androgen values are obtained using blood sample analysis during the on and off periods of the treatment by the following relation:

$$U_{\rm SA}(t) = U_{\rm SA}(t_{\rm on}) + \Big(U_{\rm SA}(t_{\rm off}) - U_{\rm SA}(t_{\rm on})\Big)e^{(t - t_{\rm off})d_{\rm U_1}}, \tag{7.18}$$

where $t_{\rm on}$ and $t_{\rm off}$ denote the on-treatment time and off-treatment time at which measurement is made, respectively, and $d_{\rm U_1}$ quantifies the elimination rate of serum androgen. The second term of (7.14) models the reduction in cell-quota (usage) of the ith cell with respect to the maximum proliferation rate $r_{\rm m}$.

In (7.15), the dynamics of PSA in blood is modeled, where r_0 denotes the baseline value of PSA production rate, r_i, $i = 1, 2$ quantify the rate of PSA production by AD and AI cells, respectively. In this model, the second and third terms in (7.15) account for the fact that both AD and AI cells respond differently to the level of androgen. These two hill functions are used to model the relation between the cell-quota of each cell population and PSA concentration, where θ is the associated steepness coefficient, ρ_{50}^i, $i = 1, 2$, denote the half-saturation level associated with

Table 7.5 Parameter values of the hormone therapy model given by (7.12)–(7.17) [8]

Parameter	Value (unit)	Parameter	Value (unit)
r_{m}	0.025–0.045 (days^{-1})	υ_{m}	0.275 (nM days^{-1})
q_1	0.175–0.45 (nM)	υ_{50}	4 (nM)
q_2	0.1–0.3 (nM)	d_3	0.09 (days^{-1})
d_1, d_2	0.015–0.02 (days^{-1})	r_0	0.004-0.04 (ag ml^{-1} cell^{-1} days)
q_{m}	5 (nM)	r_1	0.05-0.3 (ag ml^{-1} cell^{-1} days)
m_{x_1}	0.00015 (days^{-1})	r_2	0.05-0.35 (ag ml^{-1} cell^{-1} days)
m_{x_2}	0.0001 (days^{-1})	ρ_{50}^1	1.3 (nM)
m_{50_1}	0.08 (nM)	ρ_{50}^2	1.1 (nM)
m_{50_2}	1.7 (nM)	d_{U}	0.08 (days^{-1})

the production of PSA with respect to the AD and AI cells, respectively, and d_{U} is the clearance rate of PSA from the blood. Compared to (1.1)–(1.2), it can be seen that the change in cell dynamics due to proliferation, apoptosis, cell alteration, and limited resources are accounted for in this model. However, the influence of normal epithelial cells, competition between cells, and the effect of the immune system on tumor dynamics are not considered.

In [8], a comparison of the Ideta model (7.4)–(7.6) with the cell-quota-based model (7.12)–(7.15) given in [10] is presented. Specifically, clinical time-series data from 7 men is used to evaluate the model fit of the cell-quota-based model and the Ideta model. Using simulations, it is shown in [8] that the Ideta model can predict the peak value of PSA for the first treatment cycle but could not predict the peak value of PSA after the first treatment cycle. However, simulation results that compared the predicted values obtained using the cell-quota model (7.15) with that of the clinical data show an improved accuracy. The modified version of the Ideta model with additional competition term that is mentioned in Sect. 7.2 overcomes the limitation of model (7.4)–(7.6) [3, 10]. Table 7.5 summarizes the parameter values of the hormone therapy model given by (7.12)–(7.17). The initial conditions for the variables in model (7.12)–(7.17) are $A_{\mathrm{D}}(0) = 15$ (cells), $A_{\mathrm{I}}(0) = 0$ (cells), and $C_{\mathrm{Q_i}}(0) = 0.5$ (nM), $i = 1, 2$. The units of $U_{\mathrm{SA}}(t)$ and $U_{\mathrm{P}}(t)$ are ng ml^{-1} and nM, respectively.

7.4 Androgen Receptor Dynamics-Based Model of Tumor Dynamics for Hormone Therapy

In [7], a mathematical model of prostate cancer with an age-dependent parameter is presented to account for inter-patient variability. Along with the dynamics of AD and AI cells, this model also accounts for the effect of the volume of healthy epithelial cells on prostate cancer. Specifically, the model incorporates the dynamics of normal epithelial cells of prostate to account for the age-dependent increase in the volume of the prostate and its contribution to the production of prostate-specific antigen (PSA). The model is given by:

$$\frac{\mathrm{d}N(t)}{\mathrm{d}t} = r_1(t)N(t)\left(1 - \frac{N(t) + c_1\big(A_\mathrm{D}(t) + A_\mathrm{I}(t)\big)}{b_1(t)}\right) - d_1(t)N(t), \tag{7.19}$$

$$\frac{\mathrm{d}A_\mathrm{D}(t)}{\mathrm{d}t} = r_2(t)A_\mathrm{D}(t)\,(1 - m_1)\left(1 - \frac{\big(c_1N(t) + A_\mathrm{D}(t) + A_\mathrm{I}(t)\big)}{b_2}\right) - d_2(t)A_\mathrm{D}(t), \tag{7.20}$$

$$\frac{\mathrm{d}A_\mathrm{I}(t)}{\mathrm{d}t} = r_3(t)A_\mathrm{I}(t)\left(1 - \frac{\big(c_1N(t) + A_\mathrm{D}(t) + A_\mathrm{I}(t)\big)}{b_3}\right) - d_3(t)A_\mathrm{I}(t) + m_1\left(1 - \frac{\big(c_1N(t) + A_\mathrm{D}(t) + A_\mathrm{I}(t)\big)}{b_2}\right), \tag{7.21}$$

$$\frac{\mathrm{d}U_\mathrm{IP}(t)}{\mathrm{d}t} = -d_{\mathrm{U}_1}U_\mathrm{IP}(t)N_\mathrm{f}(t) - \gamma_\mathrm{P}U_\mathrm{IP}(t)\frac{(A_\mathrm{D}(t) + A_\mathrm{I}(t))^2}{K_\mathrm{P} + A_\mathrm{D}(t) + A_\mathrm{I}(t)} - d_{\mathrm{U}_2}U_\mathrm{IP}(t) + r_4(t), \tag{7.22}$$

$$\frac{\mathrm{d}U_\mathrm{P}(t)}{\mathrm{d}t} = d_{\mathrm{U}_1}U_\mathrm{IP}(t)N_\mathrm{f}(t) + \gamma_\mathrm{P}U_\mathrm{IP}(t)\frac{(A_\mathrm{D}(t) + A_\mathrm{I}(t))^2}{K_\mathrm{P} + A_\mathrm{D}(t) + A_\mathrm{I}(t)} - d_{\mathrm{U}_3}U_\mathrm{P}(t), \tag{7.23}$$

where $N(t)$ denotes the healthy epithelial cells in the prostate gland, $A_\mathrm{D}(t)$ and $A_\mathrm{I}(t)$ are the AD and AI cancer cells, respectively, $U_\mathrm{IP}(t)$ denotes the intraprostatic PSA concentration, and $U_\mathrm{P}(t)$ denotes the concentration of PSA in the serum.

In (7.19), $r_1(t)$ and $d_1(t)$ represent the growth and death rates of normal epithelial cells which are dependent on the amount of activated receptors (labeled as AR^+ in Fig. 7.1) associated with testosterone (TST) and dihydrotestosterone (DHT) in the prostate gland, c_1 quantifies the interaction between normal epithelial cells and cancer cells, and $b_1(t)$ denotes the carrying capacity and is a time-varying parameter which models the age-dependent change in the volume of the prostate gland. In (7.20) and (7.21), r_i, b_i, and d_i, $i = 2, 3$, are the growth rates, carrying capacities and death rates of the AD and AI cells, respectively, and m_1 is the mutation rate of AD cells to AI cells. The growth and death rate of AD cells are dependent on the number of activated receptors (AR^+) associated with TST and DHT in the prostate gland.

The dynamics of PSA in the intraprostatic region or in the blood is modeled in (7.22) and (7.23) (Fig. 7.1). Specifically, in (7.22), $U_\mathrm{IP}(t)$ quantifies the production of PSA in the tissues by the activation and binding of androgen receptors with TST and DHT. It is identified that both healthy epithelial cells and cancerous epithelial cells of the prostate gland produce PSA [7]. The movement of PSA protein from the normal tissues to the bloodstream is hindered by the natural barriers such as basal cell layer, prostatic stroma, basement membrane, and capillary walls. However, there can be a leakage of PSA protein to the blood via cancer tissues. This leakage which is linearly related to the number of cancer cells is modeled using the term $\gamma_{\mathrm{P}} U_{\mathrm{IP}}(t) \frac{(A_{\mathrm{D}}(t)+A_{\mathrm{I}}(t))^2}{K_{\mathrm{P}}+A_{\mathrm{D}}(t)+A_{\mathrm{I}}(t)}$ in (7.22) and (7.23), where γ_{P} and K_{P} are leakage parameters. The term $d_{\mathrm{U}_1} U_{\mathrm{IP}}(t) N_{\mathrm{f}}(t)$ quantifies the leakage proportional to the normal cells, where $N_{\mathrm{f}}(t)$ is a ratio of the volume of the normal epithelium to the total volume of the prostate, d_{U_1} is the rate of leakage of intraprostatic PSA into the blood, and d_{U_2} denotes the natural decay rate of PSA production. The time-varying changes in the prostate volume is modeled as $N_{\mathrm{f}}(t) = \frac{V_{\mathrm{c}} N(t)}{P_{\mathrm{vol}}(t)}$, where $P_{\mathrm{vol}}(t) = \frac{v_1 t^{\phi}}{v_2^{\phi}+t^{\phi}} + v_3$. The last term in (7.22) models the production rate of PSA.

Note that, $r_i(t)$ and $d_i(t), i = 1, 2, 3$ in (7.19)–(7.22) denote the growth and death rate of three cell types (i.e. $N(t)$, $A_{\mathrm{D}}(t)$, $A_{\mathrm{I}}(t)$), respectively. In [7], $r_i(t)$ and $d_i(t)$ are modeled with respect to the number of activated receptors associated with TST and DHT in the prostate gland as follows:

$$r_i\,(t) = \psi_1^i \frac{\left(U_{\mathrm{D}}^i(t)\right)^2}{\left(\psi_2^i\right)^2 + \left(U_{\mathrm{D}}^i(t)\right)^2} + \Psi_1^i \frac{\left(U_{\mathrm{T}}^i(t)\right)^2}{\left(\Psi_2^i\right)^2 + \left(U_{\mathrm{T}}^i(t)\right)^2}, \quad i = 1, 2, 3, \tag{7.24}$$

$$d_i\,(t) = \frac{\psi_3^i}{\psi_4^i + \psi_5^i U_{\mathrm{D}}^i(t) + \psi_6^i U_{\mathrm{T}}^i(t)}, \quad i = 1, 2, 3, \tag{7.25}$$

where $U_{\mathrm{T}}^i(t)$ represents the concentration of androgen receptor activated by TST in each cell type, (i.e. $N(t)$, $A_{\mathrm{D}}(t)$, $A_{\mathrm{I}}(t)$) and $U_{\mathrm{D}}^i(t)$ denotes the concentration of androgen receptor activated by DHT in each cell type. The parameters ψ_j^i, $j = 1, \ldots, 6$, Ψ_j^i, $j = 1, 2$, are associated with proliferation and death of the ith cell type, $i = 1, 2, 3$ (Supplementary material of [7], S5). Here, ψ denotes a constant associated with DHT-activated AR in each cell type and Ψ denotes a constant associated with TST-activated AR in each cell type. Similarly, the production of PSA by the normal prostate epithelial cells, AD cancer cells, and AI cancer cells is given by:

$$r_4(t) = \sum_i \beta_{\mathrm{P}_i} \left(U_{\mathrm{T}}^i(t) + U_{\mathrm{D}}^i(t) + \sigma_i\right) i, \quad i = 1, 2, 3, \tag{7.26}$$

where i denotes the cell type in which $i = 1, 2$, and 3 refer to $N(t)$, $A_{\mathrm{D}}(t)$, and $A_{\mathrm{I}}(t)$, respectively, β_{P_i} denotes a rate constant, and σ_i is a constant that accounts for the possible independent production of PSA. In (7.23), d_{U_3} is the rate at which PSA is cleared from the body.

Compared to the models discussed in earlier sections, the specialty of this model is the consideration of AR binding and age-dependent prostate volume. Research suggests that mutations that lead to the transition of AD cells to AI cells and consequent development of castration are an early event which are identified independent from the androgen deprivation [7] . The parameter m_1 in (7.20) and (7.21) accounts for this important mutation as well. Note that, the parameter m_1 can account for the heterogeneity of cells in the prostate which is a significant predictor of treatment outcome. Compared to (1.1)–(1.2), it can be seen that the change in cell dynamics due to proliferation and apoptosis are modeled using time-varying growth rates and

Table 7.6 Parameter values of the hormone therapy model (7.19)–(7.25) [7]

Parameter	Value (unit)	Parameter	Value (unit)
m_1	1×10^{-4}	d_{U_1}	1.515×10^{-3} (h^{-1})
b_2, b_3	22.4 (cells in billions)	K_P	800 (cells in billions)
d_{U_2}	$\ln(2)/12.3$ (h^{-1})	c_1	negligibly small value
V_c	5.56×10^{-6} (mm^3)	v_1	18.397 (cm^3)
v_2	63.753 (h)	v_3	28.4 (cm^3)
ϕ	12	d_{U_3}	$\ln(2)/0.12$ (h^{-1})
β_{P_1}	2.2622×10^{-3} ($nM^{-1}h^{-1}$)	β_{P_2}	0.002 ($nM^{-1}h^{-1}$)
β_{P_3}	0.003 ($nM^{-1}h^{-1}$)	σ_1	10 (nM)
ψ_1^1	1.202×10^{-4} (h^{-1})	ψ_2^1	12.355 (nM activated AR)
ψ_3^1	0.008 (nM activated AR per hour)	ψ_4^1	62.162 (nM activated AR)
ψ_1^2	10.48×10^{-4} (h^{-1})	ψ_3^2	0.150 (nM activated AR per hour)
ψ_1^3	0.98×10^{-4} (h^{-1})	ψ_3^3	0.010 (nM activated AR per hour)
Ψ_1^1	1.281×10^{-4} (h^{-1})	Ψ_2^1	49.587 (nM activated AR)
Ψ_1^2	11.100×10^{-4} (h^{-1})	γ_P	3.125×10^{-4} (per million cells per hour)
Ψ_1^3	2.790×10^{-4} (h^{-1})		

death rates as given by (7.24) and (7.25) for each cell type. Similar to the other models discussed in this subsection, even though cell alteration, limited availability of resources and the effect of competition between cells are accounted for in this model, the influence of the immune system in the overall tumor dynamics is ignored.

Table 7.6 summarizes the model parameter values of the hormone therapy model (7.19)–(7.25) [7]. Some of the parameter values are from the supplementary material of [7]. The normalized initial conditions for the variables in model (7.19)–(7.25) are $N(0) = 1.5$ (cells), $A_D(0) = 1$ (cells), and $A_I(0) = 0$ (cells). The intraprostatic PSA or tissue PSA $U_{IP}(t)$ and serum PSA $U_P(t)$ are measured in ng mL^{-1}.

7.5 Piecewise Linear Tumor Growth Model Under Intermittent Hormone Therapy

As shown in Fig. 7.2, there are three types of prostate cancer cells such as the AD cells, the adapted AI cells (reversible), and mutated AI cells (irreversible). In this section, the piecewise linear IAS (intermittent androgen suppression) model is presented for the hormone therapy with these three cell types [3, 15, 20]. First, the dynamics of the three cell types during treatment is given by [15]:

$$\frac{\mathrm{d}A_D(t)}{\mathrm{d}t} = w_{1,1}^1 A_D(t), \tag{7.27}$$

$$\frac{\mathrm{d}A_{IR}(t)}{\mathrm{d}t} = w_{2,1}^1 A_D(t) + w_{2,2}^1 A_{IR}(t), \tag{7.28}$$

$$\frac{dA_{\text{II}}(t)}{dt} = w^1_{3,1}A_{\text{D}}(t) + w^1_{3,2}A_{\text{IR}}(t) + w^1_{3,3}A_{\text{II}}(t), \tag{7.29}$$

and without treatment is given by:

$$\frac{dA_{\text{D}}(t)}{dt} = w^0_{1,1}A_{\text{D}}(t) + w^0_{1,2}A_{\text{IR}}(t), \tag{7.30}$$

$$\frac{dA_{\text{IR}}(t)}{dt} = w^0_{2,2}A_{\text{IR}}(t), \tag{7.31}$$

$$\frac{dA_{\text{II}}(t)}{dt} = w^0_{3,3}A_{\text{II}}(t), \tag{7.32}$$

where $A_{\text{D}}(t)$, $A_{\text{IR}}(t)$, and $A_{\text{II}}(t)$ denote the AD cells, reversible or adapted AI cells which can change back to AD cells in an androgen rich environment, and irreversible or mutated AI cells, respectively, $w^x_{y,z}$, $y, z = 1, 2, 3$, quantify the effect of the cell population z on the net growth of cell population y, $x = 0$ and 1 denote the value of the parameter during on-treatment period and off-treatment period, respectively. For instance, $w^1_{y,z}$ denotes the on-treatment period and $w^0_{y,z}$ denotes the off-treatment period. Here, depending upon the cell transition involved, y and z can take values $1, 2$, or 3 to represent $A_{\text{D}}(t)$, $A_{\text{IR}}(t)$, or $A_{\text{II}}(t)$, respectively. The net PSA level is assumed to be $x_1A_{\text{D}}(t) + x_2A_{\text{IR}}(t) + x_3A_{\text{II}}(t)$, where x_1, x_2, and x_3 are that model parameters that can be chosen appropriately to fit the measured PSA versus tumor growth curve.

During the androgen ablation period, since the availability of androgen is less, the reversible AI cells will not switch to AD type. This is modeled in (7.27). Next, the term $w^1_{2,1}A_{\text{D}}(t)$ in (7.28) accounts for the transition of AD cells to reversible (adapted) AI cells during on-treatment period. In (7.29), the terms $w^1_{3,1}A_{\text{D}}(t)$ and $w^1_{3,2}A_{\text{IR}}(t)$ model the transition of AD cells and reversible AI cells to irreversible AI (mutated) cells during the on-treatment period. Similarly, the term $w^0_{1,2}A_{\text{IR}}(t)$ in (7.30) accounts for the transition of reversible AI cells to AD cells during the off-treatment period. It can be noted that during the treatment period there are no cell transitions associated with irreversible AI cells.

In [15], parameter fitting is done by transforming piecewise linear model (7.27)–(7.32) to equivalent difference equation using Euler's approximation. The equivalent difference equation during treatment is given by:

$$\begin{pmatrix} A_{\text{D}}(t+\Delta t) \\ A_{\text{IR}}(t+\Delta t) \\ A_{\text{II}}(t+\Delta t) \end{pmatrix} = \begin{pmatrix} \Omega^1_{1,1} & 0 & 0 \\ \Omega^1_{2,1} & \Omega^1_{2,2} & 0 \\ \Omega^1_{3,1} & \Omega^1_{3,2} & \Omega^1_{3,3} \end{pmatrix} \begin{pmatrix} A_{\text{D}}(t) \\ A_{\text{IR}}(t) \\ A_{\text{II}}(t) \end{pmatrix}, \tag{7.33}$$

and without treatment is given by

$$\begin{pmatrix} A_{\text{D}}(t+\Delta t) \\ A_{\text{IR}}(t+\Delta t) \\ A_{\text{II}}(t+\Delta t) \end{pmatrix} = \begin{pmatrix} \Omega^0_{1,1} & \Omega^0_{1,2} & 0 \\ 0 & \Omega^0_{2,2} & 0 \\ 0 & 0 & \Omega^0_{3,3} \end{pmatrix} \begin{pmatrix} A_{\text{D}}(t) \\ A_{\text{IR}}(t) \\ A_{\text{II}}(t) \end{pmatrix}, \tag{7.34}$$

Table 7.7 Parameter values of the hormone therapy model (7.33)–(7.34) for three patient types [3, 15, 20]

Parameter	Type (i)	Type (ii)	Type (iii)
$\Omega^1_{1,1}$	0.956156	0.925733	0.931568
$\Omega^1_{2,1}$	0.00130716	0.00737385	0
$\Omega^1_{2,2}$	0.995718	0.990242	0.992614
$\Omega^1_{3,1}$	0	0.000130721	0.00083635
$\Omega^1_{3,2}$	0	0	0
$\Omega^1_{3,3}$	1.00181	1.00339	1.00242
$\Omega^0_{1,1}$	1.00223	1.00089	1.00306
$\Omega^0_{1,2}$	0.1	0.1	0.1
$\Omega^0_{2,2}$	1.00392	1.00147	1.0025
$\Omega^0_{3,3}$	0.80000	1.00079	1.00282

where $\Omega^x_{y,z} = w^x_{y,z}\Delta t$ for $y \neq z$ and $\Omega^x_{y,z} = 1 + w^x_{y,z}\Delta t$ for $y = z$. The parameters $\Omega^x_{y,z}$, $i = 1, 2, 3$ is dimensionless. Table 7.7 lists the parameter values used for the hormone therapy model (7.33)–(7.34) with value a of $\Delta t = 1$ day [3, 15, 20]. In [15], three sets of parameter values for three patient types such as: type (i) patients with no relapse under IAS treatment, type (ii) patients with delayed relapse under IAS treatment, and type (iii) patients with relapse under IAS treatment are given. Table 7.7 summarizes the parameter values of the three patient types. The initial conditions for the variables in model (7.33)–(7.34) are $A_{\mathrm{D}}(0) = 17.84$ (cells), $A_{\mathrm{IR}}(0) = 0.778$ (cells), and $A_{\mathrm{II}}(0) = 0.382$ (cells) for type (i), $A_{\mathrm{D}}(0) = 13.43$ (cells), $A_{\mathrm{IR}}(0) = 1.57$ (cells), and $A_{\mathrm{II}}(0) = 0$ (cells) for type (ii), and $A_{\mathrm{D}}(0) = 11.02$ (cells), $A_{\mathrm{IR}}(0) = 0.976$ (cells), and $A_{\mathrm{II}}(0) = 0$ (cells) for type (iii). Treatment is started when PSA > 10 ng ml^{-1}.

7.6 Cell-cycle-based Model of Tumor Dynamics for Hormone Therapy

Some subtypes of breast, ovary, and uterus cancers depend on the hormone estrogen. Such cancers whose progression is influenced by estrogen receptor (ER) alpha are referred to as ER-positive cancers. Drugs such as tamoxifen and raloxifene are examples of anti-estrogen drugs used for ER-positive cancers [21, 22]. Tamoxifen is a selective estrogen receptor modulator (SERM) that helps to prevent and treat breast cancer. This drug can alter the cell-cycle and inhibit the proliferation of ER-positive cancer cells. Tamoxifen induces a delay in the cell-cycle and thus the cells accumulate in G_1 phase which in turn reduces the fraction of cells in other phases such as the S, G_2, and M-phase [23]. The cell-cycle-based model of tumor dynamics for hormone therapy with respect to the cell-kill effect of tamoxifen (TM) and

4-hydroxytamoxifen (HTM) is given in [21] where HTM is an active metabolite of TM. The model is given by:

$$\frac{\mathrm{d}A_g(t)}{\mathrm{d}t} = -m_g A_g(t)\ln\left(\frac{A_{\mathrm{sat}}}{A(t)}\right) + 2m_m A_m(t)\ln\left(\frac{A_{\mathrm{sat}}}{A(t)}\right) - a_1 A_g(t)\left(U_X(t) + \delta_1 U_H(t)\right), \tag{7.35}$$

$$\frac{\mathrm{d}A_s(t)}{\mathrm{d}t} = -m_s A_s(t) + m_g A_g(t)\ln\left(\frac{A_{\mathrm{sat}}}{A(t)}\right), \tag{7.36}$$

$$\frac{\mathrm{d}A_m(t)}{\mathrm{d}t} = -m_m A_m(t)\ln\left(\frac{A_{\mathrm{sat}}}{A(t)}\right) + m_s A_s(t), \tag{7.37}$$

where $A_g(t)$, $A_s(t)$, and $A_m(t)$, are the volume of tumor cells in the growing phase, DNA synthesis phase, and mitotic phase, respectively, A_{sat} is the volume of the tumor at growth saturation, a_1 represents the rate of drug induced cell-kill, m_g, m_s, and m_m, are the cell transition rates of cells in the growing phase, S-phase, and M-phase, respectively, and $U_X(t)$ and $U_H(t)$ are the concentration of TM and HTM, respectively. The parameter δ_1 accounts for the difference in binding affinity of the drugs TM and HTM.

In (7.35)–(7.37), $A(t) = A_g(t) + A_s(t) + A_m(t)$, and $U_X(t) = \frac{X_2(t)}{V}$ and $U_H(t) = \frac{X_3(t)}{V}$, where $X_2(t)$ and $X_3(t)$ denote the masses of the drug in two of the compartments and V is the volume. Apart from the tumor dynamics, the pharmacokinetics and pharmacodynamics of the drug are discussed in [21]. The pharmacokinetics of the drug is captured using the following mass transfer equations defined with respect to four compartments as given by:

$$\frac{\mathrm{d}X_0(t)}{\mathrm{d}t} = -k_{01}X_0(t) + u(t), \tag{7.38}$$

$$\frac{\mathrm{d}X_1(t)}{\mathrm{d}t} = -k_{12}X_1(t) + k_{01}X_0(t), \tag{7.39}$$

$$\frac{\mathrm{d}X_2(t)}{\mathrm{d}t} = -d_{U_1}X_2(t) - k_{23}X_2(t) + k_{12}X_1(t), \tag{7.40}$$

$$\frac{\mathrm{d}X_3(t)}{\mathrm{d}t} = -d_{U_2}X_3(t) + k_{23}X_2(t), \tag{7.41}$$

where $X_i(t)$, $i = 0, 1$, and 2 are the masses of TM in the 0th, 1st, and 2nd compartment respectively, $X_3(t)$ is the mass of the HTM in the 3rd compartment, k_{01}, k_{12}, and k_{23}, are the rate of mass transfer from 0th to 1st, 1st to 2nd, and 2nd to 3rd compartment, respectively, d_{U_1} and d_{U_2} are the rate of elimination of drug from compartment 2 and 3, respectively, and $u(t)$ is the infusion rate of TM.

In this model, it is assumed that the annihilation of cancer cells is facilitated only by the therapeutic agent. The cell-killing effect of the immune system response is ignored. However, as the immune cell level is an indication of the patient's health, the pharmacodynamics of the drug is given in terms of the rate of change in the number of circulating lymphocytes ($E_{CL}(t)$) as follows:

Table 7.8 Parameter values of the hormone therapy model (7.35)–(7.42) [21]

Parameter	Value (unit)	Parameter	Value (unit)
m_g	0.0013 (h^{-1})	A_{sat}	10^4 (mm^3)
m_s	0.0390 (h^{-1})	a_1	0.0062 (mL $\mu g^{-1} h^{-1}$)
m_m	0.0169 (h^{-1})	a_2	0.010 (mL $\mu g^{-1} h^{-1}$)
k_{01}	0.048 (h^{-1})	δ_1	25
k_{12}	0.993 (h^{-1})	δ_2	25
k_{23}	35.932 (h^{-1})	s	1.21×10^5 (h^{-1})
d_{U_1}	1.145 (h^{-1})	d_1	1.20×10^{-2} (h^{-1})
d_{U_2}	39.525 (h^{-1})	V	8.592 (mL)

$$\frac{dE_{CL}(t)}{dt} = s - d_1 E_{CL}(t) - a_2 E_{CL}(t) \left(U_X(t) + \delta_2 U_H(t)\right), \qquad (7.42)$$

where s is the generation rate or constant influx rate of circulating lymphocytes, d_1 is the rate of apoptosis, δ_2 accounts for the difference in killing effect of TM and HTM, and a_2 is the cell-kill rate due to the drug.

Compared to the general model given by (1.1) and (1.2), it can be seen this model accounts for cell transition and drug-induced cell death. However, the influence of normal cells, competition between cells, and influence of immune system on tumor dynamics are assumed to be negligible. Note that, this model is similar to the cell-cycle-based compartmental model of tumor dynamics discussed in Sect. 3.5 related to chemotherapy.

Parameters related to the cell growth are derived using experimental data using mouse model reported in [24, 25] and that about circulating lymph is from [26]. Rest of the parameter values of this model are adopted from [27]. Table 7.8 summarizes the parameter values of the hormone therapy model (7.35)–(7.42) [21]. The initial conditions for the variables in model (7.35)–(7.42) are $A_g(0) = 900\,(mm^3)$, $A_s(0) = A_m(0) = 50\,(mm^3)$, $X_0(0) = X_1(0) = X_2(0) = X_3(0) = 0\,(\mu g)$, and $E_{CL}(0) = 10^7$ (cells). The unit of $U_H(t)$ and $U_X(t)$ is $\mu g\ mL^{-1}$.

7.7 Summary

In this chapter, six different mathematical models of hormone therapy are discussed. All these models assume that the effect of the immune system in cancer progression is negligible. The cell-cycle-based model for breast cancer has accounted for the side effect of drug tamoxifen on circulating lymphocyte but the immune effect on cancer dynamics is ignored. However, literature suggests that androgen deprivation-mediates T and B cell lymphopoiesis, and thymic regeneration and it can adversely affect the regulation of several cytokines and maturization of dendritic cells [28–31].

Elevated levels of cytokines IL-6, IL-8, and TNF-α are reported in prostate cancer patients [32]. Given the association of the immune system with the progression of prostate cancer and response to hormone therapy, it is imperative to develop mathematical models that portray these interactions. Extending the models discussed in this chapter with the influence of immune response will give an overall picture of the prostate cancer dynamics under hormone therapy and helps to elucidate mechanisms that cause side effects and drug resistance.

More investigation is required to understand the exact role of androgen level in the dynamics of AI cells. The cell-quota-based model hypothesize that the growth of AI cells indirectly (mutated pathway) depends on a certain minimal level of androgen [8, 33]. Hence, this model has been used to investigate further on the controversy regarding the relevance of androgen in the growth of androgen-independent cells. However, the predictability of the cell-quota-based model is under debate. Even though cell-quota models have shown improved fitting and predictability [34, 35], it is not able to predict PSA relapse profile under CAS [33].

Mathematical models of prostate cancer under hormone therapy have been widely used for deriving optimal control input for IAS therapy, forecasting the development of treatment resistance, and quantification of uncertainty of the model prediction with respect to clinical data [33]. Several hormone-based therapeutic pathways have been used for breast and ovarian cancers as well. For instance, GnRH agonist is suggested for hormone receptor-positive and HER2-negative metastatic breast cancer therapy [36]. However, mathematical models of hormone therapy for breast and ovarian cancer are scarce [2].

As mentioned earlier, hormone therapy is often used as a neoadjuvant or an adjuvant therapy and hence it is desirable to depict the related cell dynamics under combination therapy settings [37]. Such mathematical models will be discussed in Chap. 9 of this book.

References

1. E.P. Winer, C. Hudis, H.J. Burstein, R.T. Chlebowski, J.N. Ingle, S.B. Edge, E.P. Mamounas, J. Gralow, L.J. Goldstein, K.I. Pritchard et al., American society of clinical oncology technology assessment on the use of aromatase inhibitors as adjuvant therapy for women with hormone receptor-positive breast cancer: Status report 2002. J. Clin. Oncol. **20**(15), 3317–3327 (2002)
2. C. Chen, W.T. Baumann, J. Xing, L. Xu, R. Clarke, J.J. Tyson, Mathematical models of the transitions between endocrine therapy responsive and resistant states in breast cancer. J. R. Soc. Interface **11**(96), 20140206 (2014)
3. Y. Hirata, G. Tanaka, N. Bruchovsky, K. Aihara, Mathematically modelling and controlling prostate cancer under intermittent hormone therapy. Asian J. Androl. **14**(2), 270–277 (2012)
4. A. Zazoua, W. Wang, Analysis of mathematical model of prostate cancer with androgen deprivation therapy. Commun. Nonlinear Sci. Numer. Simul. **66**, 41–60 (2019)
5. E.D. Crawford, Hormonal therapy in prostate cancer: historical approaches. Rev. Urol. **6**(Suppl 7), S3 (2004)
6. C. Chen, W.T. Baumann, R. Clarke, J.J. Tyson, Modeling the estrogen receptor to growth factor receptor signaling switch in human breast cancer cells. FEBS Lett. **587**(20), 3327–3334 (2013)

7. H.V. Jain, S.K. Clinton, A. Bhinder, A. Friedman, Mathematical modeling of prostate cancer progression in response to androgen ablation therapy. Proc. Natl. Acad. Sci. **108**(49), 19701–19706 (2011)
8. T. Portz, Y. Kuang, J.D. Nagy, A clinical data validated mathematical model of prostate cancer growth under intermittent androgen suppression therapy. AIP Adv. **2**(1), 011002 (2012)
9. W. Song, V. Soni, M. Khera, Combined tests of prostate specific antigen and testosterone will improve diagnosis and monitoring the progression of prostate cancer. Asian J. Androl. **17**(5), 807–810 (2015)
10. A.M. Ideta, G. Tanaka, T. Takeuchi, K. Aihara, A mathematical model of intermittent androgen suppression for prostate cancer. J. Nonlinear Sci. **18**(6), 593 (2008)
11. Y. Hirata, K. Morino, K. Akakura, C.S. Higano, K. Aihara, Personalizing androgen suppression for prostate cancer using mathematical modeling. Nat.: Sci. Rep. **8** (2018)
12. B.J. Feldman, D. Feldman, The development of androgen-independent prostate cancer. Nat. Rev. Cancer **1**, 34–45 (2001)
13. H.I. Scher, G. Buchanan, W. Gerald, L.M. Butler, W.D. Tilley, Targeting the androgen receptor: improving outcomes for castration-resistant prostate cancer. Endocrine-related Cancer **11**(3), 459–476 (2004)
14. J. Edwards, J.M. Bartlett, The androgen receptor and signal-transduction pathways in hormone-refractory prostate cancer. Part 1: Modifications to the androgen receptor. BJU Int. **95**(9), 1320–1326 (2005)
15. Y. Hirata, N. Bruchovsky, K. Aihara, Development of a mathematical model that predicts the outcome of hormone therapy for prostate cancer. J. Theor. Biol. **264**(2), 517–527 (2010)
16. T. Shimada, K. Aihara, A nonlinear model with competition between prostate tumor cells and its application to intermittent androgen suppression therapy of prostate cancer. Math. Biosci. **214**(1), 134–139 (2008)
17. M. Droop, Some thoughts on nutrient limitation in algae 1. J. Phycol. **9**(3), 264–272 (1973)
18. R. Gibson, R. Atkinson, J. Gordon, Use, abuse, misconceptions and insights from quota models–the Droop cell quota model 40 years on. Oceanogr. Marine Biol.: An Ann. Rev. **46**, 1–23 (2008)
19. E. Litchman, C.A. Klausmeier, Trait-based community ecology of phytoplankton. Ann. Rev. Ecol. Evol. Syst. **39**, 615–639 (2008)
20. G. Tanaka, Y. Hirata, S.L. Goldenberg, N. Bruchovsky, K. Aihara, Mathematical modelling of prostate cancer growth and its application to hormone therapy. Philos. Trans. R. Soc. A: Math. Phys. Eng. Sci. **368**(1930), 5029–5044 (2010)
21. T. Chen, N.F. Kirkby, R. Jena, Optimal dosing of cancer chemotherapy using model predictive control and moving horizon state/parameter estimation. Comput. Methods Prog. Biomed. **108**(3), 973–983 (2012)
22. G. Lebedeva, A. Yamaguchi, S.P. Langdon, K. Macleod, D.J. Harrison, A model of estrogen-related gene expression reveals non-linear effects in transcriptional response to tamoxifen. BMC Syst. Biol. **6**(1), 138 (2012)
23. C.K. Osborne, D.H. Boldt, G.M. Clark, J.M. Trent, Effects of tamoxifen on human breast cancer cell cycle kinetics: accumulation of cells in early G1 Phase. Cancer Res. **43**(8), 3583–3585 (1983)
24. S.P. Robinson, S.M. Langan Fahey, D.A. Johnson, V.C. Jordan, Metabolites, pharmacodynamics, and pharmacokinetics of tamoxifen in rats and mice compared to the breast cancer patient. Drug Metabol. Dispos. **19**(1), 36–43 (1991)
25. B.A. Conley, T.S. Ramsland, D.L. Sentz, S. Wu, D.M. Rosen, M. Wollman, J.L. Eiseman, Antitumor activity, distribution, and metabolism of 13-cis-retinoic acid as a single agent or in combination with tamoxifen in established human MCF-7 xenografts in mice. Cancer Chemother. Pharmacol. **43**(3), 183–197 (1999)
26. L.G. de Pillis, W. Gu, A.E. Radunskaya, Mixed immunotherapy and chemotherapy of tumors: modeling, applications and biological interpretations. J. Theor. Biol. **238**(4), 841–862 (2006)
27. J.A. Florian Jr., J.L. Eiseman, R.S. Parker, Nonlinear model predictive control for dosing daily anticancer agents using a novel saturating-rate cell-cycle model. Comput. Biol. Med. **38**(3), 339–347 (2008)

28. Y.T. Koh, A. Gray, S.A. Higgins, B. Hubby, W.M. Kast, Androgen ablation augments prostate cancer vaccine immunogenicity only when applied after immunization. The Prostate **69**(6), 571–584 (2009)
29. J. Creemers, H. Westdorp, I. van Oort, G. Schreibelt, M. Gorris, N. Mehra, M. Simons, A. de Goede, M. van Rossum, S. Croockewit, et al., Natural dendritic cell vaccinations generate immune responses that correlate with clinical outcome in patients with chemo-naive castration-resistant prostate cancer. Ann. Oncol. **30**, v480 (2019)
30. F. Cappuccini, R. Bryant, E. Pollock, L. Carter, C. Verrill, J. Hollidge, I. Poulton, M. Baker, C. Mitton, A. Baines, et al., Safety and exceptional immunogenicity of novel 5T4 viral vectored vaccination regimes in early stage prostate cancer: a Phase I clinical trial. MedRxiv (2020)
31. E. Zhang, F. Dai, Y. Mao, W. He, F. Liu, W. Ma, Y. Qiao, Differences of the immune cell landscape between normal and tumor tissue in human prostate. Clin. Transl. Oncol. **22**(3), 344–350 (2020)
32. D.A. Galvão, K. Nosaka, D. Taaffe, J. Peake, N. Spry, K. Suzuki, K. Yamaya, M. McGuigan, L.J. Kristjanson, R. Newton, Endocrine and immune responses to resistance training in prostate cancer patients. Prostate Cancer Prostatic Dis. **11**(2), 160–165 (2008)
33. Z. Wu, T. Phan, J. Baez, Y. Kuang, E.J. Kostelich, Predictability and identifiability assessment of models for prostate cancer under androgen suppression therapy. Math. Biosci. Eng. **16**(5), 3512–3536 (2019)
34. T. Phan, K. Nguyen, P. Sharma, Y. Kuang, The impact of intermittent androgen suppression therapy in prostate cancer modeling. Appl. Sci. **9**(1), 36 (2019)
35. O.O. Mizrak, C. Mizrak, A. Kashkynbayev, Y. Kuang, The impact of fractional differentiation in terms of fitting for a prostate cancer model under intermittent androgen suppression therapy, in *Mathematical Modelling in Health, Social and Applied Sciences* (Springer, 2020), pp. 151–197
36. Y.H. Park, T.Y. Kim, G.M. Kim, S.Y. Kang, I.H. Park, J.H. Kim, K.E. Lee, H.K. Ahn, M.H. Lee, H.J. Kim et al., Palbociclib plus exemestane with gonadotropin-releasing hormone agonist versus capecitabine in premenopausal women with hormone receptor-positive, HER2-negative metastatic breast cancer (KCSG-BR15-10): A multicentre, open-label, randomised, Phase 2 trial. Lancet Oncol. **20**(12), 1750–1759 (2019)
37. E.M. Rutter, Y. Kuang, Global dynamics of a model of joint hormone treatment with dendritic cell vaccine for prostate cancer. Discret. Contin. Dyn. Syst.-B **22**(3), 1001 (2017)

Chapter 8
Miscellaneous Therapy Models

In Chaps. 3–7, five major therapeutic approaches currently in use for cancer management are discussed. In this chapter, mathematical models of cancer dynamics under gene therapy, oncolytic virotherapy, nanocarrier-based therapy, and stem cell therapy are presented. Most of these therapeutic strategies are experimental and emerging and some are interrelated to the treatment methods that have been discussed in earlier chapters. For instance, some literature categorize the gene therapy as immunotherapy, while some others discuss it as two different treatment modalities [1]. Similarly, the oncolytic virotherapy involves the use of genetically engineered viruses to mediate cell death, while the gene therapy uses genetically engineered viruses as a vector for gene delivery [2, 3]. All such treatment modalities are discussed in this chapter under the heading of miscellaneous therapy models for cancer management and their interrelations are clarified.

8.1 Gene Therapy

Gene therapy is the common word used for the treatment or prevention of diseases by altering associated genes that are responsible for the disease. Gene therapy-based approaches for cancer management include:

- using genetically altered genes that can directly annihilate cancer cells,
- gene transfer to modify the aberrant functioning and behavior of cancer cells,
- altering genetic patterns related to immunity to boost the immune response in fighting cancer, and
- inserting genes that make cancer cells more responsive to other treatment methods such as chemotherapy or radiotherapy [1, 4–6].

Figure 8.1 shows various gene therapy strategies and vectors. Treatment modalities include inserting DNA with supporting lipids or proteins, naked plasmid DNA,

R. Padmanabhan et al., *Mathematical Models of Cancer and Different Therapies*, Series in BioEngineering, https://doi.org/10.1007/978-981-15-8640-8_8

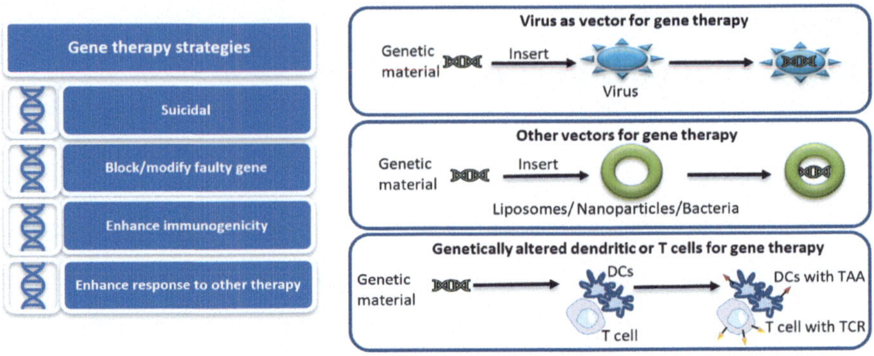

Fig. 8.1 Illustrative diagram showing various strategies adopted to facilitate gene therapy. Insertion of suicidal genes can trigger self-destruction of cancer cells. Blocking or modifying faulty genes to regulate the aberrant behavior of cancer cells is also possible by means of gene therapy. Immunogenicity of tumor cells can be enhanced by gene therapy. Viruses, liposomes, nanoparticles, and bacteria are common vectors used to facilitate gene therapy. Dendritic cells (DCs) and T cells can be genetically altered to expresses tumor-associated antigens (TAA) and T cell receptors (TCR), respectively. TAA and TCR enhance the tumor-specific immune response

fragments of RNA (siRNA), or messenger RNA (mRNA) [4, 7–9]. Vectors (elements) used for gene delivery include viruses, liposomes, nanoparticles, and bacteria. The choice of viral vectors depends on many factors such as (1) genetic combination, structure, and replication of the virus, (2) whether the transgene expression lasts for short term (transient) or long term, and (3) presence of negative/positive virion polymerase. For instance, retrovirus has an envelope while adenovirus has no envelope or coating. Adenovirus is a replication-defective vector whose certain genes are replaced by the desired genes that express therapeutic proteins for a short period of time [10]. Similarly, the choice of nanocarriers for gene therapy depends on many factors including target specificity, sustained gene delivery, bio-compatibility, etc. [11].

Even though gene therapy has been used successfully to treat many inherited genetic disorders and infections, this method is comparatively new in cancer research. Gene therapy is a very expensive method and several experiments are underway to overcome its uncertain and potentially lethal side effects [3, 4]. However, the positive side of the therapeutic approach has motivated cancer scientists to conduct clinical trials to figure out feasible ways to achieve more reliable outcomes [6, 12, 13]. The first gene therapy-based drug (Kymriah) got approval in 2015 for acute lymphoblastic leukemia. Since then, several gene therapeutic approaches have got FDA approval as well [14]. Due to its potential to enhance other modes of therapy, gene therapy is usually used as a combination therapy. Combination therapy models are discussed in the next chapter of book.

As mentioned above, gene therapy can be used to boost the immune system's capabilities to identify the tumor cells and thus facilitate targeted cancer cell-lysis. Such an immune-boosting approach is used in [7]. Specifically, short interfering

RNAs (siRNA), which are capable of altering the gene expression, and thus the behavior of a cell is used to increase the immunogenicity of cancer cells. In [15], a PDE model of molecular transport is used to predict the staphylococcus aureus α-hemolysin (SAH) efficacy in fighting cancer. This bacterial gene therapy is tested on murine tumors and the model suggests that the treatment efficacy is related to the size of the colony and rate of protein production. Here, SAH is the payload protein and it enables effective therapy due to its ability to diffuse into tissues to facilitate tumor necrosis.

Even though there exist several strategies to facilitate gene therapy, most of the mathematical modeling and analysis are done in the area on oncolytic virotherapy. Mathematical models using other vectors are scarce. In this section, two gene therapy models are discussed which can be explained as special cases of the general model given by (1.1) and (1.2), namely:

1. Modified predator-prey model for gene therapy, and
2. Model of siRNA mediated cancer management.

Tables 8.1 and 8.2 summarize the notations used for gene therapy models.

Table 8.1 Different types of cells and biochemicals in gene therapy

Var.	Description	Var.	Description
$E(t)$	Number of immune cells	$A(t)$	Number of cancer cells
$C_1(t)$	Amount of the cytokine IL-2	$C_2(t)$	Amount of the cytokine TGF-β
$G(t)$	Amount of siRNA	$s(t)$	Immune cell influx rate
$\alpha_a(t)$	Antigenicity of tumor	$a(t)$	Drug induced cell-kill rate
$r_2(t)$	Growth rate of $A(t)$	$u(t)$	siRNA input rate

Table 8.2 Parameter notations in gene therapy

Param.	Description	Param.	Description
g	Half-saturation constant related to a cell population or cytokine	μ	Critical value of $A(t)$ at which TGF-β production increases
r	Growth rate of a cell population or cytokine	d	Rate of apoptosis or depletion of a cell population or cytokine
b	Reciprocal carrying capacity	α_a	Antigenicity of tumor
a	Drug induced cell-kill rate	ρ_1	Max. rate of proliferation of $E(t)$ in the absence of TGF-β
ρ_2	Max. rate of proliferation of $A(t)$ due to TGF-β	ρ_3	Max. rate of IL-2 production
ρ_4	Max. rate of TGF-β production	γ_1	TGF-β induced inhibition of antigenicity of tumor cells
γ_2	Inhibition of IL-2 by TGF-β	γ_3	Blocking of mRNA by siRNA
ψ	Proportion of siRNA bound to mRNA		

8.1.1 Modified Predator-Prey Model for Gene Therapy

In this subsection, a modified version of the immunotherapy model discussed in Sect. 4.1 is presented which shows the enhanced immune response achieved by using genetically engineered T cells. In [6], a clinical trial is reported in which certain genes are transferred to the T cells of the blood sample drawn from patients to facilitate the expression of T cell receptor (TCR). These altered T cells with TCR are capable of recognizing and binding with the cancer cells and thus triggering an immune attack to annihilate cancer cells (Fig. 8.1). Hence, in [4], a mathematical model is developed for gene therapy using the predator-prey model of immunotherapy (4.1)–(4.3) discussed in [16]. The modified predator-prey model for gene therapy is given by:

$$\frac{\mathrm{d}E(t)}{\mathrm{d}t} = s(t) + \alpha_{\mathrm{a}}(t)A(t) - d_1 E(t) + r_1 \frac{E(t)}{E(t) + g_1}, \tag{8.1}$$

$$\frac{\mathrm{d}A(t)}{\mathrm{d}t} = r_2(t)A(t)(1 - bA(t)) - a(t)\frac{E(t)A(t)}{A(t) + g_2}, \tag{8.2}$$

where $E(t)$ and $A(t)$ represent the immune cells and cancer cells, respectively.

In (8.1), as the gene therapy mediated TCR expression can attract more effector cells to the tumor micro-environment, a time-varying variable $s(t)$ is used to model the influx rate of immune cells. Similarly, $\alpha_{\mathrm{a}}(t)$ is used to model the antigenicity of tumor, instead of α_{a} in (4.1). The last two terms account for the apoptosis and limited proliferation of the immune cells, where d_1 models the death rate of immune cells, r_1 is the growth rate, and g_1 is the half-saturation constant of $E(t)$ proliferation.

In (8.2), the term $r_2(t)A(t)(1 - bA(t))$ models the growth of cancer cells, where $r_2(t)$ and b are growth rate and reciprocal carrying capacity, respectively. As the immunogenicity of the tumor cells increases, the annihilation of the tumor cells will change considerably over time more like a step function. Consequently, the growth rate of cancer cells is also assumed to be decreasing abruptly, which is modeled using the term $r_2(t)$ in (8.2). The last term $a(t)\frac{E(t)A(t)}{A(t)+g_2}$ models the effect of gene therapy, where $a(t)$ is the treatment-induced cell-kill effect and g_2 is the related half-saturation constant. Compared to the Kirschner–Panetta (KP) model given by (4.1)–(4.3), in this model the effect of the cytokine IL-2 in (4.3) is omitted for simplicity.

Table 8.3 summarizes parameter values of the gene therapy model (8.1)–(8.2) [4]. The initial conditions for the variables in model (8.1)–(8.2) are $E(0) = A(0) = 10^3$ (cells).

8.1.2 Mathematical Model of siRNA Mediated Cancer Management

In [7], the KP model of immunotherapy is extended by adding the dynamics of cytokines (TGF-β) and siRNA. Gene therapy is used to alter the expression of the gene that is responsible for the production of TGF-β using siRNA. TGF-β is the

Table 8.3 Parameter values of the gene therapy model (8.1)–(8.2) [4]

Parameter	Value (unit)	Parameter	Value (unit)
$s(t)$	1 (cells time^{-1})	$\alpha_a(t)$	0.05 (time^{-1})
d_1	0.03 (time^{-1})	r_1	0.1245 (time^{-1})
g_1	10^{-3} (cells^{-1})	$r_2(t)$	0.18 (time^{-1})
b	10^{-9} (cells^{-1})	g_2	10^5 (cells)
$a(t)$	1 (time^{-1})		

cytokine that restricts the tumor-antigen expression and thus reduces the activation of effector cells. The model discusses the dynamics of immune cells and cancer cells under siRNA mediated cancer management.

As discussed earlier in Chap. 4, the cytokine TGF-β (Fig. 4.3) is a regulatory polypeptide that can influence multiple cellular functions such as growth, differentiation, adhesion, apoptosis, migration, angiogenesis, and immunosurveillance [17]. It should be noted that TGF-β mediates all these cellular functions with the help of other growth factors and binding receptors. Interestingly, the cytokine TGF-β is identified to have both tumor-promoting and tumor-inhibiting roles in the tumor micro-environment. An example of the tumor-inhibiting role is the inhibition of the proliferation of epithelial cells by TGF-β mediated autocrine signaling [17]. On the other hand, in the absence of autocrine action, this cytokine is identified to promote the growth of tumor cells and it aids in tumor vascularization [4, 17]. Specifically, it is found that TGF-β inhibits the cell growth and triggers apoptosis by promoting cell-cycle arrest during the initial phase of tumorigenesis. Later, when the tumor cells alter signaling pathways and become resistant to cell lysis via the action of TGF-β, then these cytokines are identified to change their role to act as tumor growth promoters. TGF-β can also promote tumor growth by reducing the immunogenicity of tumors and also by suppressing the activation of effector cells. Due to the involvement (even though contradicting) of TGF-β in the progression and regression of cancer, the signaling pathways associated with TGF-β are considered as a viable target for facilitating gene therapy-based cancer regression [17].

The mathematical model of siRNA mediated cancer management discussed in [7] is given by:

$$\frac{\mathrm{d}E(t)}{\mathrm{d}t} = \frac{\alpha_a A(t)}{1+\gamma_1 C_2(t)} - d_1 E(t) + \left(\frac{E(t)C_1(t)}{g_1 + C_1(t)}\right)\left(\rho_1 - \frac{r_{\max} C_2(t)}{g_2 + C_2(t)}\right), \tag{8.3}$$

$$\frac{\mathrm{d}A(t)}{\mathrm{d}t} = r_1 A(t)(1 - bA(t)) - a_1 \frac{E(t)A(t)}{g_3 + A(t)} + \rho_2 \frac{C_2(t)A(t)}{g_4 + C_2(t)}, \tag{8.4}$$

$$\frac{\mathrm{d}C_1(t)}{\mathrm{d}t} = \rho_3 \frac{E(t)A(t)}{\big(g_5 + A(t)\big)\big(1 + \gamma_2 C_2(t)\big)} - d_2 E(t), \tag{8.5}$$

$$\frac{\mathrm{d}C_2(t)}{\mathrm{d}t} = \frac{\rho_4 A^2(t)}{\mu^2 + \left(1 + \frac{\psi G(t)}{\gamma_3}\right)A^2(t)} - d_3 C_2(t), \tag{8.6}$$

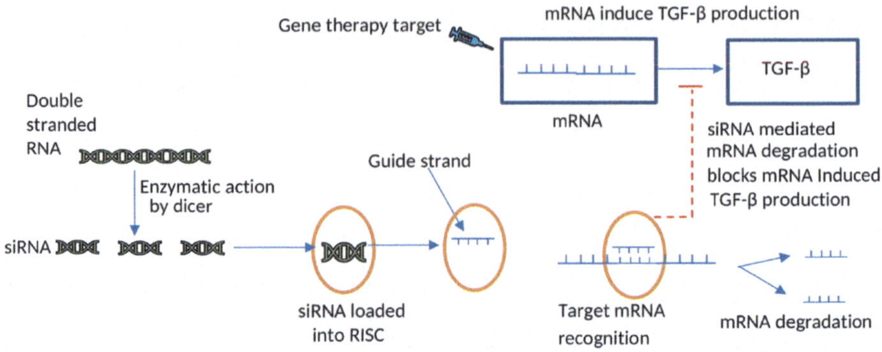

Fig. 8.2 Illustrative diagram showing siRNA (small interfering RNA) mediated degradation of mRNA (messenger RNA) that is responsible for the production of TGF-β in tumor cells. The enzyme dicer slices RNA into short nucleotides called as siRNAs. Once siRNA is loaded into the RISC (RNA-induced gene silencing complex), the double stranded RNA is unwound and a guide strand is retained. Upon target mRNA recognition by the guide strand, RISC mediates mRNA degradation. Here, the gene therapy target is mRNA whose degradation/silencing blocks production of TGF-β in tumor cells [7]

$$\frac{\mathrm{d}G(t)}{\mathrm{d}t} = u(t) - d_{\mathrm{U}}G(t), \tag{8.7}$$

where $E(t)$ and $A(t)$ are the immune and cancer cells, respectively, $C_1(t)$ and $C_2(t)$ represent IL-2 and TGF-β, respectively, and $G(t)$ denotes the siRNA.

It can be seen that the above model is similar to (4.1)–(4.3), except for the terms that account for the influence of TGF-β on the dynamics of effector cells, cancer cells, and interleukin. In (8.3), the term $\frac{\alpha_a A(t)}{1+\gamma_1 C_2(t)}$ models the recruitment of effector cells to the tumor micro-environment with respect the amount of tumor cells, where α_a is the antigenicity of the tumor. As α_a and $A(t)$ are increased, the number of the immune cell $E(t)$ is also increased. However, this increased recruitment is limited by the presence of TGF-β in the tumor micro-environment. The denominator term models the TGF-β induced restriction in the recruitment of effector cells, where γ_1 is the TGF-β induced inhibition rate of tumor antigenicity. The second term accounts for the apoptosis of effector cells, where d_1 is the death rate. The third term accounts for the increase in effector cells due to the presence of IL-2. The Michaelis–Menten term $\frac{E(t)C_1(t)}{g_1+C_1(t)}$ accounts for IL-2 induced effector recruitment and its self limiting property, where g_1 denotes the half-saturation constant. TGF-β induced reduction in the influence of IL-2 on immune cell recruitment is modeled using the term $\rho_1 - \frac{r_{\max} C_2(t)}{g_2+C_2(t)}$, where ρ_1 and $r_{\max}$ are the maximum rate of proliferation of effector cells in the absence of TGF-β and the maximum rate of growth inhibition effect of TGF-β, respectively, and g_2 is the half-saturation constant.

In (8.4), the first term accounts for the growth of tumor cells, where r_1 and b are the growth rate and reciprocal carrying capacity. The second term models the reduction of tumor growth due to the immune response, where a_1 is the effector cell mediated

Table 8.4 Parameter values of the siRNA mediated gene therapy model (8.3)–(8.7) [7]

Parameter	Value (unit)	Parameter	Value (unit)
α_a	0-0.035 (days^{-1})	γ_1	10
d_1	0.03 (days^{-1})	g_1	2×10^7 (pg L^{-1})
ρ_1	0.1245 (days^{-1})	r_{max}	0.1121 (days^{-1})
g_2	2×10^6 (pg l^{-1})	r_1	0.18 (days^{-1})
b	10^{-9} (ml cells^{-1})	a_1	1 (days^{-1})
g_3	1×10^5 (cells ml^{-1})	ρ_2	0.27 (days^{-1})
g_4	2×10^7 (pg ml^{-1})	ρ_3	5 (pg $\text{cells}^{-1}\text{days}^{-1}$)
g_5	1×10^3 (cells ml^{-1})	γ_2	1×10^{-3} (l pg^{-1})
d_2	10 (days^{-1})	ρ_4	0–3×10^8 (pg l^{-1} days^{-1})
μ	10^6 (cells ml^{-1})	d_U	0.66 (days^{-1})
ρ_3	5 (pg (cells days)$^{-1}$)	d_3	10 (days^{-1})

tumor cell-kill rate and g_3 is the half-saturation constant. The term $\rho_2 \frac{C_2(t)A(t)}{g_4+C_2(t)}$ models the increase in tumor growth due to TGF-β, where ρ_2 is the maximum rate of increase in $A(t)$ due to the effect of TGF-β and g_4 is the half-saturation constant.

In (8.5), the first term accounts for the increase in production of IL-2 due to the interaction of effector cells with the tumor cells, where ρ_3 is the maximum rate of IL-2 production, g_5 is the half-saturation associated with the self-limiting associated with IL-2 production in the absence of TGF-β, and γ_2 is the inhibition of the IL-2 production by TGF-β. The second term models depletion of IL-2, where d_2 is the depletion rate.

In (8.6), the first term models the increased production of TGF-β with respect to the growth of the tumor. During the initial phase of tumorigenesis, the production of TGF-β is less. However, as the tumor grows, an increase in the production of TGF-β is noticed to favor angiogenesis. The critical value of $A(t)$ at which TGF-β production increases considerably is modeled using the parameter μ and ρ_4 is the maximum rate of TGF-β production. As shown in Fig. 8.2, siRNA can inhibit the production of TGF-β via mRNA degradation. This is modeled in the term $\frac{\psi G(t)}{\gamma_3}$, where ψ is the proportion of $G(t)$ that is bound to the mRNA, and γ_3 is the inhibition rate or suppression rate of mRNA by the siRNA. Finally, (8.7) models the siRNA dynamics, where $u(t)$ denotes dose of siRNA and d_U is the decay rate of siRNA.

Table 8.4 summarizes the parameter values of the siRNA mediated gene therapy model (8.3)–(8.7) [7]. In model (8.3)–(8.7), the variables $E(t)$ and $A(t)$ are given in cells and $C_1(t)$ and $C_2(t)$ are given in pg ml^{-1}.

8.2 Oncolytic Virotherapy

As shown in Fig. 8.1, in the case of gene therapy, genetically modified viruses are used for the transfer of genes that can facilitate tumor suppression, apoptosis, or the release of oncolytic cytokines. In the case of oncolytic virotherapy (OV), genetically altered viruses that are capable of intruding selectively into the cancer cells to facilitate targeted annihilation of cancer cells are used (Fig. 8.3). These oncolytic viruses can then replicate within the cancer cells to cause viral burden to the cell which in turn leads to cell death [3, 18]. Moreover, the oncolytic viruses that are released from the virus-infected and lysed cancer cells can infect and kill other cancer cells. Many oncolytic viruses are used in clinical trials to evaluate their efficacy in relieving cancers of ovary, sarcoma, pancreas, prostate, and bladder [18]. Adenoviruses, retroviruses, herpes viruses, paramyxoviruses, measles, vesicular stomatitis virus, etc., are some of the oncolytic viruses used to facilitate cancer cure. Some viruses are capable of infecting and killing cancer cells with defective genes. For instance, ONYX-15, a modified adenovirus can selectively kill cancer cells with an abnormal *p53* gene. There are several ways by which a therapeutic virus mediates the regression of cancer.

Even though most of the suggested approaches in oncolytic virotherapy are premature and experimental, the fact that the FDA has already given its approval for the use of oncolytic virus therapy (T-VEC, Imlygic) in 2015 shows its potential [18]. In short, virotherapy based anti-cancer approaches make use of the potential of oncolytic viruses to [19–21]:

- replicate repeatedly in the cancer cells to eventually burden the cancer cells and cause cell death,
- produce cytotoxic protein while they are inside the cancer cells and thus cause cell death, and
- to infect the cancer cells in such a way that it will induce or boost anti-tumor immunity of the body.

Even though there exist many mathematical models of oncolytic virotherapy in the literature, in this section, the following two models are discussed:

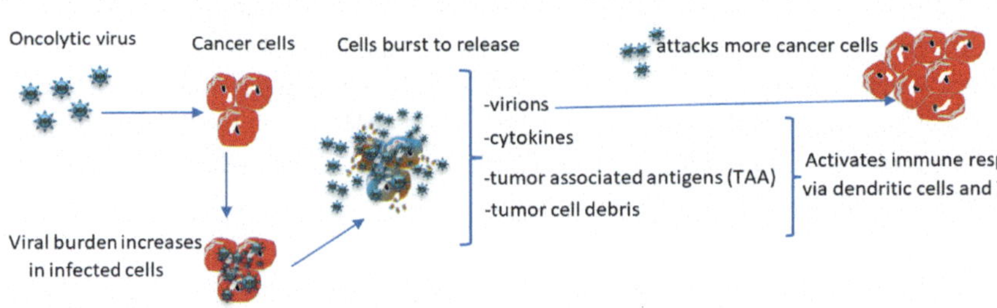

Fig. 8.3 Illustrative diagram showing oncolytic virus attacking cancer cells. These viruses replicate inside the cancer cells and they burst to release virions, cytokines, TAA, and tumor cell debris which will increase the immunogenicity of the cancer cells

Table 8.5 Different types of cells and biochemicals in oncolytic virotherapy

Var.	Description	Var.	Description
$A_U(t)$	Tumor cells that are not infected by the virus	$A_V(t)$	Tumor cells that are infected by the virus
$V(t)$	Number of viruses	$D(t)$	Number of dendritic cells
$E(t)$	Number of activated T cells	$E_N(t)$	Number of naive T cells
$A_{tot}(t)$	Total number of cells in the tumor micro-environment	$u_D(t)$	Dendritic cell input rate
$u_V(t)$	Oncolytic virus input rate		

Table 8.6 Parameter notations in oncolytic virotherapy

Param.	Description	Param.	Description
r	Growth rate of a cell population	m	Mutation or cell-transition rate of a cell population
b	Reciprocal carrying capacity of a cell population	d	Rate of apoptosis of a cell population
α_T	Transfection or infection of virus	a_0	Virus independent cell-kill rate
a	Virus or drug induced cell-kill rate	d_U	Depletion rate of a drug or virus

1. Model of cancer therapy using oncolytic virus with various modes of transmission of infection, and
2. Model of cancer therapy using oncolytic virus and dendritic cells.

Tables 8.5 and 8.6 summarize the notations used for oncolytic virotherapy models.

8.2.1 Model of Cancer Therapy Using Oncolytic Virus with Various Modes of Infection Transmission

In the case of oncolytic virotherapy, the mode of transmission of virus infection is an important factor that specifies the treatment efficacy [19]. Effect of the transfection mechanism on the cell population dynamics is similar to the mechanisms associated with competition ($\mathscr{C}(\cdot)$) and mutation ($\mathscr{M}(\cdot)$) discussed in (1.1). There are many models that depict the dynamics of tumor micro-environment under oncolytic virotherapy as discussed in [18, 19, 22–25], and the references therein. The mathematical model of transmission of infection from an infected cancer cell population under oncolytic virotherapy that is given in the literature follows the following form:

$$\frac{\mathrm{d}A_U(t)}{\mathrm{d}t} = \mathscr{G}(A_V(t), r) - \mathscr{A}(A_V(t), d) - \mathscr{T}(A_U(t), A_V(t), \alpha_T)\, A_V(t), \quad (8.8)$$

Table 8.7 Parameter values of the oncolytic virotherapy model (8.9)–(8.10) [19]

Parameter	Value	Parameter	Value	Parameter	Value
α_{T}	0.5–1.5	r	0.3–2.5	d	0.3–2

where r is the growth rate, d is the death rate, and α_{T} is the infection rate of uninfected cancer cells. The function that models the transmission of infection is denoted by $\mathscr{T}(A_{\mathrm{U}}(t), A_{\mathrm{V}}(t), \alpha_{\mathrm{T}})$, where α_{T} is the rate of transmission of infection. Note that, in the case of oncolytic virotherapy, the effect of drug is equivalent to the effect of virus infection, hence the function that denotes the transmission of infection ($\mathscr{T}(\cdot)$) in (8.8) is equivalent to the function $\mathscr{D}(\cdot)$ in (1.1) defined in Chap. 1.

In the case of direct annihilation of cancer cells due to the action of an oncolytic virus, the net infection rate of cancer cells is proportional to the product of the number of oncolytic viruses and uninfected cells. The simplest form of the infection transmission is given by $\mathscr{T}(\cdot) = \alpha_{\mathrm{T}} A_{\mathrm{U}}(t)$. Using this form of $\mathscr{T}(\cdot)$, the last term in (8.8) becomes $\alpha_{\mathrm{T}} A_{\mathrm{U}}(t) A_{\mathrm{V}}(t)$ which is similar to the predator-prey type of interaction that are discussed in earlier subsections. The mathematical model that accounts for this mechanism is given by [19]:

$$\frac{\mathrm{d}A_{\mathrm{U}}(t)}{\mathrm{d}t} = A_{\mathrm{U}}(t)(1 - (A_{\mathrm{U}}(t) + A_{\mathrm{V}}(t))) - \alpha_{\mathrm{T}} A_{\mathrm{U}}(t) A_{\mathrm{V}}(t), \tag{8.9}$$

$$\frac{\mathrm{d}A_{\mathrm{V}}(t)}{\mathrm{d}t} = r A_{\mathrm{V}}(t)(1 - (A_{\mathrm{U}}(t) + A_{\mathrm{V}}(t))) + \alpha_{\mathrm{T}} A_{\mathrm{U}}(t) A_{\mathrm{V}}(t) - d A_{\mathrm{V}}(t), \tag{8.10}$$

where r and d are the growth rate and death rate of infected cells, respectively, and α_{T} is the infection rate which quantifies the average number of infections caused by each infected cell. In (8.9) and (8.10), the term $\alpha_{\mathrm{T}} A_{\mathrm{U}}(t)$ models the infection transmission where it is assumed that free virus dynamics is significantly faster than the infected cell turnover. With this assumption, the number of virions is proportional to the number of infected cells and hence virion dynamics are not modeled separately. Table 8.7 summarizes the parameter values of the oncolytic virotherapy model (8.9)–(8.10) [19]. The initial conditions for the variables in model (8.9)–(8.10) are $A_{\mathrm{U}}(0) = 0.1$ (cells) and $A_{\mathrm{V}}(0) = 0.0001$ (cells).

However, the infection rate will remain proportional to the product of the size of populations involved only if the assumption that the contact rate is linearly related to the density $(A_{\mathrm{U}}(t) + A_{\mathrm{V}}(t))$ holds. Thus, the law of mass-action kinetics can be used to quantify the rate of infection transmission only if the size of the two populations involved are similar. If the size of one population is significantly different from the other, this approximation gives unrealistic results, i.e. when $A_{\mathrm{U}}(t) \ll A_{\mathrm{V}}(t)$ or vice versa. In the case of virotherapy, which involves the release of virions from an infected cell that will infect more cells, mass-action kinetics may not be sufficient (Fig. 8.3).

Another form of the oncolytic virotherapy model discussed in the literature is [19]:

$$\frac{dA_U(t)}{dt} = r_1(1 - b(A_U(t) + A_V(t))) - \alpha_{T'} \frac{A_U(t)A_V(t)}{A_U(t) + A_V(t)}, \tag{8.11}$$

$$\frac{dA_V(t)}{dt} = r_2(1 - b(A_U(t) + A_V(t))) - d_1 A_V(t) + \alpha_{T'} \frac{A_U(t)A_V(t)}{A_U(t) + A_V(t)}. \tag{8.12}$$

where infection transmission is modeled using the term $\mathscr{T}(A_U(t), A_V(t), \alpha_{T'}) = \alpha_{T'} \frac{A_U(t)}{A_U(t)+A_V(t)}$, which gives realistic values even when $A_U(t) \ll A_V(t)$ or vice versa. The transmission term used in [26] is $\mathscr{T}(A_U(t), A_V(t), \alpha_{T'}) = \frac{\alpha_{T'} A_U(t)}{1+a\alpha_{T'} A_V(t)}$ which models the saturation effect as well. In a holling type model given by $\mathscr{T}(z) = \alpha_{T'} \frac{z}{1+z}$, with $z = \frac{A_U(t)}{A_V(t)}$, it follows that $\mathscr{T}(\cdot) = \alpha_{T'} \frac{A_U(t)}{A_U(t)+A_V(t)}$ which is same as the density dependent or ratio dependent model [27]. The model (8.11)–(8.12) is equivalent to (8.9)–(8.10) with $\alpha_T = \frac{\alpha_{T'}}{br_1}$, $r = \frac{r_2}{r_1}$, and $d = \frac{d_1}{r_1}$.

In [18], with the help of equilibrium point analysis of the model for oncolytic virotherapy, it is point out that there is no stable equilibrium point for the model if the tumor growth is increasing or if the oncolytic virus has a positive decay rate. Hence, with a detailed investigation, in [18], it is concluded that oncolytic virotherapy alone can reduce tumor growth significantly but is insufficient to eradicate the tumor. As shown in the next subsection, combining oncolytic virotherapy with immunotherapy is a more promising approach.

8.2.2 *Model of Cancer Therapy Using Oncolytic Virus and Dendritic Cells*

In this subsection, a mathematical model of virotherapy is presented which uses oncolytic adenovirus to enhance the immune response and thus to cause cancer lysis via co-stimulatory molecule 4-1BB ligand (4-1BBL) and cytokine IL-12 [23–25]. Tumor volume data from murine experiments reported in [28], which are obtained using four different oncolytic adenoviruses are used to develop the mathematical model in [23]. The mathematical model for the oncolytic virus mediated cancer regression is given by [24]:

$$\frac{dA_U(t)}{dt} = r_1 A_U(t) - \alpha_T \frac{A_U(t)V(t)}{A_{tot}(t)} - (a_0 + a_1 A_V(t)) \frac{A_U(t)E(t)}{A_{tot}(t)}, \tag{8.13}$$

$$\frac{dA_V(t)}{dt} = \alpha_T \frac{A_U(t)V(t)}{A_{tot}(t)} - a_2 A_V(t) - (a_0 + a_1 A_V(t)) \frac{A_V(t)E(t)}{A_{tot}(t)}, \tag{8.14}$$

$$\frac{dV(t)}{dt} = u_V(t) + r_2 a_2 A_V(t) - d_{U_1} V(t), \tag{8.15}$$

$$\frac{dE(t)}{dt} = a_3 A_V(t) + m E_N(t) + a_4 D(t) - d_1 E(t), \tag{8.16}$$

$$\frac{dE_N(t)}{dt} = a_5 A_V(t) - d_2 E_N(t), \tag{8.17}$$

$$\frac{\mathrm{d}D(t)}{\mathrm{d}t} = u_{\mathrm{D}}(t) - d_{\mathrm{U}_2} D(t), \tag{8.18}$$

where $A_{\mathrm{U}}(t)$ and $A_{\mathrm{V}}(t)$ represent tumor cell volume that are not infected and infected by the adenovirus, $D(t)$ and $V(t)$ denote the number of dendritic cells and virus cells, $E(t)$ and $E_{\mathrm{N}}(t)$ are the number of activated T cells and naive T cells in the tumor micro-environment, respectively, and $A_{\mathrm{tot}}(t)$ is the total number of cells in the tumor micro-environment, i.e, $A_{\mathrm{tot}}(t) = A_{\mathrm{U}}(t) + A_{\mathrm{V}}(t) + E(t) + E_{\mathrm{N}}(t)$.

In (8.13), the first term depicts the growth of uninfected tumor cells, where r_1 is the exponential growth rate and the second term accounts for the infection of cells, where α_{T} is the rate of transition of the uninfected tumor cells to infected tumor cells. Cells that are infected by the adenovirus express 4-1BBL molecules which enhance T cell differentiation [23]. Note that 4-1BB is a receptor that belongs to the tumor necrosis factor category which is expressed on activated T cells and 4-1BBL is its ligand (Fig. 4.3 in Chap. 4). The signaling pathways associated with 4-1BBL can be used to trigger anti-tumor immunity and enhance the cytotoxicity of T cells [2]. The third term $(a_0 + a_1 A_{\mathrm{V}}(t)) \frac{A_{\mathrm{U}}(t)E(t)}{A_{\mathrm{tot}}(t)}$ in (8.13) and (8.14) is used to account for the cell-kill mediated by adenovirus-infected cancer cells via the release of 4-1BBL and the cytotoxic cytokine IL-12. Note that this term accounts for the fact that the activated T cells kill both the infected as well as uninfected cancer cells. Here, the cell-kill rate denoted by a_1 is proportional to the number of virus-infected cells and a_0 is the virus independent cell-kill rate.

In (8.14), the first term models the transition of $A_{\mathrm{U}}(t)$ to $A_{\mathrm{V}}(t)$ and the second term models the reduction in $A_{\mathrm{V}}(t)$, where a_2 represents the cell-kill rate due to the oncolytic virus and other mechanisms, and the third term models the tumor cell-kill by the immune cells.

In (8.15), the term $u_{\mathrm{V}}(t)$ denotes the infusion rate of oncolytic virus. The rate of virion production from each cell is modeled using the parameter r_2. The apparent increase in the number of the virus with respect to the number of infected tumor cells is accounted for by using the term $r_2 a_2 A_{\mathrm{V}}(t)$. The last term models the depletion of the virus in the tumor micro-environment, where d_{U_1} is the decay rate of virions due to natural death. Note that, in contrast to the general model given by (1.2) in Chap. 1, in (8.15), there exists an additional term to account for the re-infections due to the release of virions from the lysed cancer cells, where r_2 is the average rate at which virions are released from each cell.

Dynamics involved in the oncolytic virotherapy along with the dendritic cell therapy are modeled in (8.16). It can be seen that the increase in the number of the activated T cells is attributed to three T cell activation pathways such as:

- the cell transition (alteration) of naive T cells to activated T cells captured by the rate parameter m,
- the stimulation of T cells due to the increased production of 4-1BBL by the adenovirus infected cancer cells captured by the rate parameter a_3, and
- the production of T cells mediated by the injected dendritic cells captured by the rate parameter a_4.

Table 8.8 Parameter values of the oncolytic virus and dendritic cell therapy model (8.13)–(8.18) [23–25]

Parameter	Value (unit)	Parameter	Value (unit)
r_1	0.3198 (days^{-1})	α_T	0.00100854 (days^{-1})
a_1	5.954×10^{-7}	a_2	1 (days^{-1})
r_2	3500	d_{U_1}	2.3 (days^{-1})
a_3	1.6984 (days^{-1})	a_4	4.6754
d_1, d_2	0.35 (days^{-1})	a_5	0.22–1.44 (days^{-1})

These three effects are modeled using the terms $a_3 A_V(t)$, $m E_N(t)$, and $a_4 D(t)$, respectively. The last term in (8.16) models the reduction in the number of activated immune cells, where d_1 is the rate of apoptosis of activated T cells.

The infection of cancer cells by the oncolytic viruses triggers the recruitment of naive T cells to the tumor micro-environment. This is modeled in (8.17) using the term $a_5 A_I(t)$, where a_5 is a positive constant. The second term models the death of naive T cells, where d_2 is the death rate. Finally, in (8.18), $u_D(t)$ models the input rate of dendritic cells and d_{U_2} denotes the decay rate of the dendritic cells.

It can be seen that the model given by (8.13)–(8.18) is also a special case of the general model (1.1)–(1.2) with respective terms that model the growth function $\mathscr{G}(\cdot)$, cell transition function $\mathscr{M}(\cdot)$, effect of drug $\mathscr{D}(\cdot)$, drug dynamics $\mathscr{D}_c(\cdot)$, and infection transmission dynamics $\mathscr{T}(\cdot)$ as explained already. However, the changes in the dynamics of the different cell population involved, which occur due to the effect of the resource availability and competition between the cell populations (denoted as $\mathscr{K}(\cdot)$ and $\mathscr{C}(\cdot)$, respectively in (1.1)) are not considered in the model (8.13)–(8.18).

Table 8.8 summarizes the parameter values of the oncolytic virus and dendritic cell therapy model (8.13)–(8.18) [23–25]. The initial conditions for the variables in model (8.13)–(8.18) are $A_U(0) = 60\,(\text{mm}^3)$, $A_V(0) = 0\,(\text{mm}^3)$, $V(0) = 0$ (virions), $E(0) = 0$ (cells), $E_N(0) = 0$ (cells), and $D = 0$ (cells). Inputs are $u_V(t) = 2.5 \times 10^9 - 5 \times 10^9$ (virions days^{-1}) virions and $u_D(t) = 10^6$ (DCs days^{-1}), with $d_{U_2} \approx 0.35$ (days^{-1}).

8.3 Anti-cancer Drug Delivery Using Nanocarriers

This section presents the targeted delivery of anti-cancer drugs using nanocarriers. Metal-based, lipid-based, polymer-based, and biological particle-based nanoparticles can be used as carriers for precisely delivering anti-cancer drugs to the target. These nanocarriers can transfer the therapeutically active drug molecule directly to the site of action. This approach relies on the surface functionalization capability of the carrier molecules to bind with specific receptors on the surface of the cancer cells. This limits the leakage of the therapeutically active drug molecule to the surrounding areas of the cancer cells and thus impedes the development of induced drug resistance [29]. This will, in turn, reduce the amount of drug needed to achieve certain desired drug effects as well as the adverse effect on other healthy cells. Apart from these advantages, one of the unique features of nanomedicine-based treatment is that, with this method a triggered drug delivery is also possible. This means that the therapeutically active drug molecules remain encapsulated in the carriers unless certain physiological or external stimuli such as pH, temperature, enzymes, or electromagnetic radiation are used to trigger their delivery (unload) to the target. Some of the anti-cancer agents transported successfully using nanoparticles are paclitaxel, irinotecan, vincristine, asparaginase, and doxorubicin [30–32]. For example, abraxane is a combination of albumin nanoparticles with the chemotherapeutic drug paclitaxel.

Even though nanotherapy based approaches for cancer management has witnessed significant progress in the last few decades, many biophysical barriers impede the widespread use of this mode of therapy. Various challenges come in the way of nano molecules during its course to the target site. Firstly, the influence of the physiological and hemodynamics conditions during the circulation decides their fate, then comes the size-dependent challenges that influence extravasation into interstitial fluids or excretion by kidneys, next is the opsonization and phagocytosis threat due to immune activation, and finally antagonistic tumor micro-environment which hinders the transport and delivery of nanomolecules to cancer cells which are far from blood capillaries [29, 33].

Another important characteristic of the nanocarriers is the number of protein-specific binding sites on the surface of the nanoparticle. The factors that influence this number is the size, hydrophobicity, and surface chemistry of the nanoparticle. As soon as the therapeutic nanomolecules enter the bloodstream, they are covered with protein molecules (corona formation) which changes the property of the molecule. In short, a mathematical model that depicts the pharmacokinetics and pharmacodynamics of nanomedicines for cancer cure should account for the following factors:

- the course of transport of nanocarriers,
- distribution of nanocarriers,
- cellular uptake of nanoparticles,
- tumor deliverability of nanocarriers, and
- drug effect of these therapeutic agents.

A review on the molecular dynamics (ODE models) of corona formation that occurs once the nanoparticle enters the bloodstream is presented in [29]. Similarly, the transport mechanism of nanoparticle in the circulatory system is modeled using discrete, continuous, and hybrid models [34–37]. The cellular uptake of the nanoparticles after extravasation is represented using discrete models and the whole body distribution and clearance of the therapeutic nanoparticles are depicted using a compartmental model [38]. The tumor deliverability is studied via hybrid models [39, 40] and the efficacy of nanotherapy are studied [41, 42] using pharmacodynamic models.

Tables 8.9 and 8.10 summarize the notations to model cancer dynamics under nanotherapy.

Table 8.9 Different types of cells and biochemicals in nanotherapy

Var.	Description	Var.	Description
$A(t)$	Number of tumor cells	$U_{\mathrm{B}}(t)$	Concentration of the product of nanoparticle and protein
$U_{\mathrm{np}}(t)$	Concentration of therapeutic nanoparticle	$P(t)$	Concentration of protein
$U_{\mathrm{c}}(t)$	Concentration of therapeutic nanoparticle in the central compartment	$U_{\mathrm{p}}(t)$	Concentration of therapeutic nanoparticle in the peripheral compartment

Table 8.10 Parameter notation used in nanotherapy

Param.	Description	Param.	Description
a	Drug induced cell-kill rate	ϕ_{np}	Radius of the nanoparticle molecule
ϕ	Radius of protein	n	Number of binding sites of protein
α_{N}	Association rate of protein	δ	Dissociation of binded nanoparticle-protein pair
i	$i = 1, 2, 3$ represent three proteins and $i = 4$ is the target (receptor)	d_{U}	Drug uptake rate
k_{10}	Elimination rate of doxorubicin from central compartment	k_{12}	Rate of transfer of doxorubicin from central to peripheral compartment
k_{21}	Rate of transfer of doxorubicin from peripheral to central compartment		

8.3.1 *Mathematical Model for Anti-cancer Drug Delivery Using Nanocarriers*

The mathematical models in [36, 37] discuss the biochemical phenomenon of corona formation around the nanoparticle and the interaction of nanoparticle with target biomolecule (a receptor). In [37], this is modeled by assuming mass-action kinetics for human serum albumin (HSA), high-density lipoprotein (HDL), and fibrinogen (Fib) as:

$$\frac{\mathrm{d}U_{\mathrm{B}i}(t)}{\mathrm{d}t} = n_i \alpha_{Ni} U_{\mathrm{np}}(t) P_i(t) - \delta_{Ni} U_{\mathrm{B}i}(t), \quad i = 1, 2, 3, \tag{8.19}$$

where $U_{\mathrm{B}i}(t)$, $i = 1, 2, 3$, denote the time-varying concentration of the product of binding between nanoparticle and the protein HSA, HDL, and Fib, respectively, $U_{\mathrm{np}}(t)$ denotes the concentration of therapeutic nanoparticle, $P_i(t)$, $i = 1, 2, 3$, are the concentration of HSA, HDL, and Fib, respectively, and α_{Ni}, $i = 1, 2, 3$, quantify the association rate of HSA, HDL, and Fib, respectively. Here, δ_{Ni}, $i = 1, 2, 3$, denote the dissociation of bound nanoparticle-protein pair. The number of protein-specific binding sites on the surface of a nanoparticle is a significant factor that influences the corona formation around it. This parameter is denoted by n_i, $i = 1, 2, 3$, representing the number of binding site for each of the protein HSA, HDL, and Fib, respectively. Assuming a spherical shape for the nanoparticle-protein pair, this parameter is given by $n_i = \frac{4\pi(\phi_{\text{np}}+\phi_i)^2}{\pi\phi_i^2}$, where ϕ_{np} is the radius of the nanoparticle molecule and ϕ_i, $i = 1, 2, 3$, is the radius of each of the three proteins. In (8.19), the equation with $i = 4$ represents the interaction of the nanoparticle with the target and n_4 denotes the number of peptides attached on the nanoparticle. Given the biophysical barriers associated with the pharmacokinetics of nanomedicines, the development of associated mathematical models is essential to assess the efficacy of drug transport and to predict the fate of the nanomolecules.

The model (8.19) is not complete as it accounts only for the initial corona formation. In [29], a model that involves absorption, distribution, and metabolism of therapeutic contents embedded in nanoparticles and the excretion of the same using compartmental kinetics is presented as follows:

$$\frac{\mathrm{d}U_{\text{c}}(t)}{\mathrm{d}t} = k_{21}U_{\text{p}}(t) - (k_{10} + k_{12})\,U_{\text{c}}(t), \quad U_{\text{c}}(0) = c_0 \tag{8.20}$$

$$\frac{\mathrm{d}U_{\text{p}}(t)}{\mathrm{d}t} = k_{12}U_{\text{c}}(t) - k_{21}U_{\text{p}}(t), \quad U_{\text{p}}(0) = 0, \tag{8.21}$$

where $U_{\text{c}}(t)$ and $U_{\text{p}}(t)$ are the concentrations of therapeutic nanoparticles in the central and peripheral compartments, respectively, and k_{12}, and k_{21} are rate constants that quantify the rate of transfer of therapeutic nanoparticles between central and peripheral compartments and k_{10} denotes the elimination rate of therapeutic nanoparticles from the central compartment.

In [29], a pharmacodynamic model for therapeutic nanomedicines given in [41] is also reviewed. The reliability of this pharmacodynamic model for the prediction of drug-induced cell-kill profile is validated by assessing the viability of cells in vitro which are treated with free-doxorubicin and nanoparticle loaded doxorubicin. This pharmacodynamic model which quantifies the cytotoxicity of therapeutic nanoparticles is given by:

$$\frac{A(t)}{A_0} \approx 1 - \frac{1}{2}aU_{\text{np0}}d_{\text{U}}A_0t^2, \quad \frac{U_{\text{np}}(t)}{U_{\text{np0}}} = e^{-d_{\text{U}}A_0t}, \quad \text{for} \quad d_{\text{U}}A_0t \ll 1 \tag{8.22}$$

$$\frac{A(t)}{A_0} \approx e^{-a(U_{\text{np0}}-U_{\text{np}\infty})t}, \quad U_{\text{np}}(t) \approx U_{\text{np}\infty}, \quad \text{for} \quad d_{\text{U}}A_0t \gg 1, \tag{8.23}$$

where $A(t)$ is the number of cancer cells (or concentration of cells), A_0 is the value at time $t = 0$, a is the drug induced cell-kill rate, d_{U} is the rate of drug uptake, $U_{\text{np}}(t)$, U_{np0}, and $U_{\text{np}\infty}$ are the concentrations of drug at time t, $t = 0$, and $t = \infty$. Note that, in (8.22) the term $e^{-d_{\text{U}}A_0t}$ quantifies the exponential decay of the drug due to cellular uptake of drugs at a the rate of $d_{\text{U}}A_0$.

Note that, as cited above, the model equations discussed in this subsection are not from a single literature. There is no complete ODE-based mathematical models

Table 8.11 Parameter values of the nanomedicine corona model (8.19) [36]

Parameter	Value (unit)	Parameter	Value (unit)
α_{N1}	2.4×10^3 ($M^{-1}s^{-1}$)	ϕ_{np}	35 (nm)
α_{N2}	3×10^4 ($M^{-1}s^{-1}$)	U_{np0}	18×10^{-9} (M)
α_{N3}	2×10^3($M^{-1}s^{-1}$)	α_{N4}	$10^4 - 10^7$ ($M^{-1}s^{-1}$)
δ_{N1}	2×10^{-3}(s^{-1})	ϕ_1	5 (nm)
δ_{N2}	3×10^{-5} (s^{-1})	ϕ_2	4 (nm)
δ_{N3}	2×10^{-3} (s^{-1})	ϕ_3	8.3 (nm)
δ_{N4}	$10^{-3} - 10^{-12}$(M)		

Table 8.12 Parameter values of the pharmacokinetic model (8.20)–(8.21) for the drug doxorubicin [39]

Param.	Value (unit)	Param.	Value (unit)	Param.	Value (unit)
k_{10}	0.0820 (min^{-1})	k_{12}	0.0475 (min^{-1})	k_{21}	0.00125 (min^{-1})

pertaining to the overall dynamics of nanotherapy towards tumor regression. Most of the literature that deals with the mathematical modeling of nanotherapy discuss the spatio-temporal distribution of nanoparticles rather than the effect on the tumor micro-environment. Being an emerging area in cancer therapy, there is much more to be known regarding the drug and carrier-specific pharmacokinetics, pharmacodynamics, and cell dynamics under nanotherapy.

Tables 8.11 and 8.12 summarize the parameter values of the nanomedicine corona model (8.19) and pharmacokinetic model of doxorubicin given by (8.20)–(8.21) [36, 39]. The initial conditions for the variables in model (8.19) are $U_{B1}(0) = 1.4 \times 10^{-8}$ (M), $U_{B2}(0) = 0.4 \times 10^{-8}$ (M), $U_{B3}(0) = 0$ (M), $U_{np}(0) = 18 \times 10^{-9}$ (M), $P_1(0) = 6 \times 10^{-4}$ (M), $P_2(0) = 1.5 \times 10^{-5}$ (M), and $P_3(0) = 8.8 \times 10^{-6}$ (M).

8.4 Mathematical Models for Stem Cell Therapy

The important therapeutic advantage of stem cell therapy compared to other therapeutic modes is its potential to restrict the relapse of disease as well as the development of drug resistance [43, 44]. However, this approach is in a developing stage and most of the reported mathematical models explore the dynamics of the stem cells, with respect to their self-renewal, differentiation, and migration patterns. Stem cells are basically of two types: (1) the embryonic stem cells that are present in the initial stages of development (blastocyst), which divide, differentiate, and develop into various cell types to form tissues, organs and body (organism), and (2) the somatic stem cells which are maintained in the body for routine repair of various organs. Stem cells exhibit peculiar cell division and gene expression patterns. Depending upon their differentiation patterns, they are categorized into three types: (I) unipotent stem cells that differentiate to one type of specialized cells, (II) multipotent stem cells that

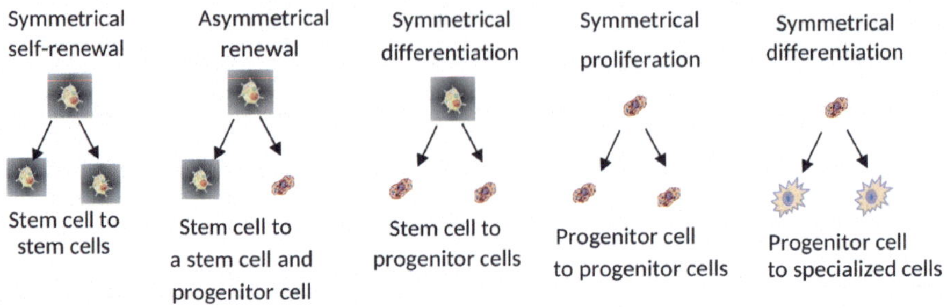

Fig. 8.4 Various types of cell division involved in the proliferation and differentiation of stem cells and progenitor cells

can differentiate to different types of stem cells, and (III) pluripotent stem cells that can produce any types of cells in the body [45]. For instance, hematopoietic stem cells (HSCs) are multipotent and can generate and maintain the cell count of white blood cells, red blood cells, and platelets in the blood. Examples of unipotent and pluripotent cells are skin cells and embryonic cells, respectively.

Cellular plasticity of stem cells is defined as the ability of a parent stem cell to switch to new identities. Figure 8.4 shows various types of stem cell division. If a stem cell divides to give two daughter stem cells, then it is symmetrical cell division (symmetrical self-renewal). Stem cell division can also be obligate-asymmetric replication (asymmetrical renewal) which results in a daughter stem cell and another cell that differentiates and specializes into specific cell type [46]. The stem cells exhibit stochastic differentiation (symmetrical differentiation) which results in two progenitor cells that differentiate into specialized cells. Stochastic cell division which uses up stem cells is often compensated by self-renewal of other stem cells. The symmetrical proliferation of progenitor cells and their differentiation to special cells are also shown in Fig. 8.4. In general, the number of stem cells is kept marginal and they usually do not proliferate too much.

Induced pluripotency of stem cells (iPSCs) is a milestone achievement that has enhanced the scope of application of stem cell oriented therapy in regenerative medicine to reconstruct a damaged organ or body part [47]. It allows reprogramming of the cells to revert specialized somatic cells to pluripotent cells by inducing certain genes. The main attraction of this method is that since the cells are derived from the patient's own body, there is less fear of immune rejection and associated complications. Thus, this method can be used for stem cell regeneration after chemotherapy for leukemia to reproduce all types of blood cells. Stem cells are organ-specific and are present in every organ. Even though stem cells as such do not perform any organ-specific function, they can serve as a reservoir to replenish the worn-out cells of the respective organ which they represent.

Similar to the normal (non-malignant) stem cells, some of the cancer cells can differentiate into every other type of cells in a neoplasm. Such cells are called cancer stem cells (CSC)s. The malignant counterpart of hematopoietic stem cell which is associated with leukemia is called a leukemia stem cell (LSC). In the case of patients with diseases like leukemia or lymphoma, the impaired generation of normal cells will hinder body functions. In such cases, stem cell transplants are recommended as a treatment. Depending upon the donor of the stem cells there are two types of stem cell transplants that are used for therapeutic purposes, namely allogeneic stem cell transplant and autologous stem cell transplant. In the allogeneic stem cell transplant, the stem cells from a matching donor are used and in the autologous stem cell transplant, the stem cells taken from the patient's own body is used. Due to immunological incompatibility, allogeneic stem cell transplants have a comparatively lesser success rate.

Most of the therapy methods used currently for the annihilation of the tumor are believed to leave some of the CSCs undamaged which later on causes the relapse of the disease. For instance, CSCs are identified to be resistant to many conventional therapies [48, 49]. This is mainly due to the fact that the stem cells are identified to have an inherent protective niche that keeps harmful drugs away from them. For instance,

- they have characteristic signaling pathways for facilitating repair of damaged DNA as well as hindering apoptosis [50], and
- they multiply slowly and behave like noncancerous cells and hence drugs that target highly proliferative cells will not damage these cells [50].

Interestingly, cancer and normal stem cells show many similar characteristic behaviors such as asymmetric cell division and indefinite self-replication. Both malignant and nonmalignant stem cells are capable of producing a large number of differentiated cells, expressing specific proteins, and self-renewal (Fig. 8.4). The self-renewed stem cells help to maintain the number of cells in the stem cell pool and the differentiated cells develop to specific cell types [51]. As pointed out in [43, 52] and the references therein, many clinical trials support the notion of the possible presence of cancer stem cells that acts as a source of support for the progression of different types of cancers such as leukemia, lung, ovarian, colon, breast, and prostate cancer to name some. Hence, the main focus of many consequent research works are to figure out the exact mechanism of action of these CSCs to develop countermeasures that alter these pathways to facilitate cancer regression and prevent relapse [52, 53]. As shown in Fig. 8.5, targeted annihilation of CSCs can curtail cancer relapse [52].

Similar to the nonmalignant stem cells, CSCs are capable of self-renewal. CSCs can convert to tumorigenic or nontumorigenic cell progenitors. The findings that the stem cells and CSCs share several common properties like self-renewal, quiescence, presence of similar surface biomarkers have all lead to the assumption that the CSCs might have arisen from a mutated stem cell [43]. The capability of CSCs to initiate tumors when transplanted to animals is well studied and established. Thus, one can say CSCs are tumorigenic. Some studies suggest that miRNAs are responsible for the regulation properties of CSCs.

Even though the therapeutic implications of stem cells are apparent, more clear knowledge of the exact mechanism of action is imperative to formulate stem cell-

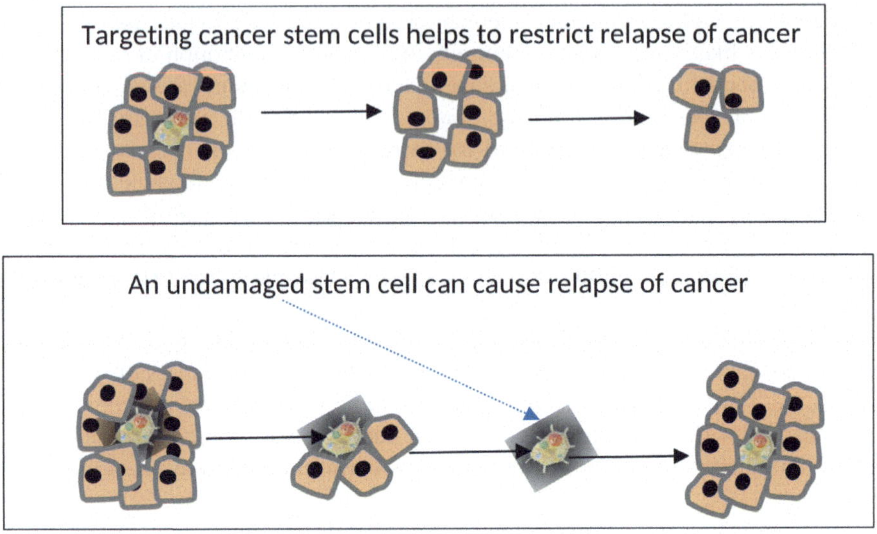

Fig. 8.5 Illustrative diagram showing restriction of cancer relapse by the targeted annihilation of cancer stem cells (CSCs). Targeted annihilation of CSCs along with non-stem cancer cells restrict relapse of cancer. Otherwise, undamaged CSCs can cause a relapse of cancer even if all non-stem cancer cells are killed by therapy

based therapies. The following are some of the possibly useful stem cell oriented pathways suggested in literature [51, 52]:

1. Destroying CSC niche by using a targeted therapeutic approach.
2. Interfering with self-renewal pathways.
3. Inducing differentiation of CSC cells in a useful way is also a suggested method of developing stem cell-based therapy. For instance,
   - evidence suggests that IL-15 can induce the differentiation of chemotherapy-resistant renal CSCs into epithelial cells which are identified to be sensitive to chemotherapy [52].
   - the knockdown of the antigen CD44 from certain breast CSCs induced differentiation to non-breast cancer stem cells with reduced tumorigenesis and increased treatment susceptibility [52].
4. To mediate the restoration of drug sensitivity. For instance, a therapeutic drug, salinomycin can be used to restore drug sensitivity of multiple drug-resistant (MDR) cell lines.

In [51], a model of six cell populations namely, normal stem cells, normal early progenitors, normal late progenitors, malignant stem cells (or CSCs), malignant early progenitors, and malignant late progenitors is presented. Instead of the usual growth rates and mutation rates used for different compartmental models, the probability of renewal to the same cell type, differentiation to other cell lineages, or mutation to other cell types (Fig. 8.4) are modeled. It is highlighted that the trigger/stimulus for mutation can be depletion of mature cells due to injury or radiation [51, 54]. Two diverse scenarios pertaining to stem cell dynamics are: (1) regulated growth (homeostasis) of stem cells and somatic cells and (2) abnormal growth of cells leading to tumorigenesis. As mentioned in [54], one of the key challenges is to account for these two diverse scenarios in one model.

Even though the therapeutic approaches that target CSC are promising, cancer scientists are looking for deciphering the signaling pathways and more in-depth knowledge to design targeted therapy protocols. Hence, mathematical and experimental studies are used to investigate the related hypothesis and contradictions. In [55], using a mathematical model and experimental evidence, the association of the proportion of CSCs in the tumor micro-environment and cancer dynamics is investigated. The study suggests that with a higher proportion of CSCs in a tumor the disease can be more aggressive. In [43], a mathematical model that accounts for the delay involved in the evolution and differentiation of cells is presented. Using the model, the possible complications that arise due to the stem cell transplant and also the therapeutic benefits are investigated. Out of the many mathematical models of stem cell therapy, here the following three mathematical models for the stem cell dynamics are discussed:

1. An 8-compartmental model of stem cell dynamics.
2. Model of stem cell dynamics in the bone marrow and peripheral blood.
3. Model of leukemia stem cell dynamics.

Tables 8.13 and 8.14 summarize the notations used in the stem cell therapy.

Table 8.13 Different types of cells and biochemicals in stem cell therapy

Var.	Description	Var.	Description
$N_{\mathrm{BM}}(t)$	Non-malignant bone marrow cells	$N_{\mathrm{Bs}}(t)$	Non-malignant basal cells
$A_{\mathrm{BM}}(t)$	Malignant bone marrow cells	$N_{\mathrm{Sq}}(t)$	Non-malignant quiescent stem cells
$A_{\mathrm{S}}(t)$	Cancer stem cells or leukemia stem cells	$A_{\mathrm{PM}}(t)$	Malignant peripheral blood cells
$N_{\mathrm{Pr}}(t)$	Non-malignant progenitor stem cells	$N_{\mathrm{PM}}(t)$	Non-malignant peripheral blood cells
$N_{\mathrm{D}}(t)$	Non-malignant differentiated cells	$A_{\mathrm{Sq}}(t)$	Malignant quiescent stem cells
$A_{\mathrm{Pr}}(t)$	Malignant progenitor stem cells	$A_{\mathrm{Bs}}(t)$	Malignant basal cells
$A_{\mathrm{D}}(t)$	Malignant differentiated cells	$N_{\mathrm{S}}(t)$	Normal hematopoietic stem cells
$d_{\mathrm{i}}'(t)$	Therapy induced apoptotic rate	$\psi(t)$	Feedback due to CSCs and LSCs

Table 8.14 Parameter notations in stem cell therapy

Param.	Description	Param.	Description
d	Death rate	r	Growth rate
m	Mutation rate	β_0	Feedback constant
$N_{b_{max}}$	Max. number of non-malignant basal cells	$A_{P_{max}}$	Max. number of malignant progenitor cells
k_{ij}	Cell transition rate of cells from ith to jth compartment	$A_{b_{max}}$	Max. number of malignant basal cells
κ_0	Cell limitation on size	δ	Dosage variation constant
u_c	Drug dose for pulsed therapy	u_p	Drug dose for continuous therapy

8.4.1 An 8-Compartmental Model for Stem Cell Dynamics

In [49], the concept of carcinogenesis in relation to cell differentiation is discussed. It is well agreed that carcinogenesis is a result of multiple events including overexpression, silencing, and mutation of associated genes. Stem cells may require lesser genetic alterations to convert to or transform into a cancer cell. Understanding the mechanisms involved in these mutations or differentiation or transformation may help to develop better approaches to tackle this disease and the differentiation therapy targets the final differentiation mechanism to facilitate cancer cure. The concept of feedback in biological elements is used in [56, 57] to explain memory, oscillations, and regulation involved in many biological mechanisms.

Each stem cell in the quiescent state can either differentiate into other cells with specific functions, self-renew, or die (Figs. 8.4 and 8.6). Note that compared to the parameters introduced in (1.1), since self-renewal contributes to the number of the same cell population, the renewal rate is considered similar to the growth rate and is denoted by r. The differentiation is similar to cell transformation, which is modeled using the function $\mathscr{M}\left(m, C_{p1}(t)\right)$, where the parameter m denotes the rate of cell differentiation or the rate of moving out of cells from a defined compartment. The elimination rate or death rate of cells with respect to each defined compartments are denoted using the parameter d. The model is given by [49]:

$$\frac{\mathrm{d}N_{\mathrm{Sq}}(t)}{\mathrm{d}t} = -d_1 N_{\mathrm{Sq}}(t) - k_{12} N_{\mathrm{Sq}}(t) + K_{21}\left(N_{\mathrm{Pr}}(t)\right) N_{\mathrm{Pr}}(t), \tag{8.24}$$

$$\begin{aligned}\frac{\mathrm{d}N_{\mathrm{Pr}}(t)}{\mathrm{d}t} &= -d_2 N_{\mathrm{Pr}}(t) + \left(r_1 + \beta\left(N_{\mathrm{D}}(t)\right)\right)\left(1 - \frac{N_{\mathrm{Pr}}(t)}{N_{\mathrm{P_{max}}}}\right) N_{\mathrm{Pr}}(t) + k_{12} N_{\mathrm{Sq}}(t) - m_1 N_{\mathrm{Pr}}(t) \\ &\quad - K_{21}\left(N_{\mathrm{Pr}}(t)\right) N_{\mathrm{Pr}}(t) - k_{23} N_{\mathrm{Pr}}(t),\end{aligned} \tag{8.25}$$

$$\frac{\mathrm{d}N_{\mathrm{Bs}}(t)}{\mathrm{d}t} = -d_3 N_{\mathrm{Bs}}(t) + k_{23} N_{\mathrm{Pr}}(t) - k_{34} N_{\mathrm{Bs}}(t) + r_2\left(1 - \frac{N_{\mathrm{Bs}}(t)}{N_{\mathrm{b_{max}}}}\right) N_{\mathrm{Bs}}(t), \tag{8.26}$$

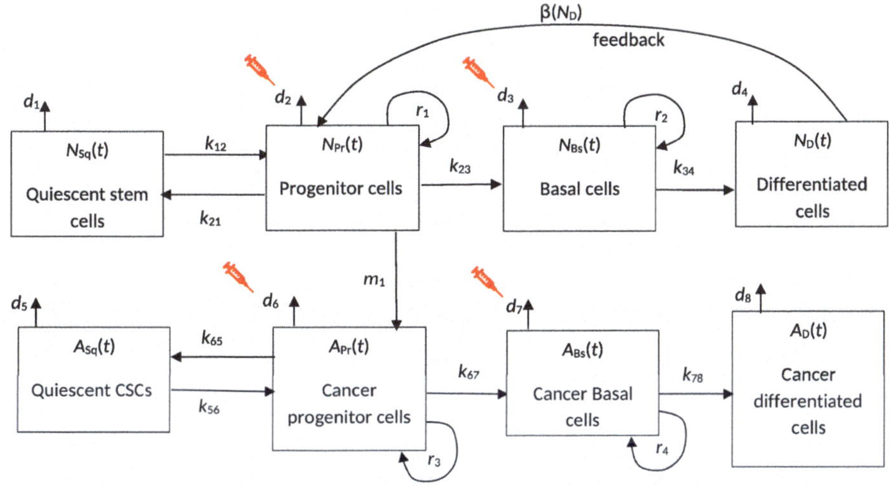

Fig. 8.6 An 8-compartmental model which shows the dynamics of normal and malignant stem cells. The overall dynamics involves apoptosis or therapy induced cell-death, cell transitions or cell differentiations, cell alterations, and self-renewal [49]. Feedback mechanism for the regulation of the number of cells are also shown

$$\frac{\mathrm{d}N_{\mathrm{D}}(t)}{\mathrm{d}t} = -d_4 N_{\mathrm{D}}(t) + k_{34} N_{\mathrm{Bs}}(t), \tag{8.27}$$

$$\frac{\mathrm{d}A_{\mathrm{Sq}}(t)}{\mathrm{d}t} = -d_5 A_{\mathrm{Sq}}(t) - k_{56} A_{\mathrm{Sq}}(t) + K_{65}\left(A_{\mathrm{Pr}}(t)\right) A_{\mathrm{Pr}}(t), \tag{8.28}$$

$$\begin{aligned}\frac{\mathrm{d}A_{\mathrm{Pr}}(t)}{\mathrm{d}t} &= -d_6 A_{\mathrm{Pr}}(t) + r_3\left(1 - \frac{A_{\mathrm{Pr}}(t)}{A_{\mathrm{Pmax}}}\right) A_{\mathrm{Pr}}(t) + k_{56} A_{\mathrm{Sq}}(t) - K_{65}\left(A_{\mathrm{Pr}}(t)\right) A_{\mathrm{Pr}}(t) \\ &\quad - k_{67} A_{\mathrm{Pr}}(t) + m_1 N_{\mathrm{Pr}}(t),\end{aligned} \tag{8.29}$$

$$\frac{\mathrm{d}A_{\mathrm{Bs}}(t)}{\mathrm{d}t} = -d_7 A_{\mathrm{Bs}}(t) + k_{67} A_{\mathrm{Pr}}(t) - k_{78} A_{\mathrm{Bs}}(t) + r_4\left(1 - \frac{A_{\mathrm{Bs}}(t)}{A_{\mathrm{bmax}}}\right) A_{\mathrm{Bs}}(t), \tag{8.30}$$

$$\frac{\mathrm{d}A_{\mathrm{D}}(t)}{\mathrm{d}t} = -d_8 A_{\mathrm{D}}(t) + k_{78} A_{\mathrm{Bs}}(t), \tag{8.31}$$

where $N_{\mathrm{Sq}}(t)$, $N_{\mathrm{Pr}}(t)$, $N_{\mathrm{Bs}}(t)$, and $N_{\mathrm{D}}(t)$ are non-malignant stem cell variants named according to their stages of differentiation and $A_{\mathrm{Sq}}(t)$, $A_{\mathrm{Pr}}(t)$, $A_{\mathrm{Bs}}(t)$, and $A_{\mathrm{D}}(t)$ are malignant stem cell variants named according to their stages of differentiation. As shown in Fig. 8.6, the non-malignant quiescent stem cells transition to active progenitor cells which are also called as transit cells. These cells become immature specialized cells, which are also known as early differentiating cells or basal cells which finally mature to specialized cells or differentiated cells. Similarly, the malignant quiescent stem cells or cancer stem cells (CSCs) transition to cancer progenitor cells, which then become immature cancer basal cells that finally mature to cancer differentiated cells. Here, k_{ij}, $i \neq j$, $i, j = 1, \ldots, 8$, denotes the cell transition rate of cells in the ith compartment to the jth compartment. Note that $K_{21}\left(N_{\mathrm{Pr}}(t)\right)$ and $K_{65}\left(A_{\mathrm{Pr}}(t)\right)$ are time-varying and are given by:

$$K_{21}\left(N_{\mathrm{Pr}}(t)\right)=k_{21}\left(1-\frac{N_{\mathrm{Pr}}(t)}{N_{\mathrm{Pr}}(t)+N_{\mathrm{Pr}\infty}}\right), \tag{8.32}$$

$$K_{65}\left(A_{\mathrm{Pr}}(t)\right)=k_{65}\left(1-\frac{A_{\mathrm{r}}(t)}{A_{\mathrm{Pr}}(t)+A_{\mathrm{Pr}\infty}}\right), \tag{8.33}$$

where $N_{\mathrm{Pr}\infty}$ and $A_{\mathrm{Pr}\infty}$ are saturation coefficients used to model the limitations in the transfer of normal and malignant progenitor cells to the quiescent compartment.

In (8.24)–(8.31), the first term accounts for the death of respective cell population, where d_i, $i=1,\ldots,7$, denotes the death rate when there is no treatment. In (8.24), the second term models the transition to progenitor cells and the last term $K_{21}\left(N_{\mathrm{Pr}}(t)\right)N_{\mathrm{Pr}}(t)$ models the increase in quiescent stem cells population in a logistical fashion as given by (8.32).

In (8.25), the second term accounts for the self-renewal and feedback, where r_1 is the rate of self renewal and $N_{\mathrm{p_{max}}}$ is the maximum number of progenitor cells (Fig. 8.6). The feedback term in (8.25) is given by $\beta\left(N_{\mathrm{D}}(t)\right)=\beta_0\left(1-\frac{N_{\mathrm{D}}(t)}{N_{\mathrm{D}}(t)+\kappa_0}\right)$, where β_0 denotes the feedback constant and κ_0 is a coefficient that limits the size of the differentiating cells. The term $m_1N_{\mathrm{Pr}}(t)$ in (8.25) and (8.29) model the mutation of normal progenitor cells to malignant ones, where m_1 is the mutation rate which oscillates randomly as captured by $m_1=m_0(1+w)$, m_0 is a constant, and $0<w<1$ is a random number. The last two terms in (8.25) model the cell transition of progenitor cells to quiescent and basal types.

In (8.26), the second and third terms account for the transitions of progenitor cells to basal cells and basal cells to specialized cells, respectively. The last term models the self-renewal of basal cells at a rate of r_2. The rate of self-renewal is limited by the maximum number of basal cells denoted as $N_{\mathrm{b_{max}}}$. In (8.27), the second term accounts for the differentiation of basal cells to specialized cell type. The term $k_{56}A_{\mathrm{Sq}}(t)$ in (8.28) and (8.29) accounts for the cell transition of quiescent cancer cells to cancer progenitor cells and the term $K_{65}\left(A_{\mathrm{Pr}}(t)\right)A_{\mathrm{Pr}}(t)$ in (8.28) and (8.29) models the increase in the number of quiescent CSCs in a logistical fashion as given by (8.33). The second term in (8.29) models the self-renewal of malignant progenitor cells at a rate of r_3 and $A_{\mathrm{p_{max}}}$ is the maximum number of progenitor cells. The term $k_{67}A_{\mathrm{Pr}}(t)$ in (8.29) and (8.30) models the cell transition of malignant progenitor cells to basal type and the term $r_4\left(1-\frac{A_{\mathrm{Bs}}(t)}{A_{\mathrm{b_{max}}}}\right)A_{\mathrm{Bs}}(t)$ in (8.29) models the self-renewal of malignant basal cells at a rate of r_4. The rate of self-renewal limited by the maximum number of malignant basal cells denoted as $A_{\mathrm{b_{max}}}$ and the term $k_{78}A_{\mathrm{Bs}}(t)$ in (8.30) and (8.31) accounts for the differentiation of malignant basal cells.

Note that, the model (8.24)–(8.31) does not have parameters that account for the effect of therapeutic intervention. In [49], the change in the cell dynamics under pulsed and continuous modes of treatment are also discussed by using time-varying parameters for the death rates such as $d_i'(t)$, $i=2,3,6,7$ instead of constant rates d_i, $i=2,3,6,7$ (Fig. 8.6). Time-varying death rates are defined for a pulsed mode of therapy during an interval $[t_{\mathrm{on}},t_{\mathrm{off}}]$ as follows:

$$d_2'(t) = \begin{cases} d_2 u_\mathrm{p}\left[1 + \delta\left(r_1 + \beta(N_\mathrm{D}(t))\right)\left(1 - \frac{N_\mathrm{Pr}(t)}{N_\mathrm{Pmax}}\right)\right], & t \in [t_\mathrm{on}, t_\mathrm{off}], \\ d_2 u_\mathrm{p}, & \text{otherwise}, \end{cases} \tag{8.34}$$

$$d_i'(t) = \begin{cases} 4 d_i u_\mathrm{p}, & t \in [t_\mathrm{on}, t_\mathrm{off},] \\ d_i u_\mathrm{p}, & \text{otherwise}, \end{cases} \quad i = 3, 6, 7, \tag{8.35}$$

and for the continuous mode of therapy as given by:

$$d_2'(t) = d_2 u_\mathrm{c}\left[1 + \delta\left(r_1 + \beta(N_\mathrm{D}(t))\right)\left(1 - \frac{N_\mathrm{Pr}(t)}{N_{\mathrm{P}_\mathrm{max}}}\right)\right], \tag{8.36}$$

$$d_i'(t) = d_i u_\mathrm{c}, i = 3, 6, 7, \tag{8.37}$$

where u_p and u_c denote the drug dose used for the pulsed and continuous modes of therapy. In (8.34) and (8.36), the term $1 + \delta\left(r_1 + \beta(N_\mathrm{D}(t))\right)\left(1 - \frac{N_\mathrm{Pr}(t)}{N_\mathrm{Pmax}}\right)$ is used to account for the effect of feedback in the treatment induced death rate, where δ is the dosage variation coefficient related to therapy. In the pulsed mode, treatment is applied only during $t = [t_\mathrm{on}, t_\mathrm{off}]$ and the increased cell-kill rate due to the application of drug during this interval is reflected in (8.35).

The main highlight of the model (8.24)–(8.31) is that this model accounts for the effect of treatment. However, the parameters are not validated against experimental data. While many positive and negative feedback paths are believed to regulate stem cell dynamics, only one is considered in this model [8]. Moreover, only the cytotoxic effects is accounted for in the cell-kill rate of the model parameter, the cytostatic effect of therapy such as inhibition of growth and proliferation are ignored.

Table 8.15 summarizes the parameter values of the stem cell therapy model (8.24)–(8.37) [49]. The initial conditions for the variables in model (8.24)–(8.37) are $N_\mathrm{Sq}(0) = 100$, $N_\mathrm{Pr}(0) = 1000$, $N_\mathrm{Bs}(0) = N_\mathrm{D}(0) = 2000$, $A_\mathrm{Sq}(0) = 5$, and $A_\mathrm{Pr}(0) = A_\mathrm{Bs}(0) = A_\mathrm{D}(0) = 0$.

Table 8.15 Parameter values of the stem cell therapy model (8.24)–(8.37) [49]

Param.	Value	Param.	Value	Param.	Value	Param.	Value
k_{21}	0.05	d_4	0.001	k_{12}	0.5	d_5	0.001
k_{23}	0.5	d_6	0.01	k_{34}	0.06	d_7	0.01
k_{65}	0.9	d_8	0.01	k_{56}	0.1	r_1	0.1
k_{67}	0.3	r_2	0.001	k_{78}	0.05	r_3	0.001
m_1	0.005–0.2	r_4	0.001	d_1	0.0001	$N_{\mathrm{Pr}\infty}$	100
d_2	0.001	$A_{\mathrm{Pr}\infty}$	100	d_3	0.01	N_Pmax	10000
A_Pmax	50000	N_bmax	10000	A_bmax	5000	k_{78}	0.05
κ_0	2000	β_0	1–5	u_p	30	u_c	10

8.4.2 Mathematical Model of Stem Cell Dynamics in the Bone Marrow and Peripheral Blood

In this subsection, a model of stem cell dynamics is presented which accounts for the differentiation and maturation of stem cells in the bone marrow (BM) and their movement to peripheral blood (PB) [43]. The potential starting point of many cancers is believed to be the stem cells. As shown in Fig. 8.7, in this model a small proportion of CSCs is derived from normal cells by mutation. Normal cells, blasts, and CSCs exist together in the BM. However, in the PB, normal cells and blasts exist together without any CSCs. There is a negligible loss of CSCs and blasts from BM and the blast cells are lost mainly in the PB. The model is given by [43]:

$$\frac{dN_{BM}(t)}{dt} = r_1 N_{BM}(t) \ln\left(\frac{b_1+b_2}{\theta_1 + N_{BM}(t)}\right) - m_1 N_{BM}(t) - \frac{m_2 N_{BM}(t) e^{-r_2 A_{PB}(t)}}{\theta_2 + N_{PB}(t)} - m_3 N_{BM}(t) - c_1 N_{BM}(t) A_{BM}(t), \tag{8.38}$$

$$\frac{dN_{PB}(t)}{dt} = -\frac{m_2 N_{BM}(t-\tau_1) e^{-\psi_1(t)}}{\theta_2 + N_{PB}(t-\tau_1)} - c_2 N_{PB}(t) A_{PB}(t) - d_1 N_{PB}(t), \tag{8.39}$$

$$\frac{dA_{BM}(t)}{dt} = r_3 A_{BM}(t) \ln \frac{b_3}{\theta_3 + A_{BM}(t)} + m_1 N_{BM}(t) - m_4 A_{BM}(t) + m_5 e^{-\psi_2(t)} A_S(t-\tau_2), \tag{8.40}$$

$$\frac{dA_{PB}(t)}{dt} = m_4 A_{BM}(t) - d_2 A_{PB}(t), \tag{8.41}$$

$$\frac{dA_S(t)}{dt} = r_5 A_S(t)\left(1 - b_4 A_S(t)\right) - m_5 e^{-r_4 A_{PB}(t)} A_S(t) + m_3 N_{BM}(t), \tag{8.42}$$

where $N_{BM}(t)$ and $N_{PB}(t)$ are the normal BM and PB cells, respectively, $A_{BM}(t)$ is the number of malignant BM cells (blasts), $A_{PB}(t)$ is the number of malignant PB cells, and $A_S(t)$ is the number of cancer stem cells.

In (8.38), the term $r_1 N_{BM}(t) \ln\left(\frac{b_1+b_2}{\theta_1+N_{BM}(t)}\right)$ accounts for the regulation of the number of healthy cells in the BM ($N_{BM}(t)$) by the growth and renewal of stem cells, where r_1 is the growth rate of the normal BM cells, b_1 and b_2 denote the carrying capacities of healthy cells in BM and PB, respectively, the constant θ_1 denotes the threshold population level of healthy BM cells that ensures the cell growth and cell renewal for maintaining a healthy number of cells within the total carrying capacity $b_1 + b_2$. The second term in (8.38) models the possible mutation of normal BM cells into blasts, where m_1 is the rate of mutation. The term $\frac{m_2 N_{BM}(t) e^{-r_2 A_{PB}(t)}}{\theta_2 + N_{PB}(t)}$ accounts for the movement of normal BM cells to normal PB cells, where m_2 is the rate of movement, the constant θ_2 denotes the threshold population level of healthy BM cells at which the rate of movement is half of the maximal release of BM cells to PB, and r_2 is the growth rate of PB cells after time-lag of τ_1. The term $m_3 N_{BM}(t)$ accounts for the probabilistic mutation of the normal cells in the BM to CSCs, where m_3 is the mutation rate. The last term in (8.38) models the inhibition of malignant BM cells over healthy BM cells, where c_1 is the inhibition rate or competition rate.

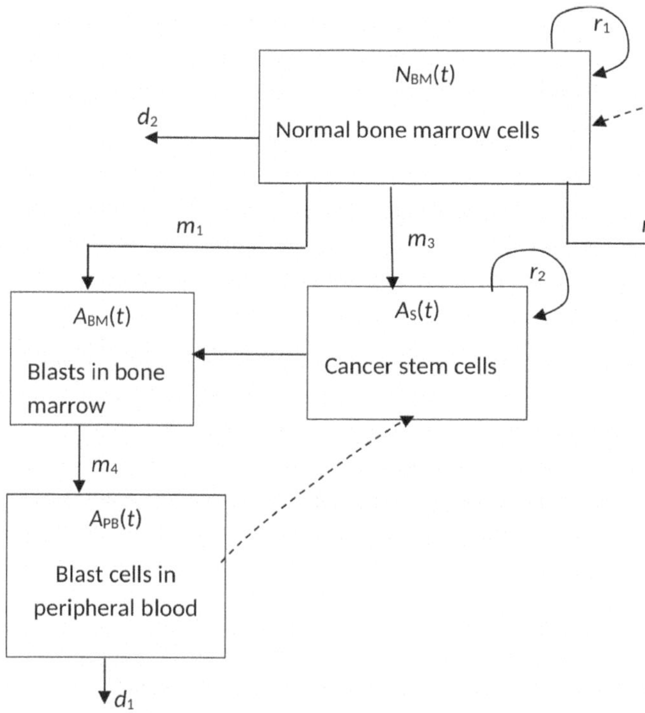

Fig. 8.7 Illustrative diagram showing various cell alterations (transitions) in bone marrow (BM) and peripheral blood (PB) as given by model (8.38)–(8.41). Normal cells, blasts, and CSCs exist together in the BM. However, in the PB, normal cells and blasts exist together without any CSCs. Normal BM cells and CSCs are capable of self-renewal. The dotted lines show the feedback paths [43]

In (8.39), the first term is similar to the third term in (8.38) except for the additional time-lag τ_1 and the exponent ψ_1. Here, τ_1 accounts for the time required for the maturation of BM cells before they transit to PB and $\psi_1(t) = \alpha_1\tau_1 + r_2 A_{PB}(t - \tau_1)$, where α_1 models the arrival rate of healthy BM cells after the maturation and transit time. The term $c_2 N_{PB}(t) A_{PB}(t)$ in (8.39) models the inhibition of malignant PB cells over healthy PB cells, where c_2 is the inhibition rate or competition rate. The last term in (8.39) models death or disappearance of healthy PB cells, where d_1 is the death rate.

Blast cells are assumed to arise as a result of the mutation of normal cells and these cells have no self-renewal capability and they grow with normal cells and hinder the latter's growth. This fact is modeled in (8.40), where the term $r_3 A_{BM}(t) \ln \frac{b_3}{\theta_3 + A_{BM}(t)}$ accounts for the growth of BM, with b_3 as the carrying capacity of all cells in BM and PB, and θ_3 as the threshold population-level related to malignant BM cells that favors malignant cell growth towards the maximum allowable value b_3. The term $m_1 N_{BM}(t)$ in (8.38) and (8.40) denotes the mutation of normal BM cells into blasts and the term $m_4 A_{BM}(t)$ in (8.40) and (8.41) denotes the transition of blasts in BM cells into blasts in PB. The cells in the BM divide and differentiate to compensate for all depleted cells in the PB. The cells in the BM restrain replication if there is an excess of or accumulation of certain cell types. Thus, the researchers suggest the existence of a feedback mechanism between PB and BM and CSCs may be converted into blasts due to this feedback mechanism [43]. The term $m_5 e^{-\psi_2(t)} A_S(t-\tau_2)$ in (8.40) accounts for this conversion of CSCs to malignant blasts, where m_5 is the transition rate. Here, $\psi_2(t) = \alpha_2\tau_2 + r_4 A_{PB}(t-\tau_2)$, where α_2 is the conversion rate, τ_2 is the time for conversion of CSCs to non-stem malignant cells, and r_4 is the growth rate of PB cells after a time lag of τ_2.

In (8.41), the term $d_2 A_{PB}(t)$ accounts for the cell loss, where d_2 is the rate of loss. In (8.42), the term $r_5 A_S(t)\,(1 - b_4 A_S(t))$ accounts for the self renewal and growth of CSCs, where r_5 is the increase rate, b_4 is the reciprocal carrying capacity of CSCs and the term $m_5 e^{-r_4 A_{PB}(t)} A_S(t)$ models the conversion of CSCs to blast cells.

This model accounts for two feedback mechanisms as shown in Fig. 8.7, one which regulates the healthy PB cells that triggers or inhibits the production of $N_{PB}(t)$ from $N_{BM}(t)$, and the second one is the feedback from $A_{PB}(t)$ to $A_S(t)$ which is believed to regulate the number of blast cells in the PB [43]. This model accounts for two time-lags involved in the cell transitions phases of cells. Here, the term τ_1 used to denote the maturation transit time of the normal cells from the BM to specialized cells in the PB (i.e. $N_{BM}(t)$ to $N_{PB}(t)$) and the term τ_2 models the time lag between the conversion of CSCs to blast cells (non-stem malignant cells) in the BM (i.e. $A_S(t)$ to $A_{BM}(t)$).

Table 8.16 summarizes the parameter values of the stem cell therapy model (8.38)–(8.42) [43]. The initial conditions for the variables in model (8.38)–(8.42) are $N_{BM}(0) = 10 \times 10^{12}$ (cells), $N_{PB}(0) = 3.5 \times 10^9$ (cells), $A_{BM}(0) = 0.4 \times 10^{12}$ (cells), $A_{PB}(0) = 0.05 \times 10^{11}$ (cells), and $A_S(0) = 10^5$ (cells).

8.4.3 Model of Leukemia Stem Cell Dynamics

In this subsection, a five cell population model is presented which includes hematopoietic stem cells (HSCs), progenitor cells, differentiated blood cells, leukemia stem cells (LSCs), and differentiated leukemia cells [44]. In this model, like the normal HSCs, LSCs, and their respective progenitors are assumed to reside in the BM (ecological niche) and migrate to PB after differentiation and maturation. Similar to the models (8.24)–(8.31) and (8.38)–(8.42) discussed in the earlier subsections, which account for the cell transition between BM and PB, the model discussed in this subsection presents the dynamics of LSCs in terms of their differentiation patterns. Moreover, three feedback pathways involved in the regulation of LSCs are also discussed. As shown in Figs. 8.4 and 8.7, the model discussed in [44] accounts for the self-renewal, symmetrical differentiation, and feedback associated with HSCs and LSCs. The model is given by:

Table 8.16 Parameter values of the stem cell therapy model (8.38)–(8.42) [43]

Parameter	Value (unit)	Parameter	Value (unit)
r_1	0.002–0.149 (hours^{-1})	b_1	1×10^{10}–5.8×10^{13} (cells L^{-1})
$\theta_1, \theta_2, \theta_3$	1×10^{10}–5×10^{11} (cells L^{-1})	b_2	1×10^{12}–1×10^{13} (cells L^{-1})
m_1	0.0013–0.0154 (hours^{-1})	m_2	9×10^{2}–1.23×10^{5} (hours^{-1})
r_2	1×10^{-13}–1×10^{-12} (L cells^{-1})	m_3	1×10^{-7}–1×10^{-3} (hours^{-1})
c_1, c_2	1×10^{-14}–5×10^{-6}	α_1	0.02–0.11 (hours^{-1})
τ_1	96–144 (hours)	d_1	0.00001–0.0083 (hours^{-1})
r_3	0.00396 ± 0.04825 (hours^{-1})	b_3	6×10^{12}–3.688×10^{14} (cells L^{-1})
m_4	0.0065-0.0565 (hours^{-1})	m_5	0.0001–0.05 (hours^{-1})
α_2	0.002–0.02 (hours^{-1})	τ_2	576–1440 (hours)
d_2	0.001–0.2 (hours^{-1})	r_5	0.0001–0.05 (hours^{-1})
b_4	1×10^{-6}–0.33×10^{-4} (L cells^{-1})	r_4	1×10^{-13}–1×10^{-12} (L cells^{-1})

$$\frac{\mathrm{d}N_{\mathrm{S}}(t)}{\mathrm{d}t} = N_{\mathrm{S}}(t)e^{-\psi_1(t)}\left(r_1 - m_1e^{-\psi_3(t)}\right) - d_1N_{\mathrm{S}}(t), \tag{8.43}$$

$$\frac{\mathrm{d}N_{\mathrm{Pr}}(t)}{\mathrm{d}t} = N_{\mathrm{S}}(t)e^{-\psi_1(t)}\left(r_2e^{-\psi_2(t)} + 2m_1e^{-\psi_3(t)}\right) + (r_3 - d_2)\,N_{\mathrm{Pr}}(t), \tag{8.44}$$

$$\frac{\mathrm{d}N_{\mathrm{D}}(t)}{\mathrm{d}t} = m_2d_2N_{\mathrm{Pr}}(t) - d_3N_{\mathrm{D}}(t), \tag{8.45}$$

$$\frac{\mathrm{d}A_{\mathrm{S}}(t)}{\mathrm{d}t} = A_{\mathrm{S}}(t)e^{-\psi_1(t)}\left(r_4 - m_3e^{-\psi_3(t)}\right) - d_4A_{\mathrm{S}}(t), \tag{8.46}$$

$$\frac{\mathrm{d}A_{\mathrm{D}}(t)}{\mathrm{d}t} = A_{\mathrm{S}}(t)e^{-\psi_1(t)}\left(r_5e^{-\psi_2(t)} + 2m_3e^{-\psi_3(t)}\right) - d_5A_{\mathrm{D}}(t), \tag{8.47}$$

where $N_{\mathrm{S}}(t)$, $N_{\mathrm{Pr}}(t)$, $N_{\mathrm{D}}(t)$, $A_{\mathrm{S}}(t)$, and $A_{\mathrm{D}}(t)$ are normal HSCs, normal progenitors derived from HSCs, normal differentiated cells, LSCs, and differentiated leukemia cells, respectively. The number of cells in each type are incorporated in the feedback term used to regulate the replication, self-renewal, and differentiation of associated stem cells. Accordingly, in the model (8.43)–(8.47), the feedback gains β_i, $i = 1, 2, 3$, are used to as follows:

$$\psi_1(t) = \beta_1 \left(N_S(t) + A_s(t)\right), \tag{8.48}$$
$$\psi_2(t) = \beta_2 \left(N_{Pr}(t) + N_D(t) + A_D(t)\right), \tag{8.49}$$
$$\psi_3(t) = \beta_3 \left(N_{Pr}(t) + N_D(t) + A_D(t)\right). \tag{8.50}$$

Here, $\psi_1(t)$ models the influence of normal CSCs and LSCs on the self-renewal ((8.43) and (8.46)) as well as in the production of the normal progeny and differentiated leukemia cells. In (8.43), the first term accounts for feedback, self-renewal, and cell differentiation, where $\psi_1(t)$ and $\psi_3(t)$ model the feedback mechanisms, r_1 denotes the symmetrical renewal rate, and m_1 is the rate of symmetric cell differentiation (HSC to two progenitor cells). The last term in (8.43) models the cell-loss, where d_1 is the death rate.

Similar to (8.43), the term $N_S(t)e^{-\psi_1(t)}r_2e^{-\psi_2(t)}$ in (8.44) accounts for the increase in the number of progenitors derived from HSCs, where r_2 denotes the rate of replication of HSC to one HSC and one progenitor cell. This is shown as asymmetrical renewal in Fig. 8.4. The term $N_S(t)e^{-\psi_1(t)}2m_1e^{-\psi_3(t)}$ in (8.44) accounts for the increase in the number of progenitors derived from HSCs via symmetrical differentiation. As shown in Fig. 8.4, one HSC can replicate to give two progenitors. The parameter r_3 accounts for the rate of proliferation of progenitors. As mentioned earlier, the change in the number of each cell population may be due to replication, migration from BM to PB, differentiation, or apoptosis. The parameter d_2 denotes the rate of disappearance of progenitor cells due to cell differentiation, migration, or apoptosis.

In (8.45), the rate of transition of progenitors to specific normal cells is modeled in terms of the transition rate m_2 and the death rate d_3. Similar to (8.43), in (8.46) the symmetrical self-renewal, symmetrical differentiation, and migration/death is modeled in terms of r_4, m_3, and d_4, respectively. Finally, in (8.47), increase in the number of differentiated cancer cells due to asymmetrical renewal and symmetrical differentiation of LSCs is modeled in terms of r_5 and m_3, where r_5 accounts for the uncontrolled growth rate of leukemia cells. The last term in (8.47) models the migration/death of differentiated leukemia cells.

Table 8.17 summarizes the parameter values of the stem cell therapy model (8.43)–(8.50). The values are from [44] and the supplementary material of [44].

Table 8.17 Parameter values of the stem cell therapy model (8.43)–(8.50) [44]

Parameter	Value	Parameter	Value
r_1, r_3	0.0–1.5	m_1	0.0–1.0
d_1	0.0–2.0	r_2, r_4, r_5	0.0–0.8
d_2	0.0–1.5	m_2, m_3	0.0–0.8
d_3, d_4, d_5	0.0–0.8	$\beta_1, \beta_2, \beta_3$	0.01

8.5 Summary

In this chapter, several mathematical models in the areas of gene therapy, oncolytic virotherapy, nanocarrier-based therapy, and stem cell therapy are discussed. Targeted treatment can particularly annihilate cancer cells and cause comparatively less systemic toxicity. Out of the many possible vectors for gene therapy, virus-mediated therapy is the most discussed type. Mathematical models of gene therapy mediated by non-viral vectors such as bacteria, liposome, and nanoparticles are scarce [58]. Even though gene therapy using plasmid DNA encoding INF-α and TGF-β gene silencing have been investigated experimentally, mathematical models of such methods are yet to be devised [7, 59–61]. Similarly, there exist some mathematical model-based investigations on nanocarrier-based cancer therapy, those models mainly focus on the use of nanoparticle drug pair for targeted drug delivery. Mathematical models of liposome-mediated drug release kinetics various gene therapeutic approaches are reported in [62, 63]. However, the dynamics of various cell types in the tumor microenvironment and immune response concerning nanocarrier-based therapy are yet to be investigated using mathematical models.

As mentioned earlier, even though many mathematical models discussed stem cell dynamics, most of the models do not study the effect of stem cell-based therapeutic interventions in curtailing cancer progression. Instead, stem cell differentiation and its regulation mechanisms are investigated. Out of the three stem cell-based models discussed in this chapter, only one model accounts for the drug effect. The model that accounted for the effects of therapy ((8.24)–(8.37)) replaced the death rate of respective cells in no treatment case by a time-varying death rate when treatment is involved. This model considers only the apoptotic effects of the drug and ignores cancer regression by inhibition of proliferation. Moreover, this model is not validated using experimental data. In [64], it is pointed out that, there exist a paradoxical relationship between the overall stem cell count and the death rate of stem cells. More investigations are imperative in this area to understand important feedback mechanisms related to stem cell dynamics [65, 66]. Gene therapy, nanocarrier mediated therapy, and stem cell-based therapy are novel areas of cancer research that need elaborate theoretical and experimental support to expand to their full potential.

References

1. D. Pardoll, Immunotherapy with cytokine gene-transduced tumor cells: the next wave in gene therapy for cancer. Curr. Opin. Oncol. **4**(6), 1124–1129 (1992)
2. A.T.C. Cheuk, G.J. Mufti, B.A. Guinn, Role of 4-1BB:4-1BB ligand in cancer immunotherapy. Cancer Gene Ther. **11**, 215–226 (2004)
3. M.M. Hulou, C.F. Cho, E.A. Chiocca, R. Bjerkvig, Chapter 11 - Experimental therapies: gene therapies and oncolytic viruses, in *Gliomas. Handbook of Clinical Neurology*, vol. 134 (Elsevier, Amsterdam, 2016), pp. 183–197

4. A. Tsygvintsev, S. Marino, D.E. Kirschner, A mathematical model of gene therapy for the treatment of cancer, in *Mathematical Methods and Models in Biomedicine* (2013)
5. S.A. Kaliberov, D.J. Buchsbaum, Cancer treatment with gene therapy and radiation therapy, *Advances in Cancer Research*, vol. 115 (Elsevier, Amsterdam, 2012), pp. 221–263
6. P.F. Robbins, R.A. Morgan, S.A. Feldman, J.C. Yang, R.M. Sherry, M.E. Dudley, J.R. Wunderlich, A.V. Nahvi, L.J. Helman, C.L. Mackall, U.S. Kammula, M.S. Hughes, N.P. Restifo, M. Raffeld, C.C.R. Lee, C.L. Levy, Y.F. Li, M. El Gamil, S.L. Schwarz, C. Laurencot, S.A. Rosenberg, Tumor regression in patients with metastatic synovial cell sarcoma and melanoma using genetically engineered lymphocytes reactive with NY-ESO-1. J. Clin. Oncol. **29**(7), 917–924 (2011)
7. J. Arciero, T. Jackson, D. Kirschner, A mathematical model of tumor-immune evasion and siRNA treatment. Discret. Contin. Dyn. Syst. - B **4**, 39 (2004)
8. B.D. Aguda, Y. Kim, M.G. Piper-Hunter, A. Friedman, C.B. Marsh, MicroRNA regulation of a cancer network: consequences of the feedback loops involving miR-17-92, E2F, and Myc. Proc. Natl. Acad. Sci. **105**(50), 19678–19683 (2008)
9. M. Sedighi, A. Zahedi Bialvaei, M.R. Hamblin, E. Ohadi, A. Asadi, M. Halajzadeh, V. Lohrasbi, N. Mohammadzadeh, T. Amiriani, M. Krutova et al., Therapeutic bacteria to combat cancer; current advances, challenges, and opportunities. Cancer Med. **8**(6), 3167–3181 (2019)
10. M.F. Naso, B. Tomkowicz, W.L. Perry, W.R. Strohl, Adeno-associated virus (AAV) as a vector for gene therapy. BioDrugs **31**(4), 317–334 (2017)
11. Z. Li, W. Ho, X. Bai, F. Li, Y.-J. Chen, X.-Q. Zhang, X. Xu, Nanoparticle depots for controlled and sustained gene delivery. J. Control. Release (2020)
12. A. Nyamay'Antu, M. Dumont, V. Kedinger, P. Erbacher, Non-viral vector mediated gene delivery: the outsider to watch out for in gene therapy. Cell Gene Ther. Insights **5**, 51–57 (2019)
13. S.F. Kruger, B.L. Cadilha, M.V. Bergwelt Baildon, S. Endres, S. Kobold, Challenges in clinical trial design for T cell-based cancer immunotherapy. Clin. Pharmacol. Ther. (1), 47–49 (2020)
14. J.E. Talmadge, K.H. Cowan, Gene therapy in oncology, in *Abeloff's Clinical Oncology* (Elsevier, Amsterdam, 2020), pp. 470–485
15. T. Adam, A.S. Charles, J.T. Panteli, Z.J. Brentzel, N.S. Forbes, Bacterial delivery of staphylococcus aureus α-hemolysin causes regression and necrosis in murine tumors. Mol. Ther. **22**(7), 1266–1274 (2014)
16. D. Kirschner, J.C. Panetta, Modeling immunotherapy of the tumor-immune interaction. J. Math. Biol. **37**(3), 235–252 (1998)
17. S.B. Jakowlew, Transforming growth factor-β in cancer and metastasis. Cancer Metastasis Rev. **25**(3), 435 (2006)
18. A.L. Jenner, A.C.F. Coster, P.S. Kim, F. Frascoli, Treating cancerous cells with viruses: insights from a minimal model for oncolytic virotherapy. Lett. Biomath. **5**(sup1), S117–S136 (2018)
19. A.S. Novozhilov, F.S. Berezovskaya, E.V. Koonin, G.P. Karev, Mathematical modeling of tumor therapy with oncolytic viruses: regimes with complete tumor elimination within the framework of deterministic models. Biol. Direct **1**, 6 (2006)
20. L. Li, S. Liu, D. Han, B. Tang, J. Ma, Delivery and biosafety of oncolytic virotherapy. Front. Oncol. **10**, 475 (2020)
21. M. Farrera Sal, C. Fillat, R. Alemany, Effect of transgene location, transcriptional control elements and transgene features in armed oncolytic adenoviruses. Cancers **12**(4), 1034 (2020)
22. G.P. Karev, A.S. Novozhilov, E.V. Koonin, Mathematical modeling of tumor therapy with oncolytic viruses: effects of parametric heterogeneity on cell dynamics. Biol. Direct **1**, 30 (2006)
23. P.S. Kim, J.J. Crivelli, I.K. Choi, C.O. Yun, J.R. Wares, Quantitative impact of immunomodulation versus oncolysis with cytokine-expressing virus therapeutics. Math. Biosci. Eng. **12**, 841 (2015)
24. J.L. Gevertz, J. Wares, Developing a minimally structured mathematical model of cancer treatment with oncolytic viruses and dendritic cell injections. Comput. Math. Methods Med. **2018**, 1–14 (2018)

25. J.R. Wares, J.J. Crivelli, C.O. Yun, I.K. Choi, J.L. Gevertz, P.S. Kim, Treatment strategies for combining immunostimulatory oncolytic virus therapeutics with dendritic cell injections. Math. Biosci. Eng. **12**, 1237 (2015)
26. C.S. Holling, The components of predation as revealed by a study of small-mammal predation of the European pine sawfly. Can. Entomol. **91**(5), 293–320 (1959)
27. R. Arditi, L.R. Ginzburg, Coupling in predator-prey dynamics: Ratio-dependence. J. Theor. Biol. **139**(3), 311–326 (1989)
28. J.H. Huang, S.N. Zhang, K.J. Choi, I.K. Choi, J.H. Kim, M. Lee, H. Kim, C.O. Yun, Therapeutic and tumor-specific immunity induced by combination of dendritic cells and oncolytic adenovirus expressing IL-12 and 4–1BBL. Mol. Ther. **18**(2), 264–274 (2010)
29. P. Dogra, J. Butner, Y.l. Chuang, S. Caserta, S. Goel, C. Brinker, V. Cristini, Z. Wang, Mathematical modeling in cancer nanomedicine: a review. Biomed. Microdevices **21** (2019)
30. L. Gianni, M. Mansutti, A. Anton, L. Calvo, G. Bisagni, B. Bermejo, V. Semiglazov, M. Thill, J.I. Chacon, A. Chan et al., Comparing neoadjuvant nab-paclitaxel vs paclitaxel both followed by anthracycline regimens in women with ERBB2/HER2-negative breast cancer-the evaluating treatment with neoadjuvant abraxane (ETNA) trial: A randomized Phase 3 clinical trial. JAMA Oncol. **4**(3), 302–308 (2018)
31. A. Singh, Evaluation of magnetic nanoparticle of irinotecan for personalized treatment of colorectal cancer. Ann. Oncol **30**(Sup1) (2019)
32. A.L.C. Maia, C.A. Ferreira, A.L.B. Barros, A.T.M. Silva, G.A. Ramaldes, A. Silva Cunha Júnior, D.C.P. Oliveira, C. Fernandes, D.C. Ferreira Soares, Vincristine-loaded hydroxyapatite nanoparticles as a potential delivery system for bone cancer therapy. J. Drug Target. **26**(7), 592–603 (2018)
33. T. Brocato, E. Coker, P. Durfee, Y.S. Lin, J. Townson, E.F. Wyckoff, V. Cristini, C. Brinker, Z. Wang, Understanding the connection between nanoparticle uptake and cancer treatment efficacy using mathematical modeling. Sci. Rep. **8** (2018)
34. F. Gentile, M. Ferrari, P. Decuzzi, The transport of nanoparticles in blood vessels: the effect of vessel permeability and blood rheology. Ann. Biomed. Eng. **36**, 254–261 (2008). Feb
35. K.M. Tsoi, S.A. MacParland, M. Ma, V. Spetzler, J. Echeverri, B. Ouyang, S.M. Fadel, E. Sykes, N. Goldaracena et al., Mechanism of hard-nanomaterial clearance by the liver. Nat. Mater. **15** (2016)
36. D. Dell'Orco, M. Lundqvist, T. Cedervall, S. Linse, Delivery success rate of engineered nanoparticles in the presence of the protein corona: a systems-level screening. Nanomedicine: Nanotechnol. Biol. Med. **8**(8), 1271–1281 (2012)
37. D. Dell'Orco, M. Lundqvist, C. Oslakovic, T. Cedervall, S. Linse, Modeling the time evolution of the nanoparticle-protein corona in a body fluid. PloS One **5**, e10949 (2010)
38. N.L. Adolphi, Z. Wang, Y.S. Lin, K.S. Butler, P.N. Durfee, J.G. Croissant, A. Noureddine, E.N. Coker, E.L. Bearer, V. Cristini, C.J. Brinker, Establishing the effects of mesoporous silica nanoparticle properties on in vivo disposition using imaging-based pharmacokinetics. Nat. Commun. **9**(1), 4551 (2018)
39. B.S Hendriks, J.G. Reynolds, S. Klinz, E. Geretti, H. Lee, S. Leonard, D. Gaddy, C. Espelin, U. Nielsen, T. Wickham, Multiscale kinetic modeling of liposomal doxorubicin delivery quantifies the role of tumor and drug-specific parameters in local delivery to tumors. CPT: Pharmacomet. Syst. Pharmacol. **1**, e15 (2012)
40. S. Stapleton, M. Milosevic, C. Allen, J. Zheng, M. Dunne, I. Yeung, D.A. Jaffray, A mathematical model of the enhanced permeability and retention effect for liposome transport in solid tumors. PloS One **8**, e81157 (2013)
41. J. Pascal, C. Ashley, Z. Wang, T. Brocato, J. Butner, E. Carnes, E. Koay, C. Brinker, V. Cristini, Mechanistic modeling identifies drug-uptake history as predictor of tumor drug resistance and nano-carrier-mediated response. ACS Nano **7** (2013)
42. H.A. Miller, H.B. Frieboes, Evaluation of drug-loaded gold nanoparticle cytotoxicity as a function of tumor vasculature-induced tissue heterogeneity. Ann. Biomed. Eng. **47**, 257–271 (2019). Jan

43. E.K. Afenya, R. Ouifki, S.D. Mundle, Mathematical modeling of bone marrow-peripheral blood dynamics in the disease state based on current emerging paradigms, Part II. J. Theor. Biol. **460**, 37–55 (2019)
44. A.L. MacLean, C.L. Celso, M.P.H. Stumpf, Population dynamics of normal and leukaemia stem cells in the haematopoietic stem cell niche show distinct regimes where leukaemia will be controlled. J. R. Soc. Interface **10**(81) (2013)
45. E. Papapetrou, Patient-derived induced pluripotent stem cells in cancer research and precision oncology. Nat. Med. **22**, 1392–1401 (2016)
46. R. Molina-Peña, M. Alvarez, A simple mathematical model based on the cancer stem cell hypothesis suggests kinetic commonalities in solid tumor growth. PloS One **7**, e26233 (2012)
47. S.N. Gentry, T. Jackson, A mathematical model of cancer stem cell driven tumor initiation: implications of niche size and loss of homeostatic regulatory mechanisms. PloS One **8**, e71128 (2013)
48. S.L. Elliott, E. Kose, A.L. Lewis, A.E. Steinfeld, E.A. Zollinger, Modeling the stem cell hypothesis: investigating the effects of cancer stem cells and TGF- β on tumor growth (2019)
49. C. Calmelet, A. Prokop, J. Mensah, L. McCawley, P. Crooke, Modeling the cancer stem cell hypothesis. Math. Model. Nat. Phenom. **5**(3), 40–62 (2010)
50. J. Zhao, Cancer stem cells and chemoresistance: the smartest survives the raid. Pharmacol. Ther. **160** (2016)
51. R. Ganguly, I. Puri, Mathematical model for the cancer stem cell hypothesis. Cell Prolif. **39**, 3–14 (2006)
52. W. Jiang, J. Peng, Y. Zhang, W.C.S. Cho, K. Jin, The implications of cancer stem cells for cancer therapy. Int. J. Mol. Sci. **13**(12), 16636–16657 (2012)
53. A.A. Barkal, R.E. Brewer, M. Markovic, M. Kowarsky, S.A. Barkal, B.W. Zaro, V. Krishnan, J. Hatakeyama, O. Dorigo, L.J. Barkal, I.L. Weissman, CD24 signalling through macrophage Siglec-10 is a target for cancer immunotherapy. Nature 1476–4687 (2019)
54. M.D. Johnston, C. Dunlop, W. Bodmer, P. Maini, S. Chapman, Examples of mathematical modeling: tales from the crypt. Cell Cycle **6**, 2106–12 (2007)
55. M.D. Johnston, P.K. Maini, S.J. Chapman, C.M. Edwards, W.F. Bodmer, On the proportion of cancer stem cells in a tumour. J. Theor. Biol. **266**(4), 708–711 (2010)
56. J. Demongeot, M. Kaufman, R. Thomas, Positive feedback circuits and memory. Comptes Rendus de l'Académie des Sciences. Série III, Sciences de la vie **323**, 69–79 (2000)
57. A.B. Pardee, Regulatory molecular biology. Cell Cycle **5**, 846–52 (2006)
58. G. Banks, R. Roselli, R. Chen, T. Giorgio, A model for the analysis of nonviral gene therapy. Gene Ther. **10**(20), 1766–1775 (2003)
59. H.M. Horton, D. Anderson, P. Hernandez, K.M. Barnhart, J.A. Norman, S.E. Parker, A gene therapy for cancer using intramuscular injection of plasmid DNA encoding interferon α. Proc. Natl. Acad. Sci. **96**(4), 1553–1558 (1999)
60. H. Yoshizawa, Y. Morishita, M. Watanabe, K. Ishibashi, S. Muto, E. Kusano, D. Nagata, TGF-β 1-siRNA delivery with nanoparticles inhibits peritoneal fibrosis. Gene Ther. **22**(4), 333–340 (2015)
61. F.O. Aval, S.A. Amiri, A. Azadmehr, M. Oladnabi, P. Saadat, H. Ebrahimi, B. Baradaran, B. Mansoori, F. Pourabdolhossein, P. Torabian et al., Gene silencing of TGFβRII can inhibit glioblastoma cell growth. Asian Pac. J. Cancer Prev. **19**(9), 2681 (2018)
62. Z.P. Parra-Guillén, G. González-Aseguinolaza, P. Berraondo, I.F. Trocóniz, Gene therapy: a pharmacokinetic/pharmacodynamic modelling overview. Pharm. Res. **27**(8), 1487–1497 (2010)
63. F. Haghiralsadat, G. Amoabediny, M.N. Helder, S. Naderinezhad, M.H. Sheikhha, T. Forouzanfar, B. Zandieh-doulabi, A comprehensive mathematical model of drug release kinetics from nano-liposomes, derived from optimization studies of cationic PEGylated liposomal doxorubicin formulations for drug-gene delivery. Artif. Cells Nanomedicine Biotechnol. **46**(1), 169–177 (2018)

64. T. Hillen, H. Enderling, P. Hahnfeldt, The tumor growth paradox and immune system-mediated selection for cancer stem cells. Bull. Math. Biol. **75**, 11 (2012)
65. T. Stiehl, N. Baran, A.D. Ho, A. Marciniak Czochra, Cell division patterns in acute myeloid leukemia stem-like cells determine clinical course: a model to predict patient survival. Cancer Res. **75**(6), 940–949 (2015)
66. B. Werner, J.G. Scott, A. Sottoriva, A.R. Anderson, A. Traulsen, P.M. Altrock, The cancer stem cell fraction in hierarchically organized tumors can be estimated using mathematical modeling and patient-specific treatment trajectories. Cancer Res. **76**(7), 1705–1713 (2016)

Chapter 9
Combination Therapy Models

Experimental and clinical evidence suggest that many single agent-based therapeutic approaches that are discussed in Chaps. 3–8 show an improved potency (additive or synergistic effects) when used in combination [1–5]. Such combination therapy approaches can bring together the positive aspects of each therapy method involved to improve the overall therapeutic efficacy and patient outcome. For instance, ionizing radiations are capable of increasing the immunogenicity of the tumor micro-environment [6]. Hence, using radiotherapy before or along with immunotherapy enhances the efficacy of immunotherapy [7]. Specifically, during radiation-induced apoptosis, the tumor cells release certain antigens, and these antigens help the immune cells to identify the otherwise hiding tumor cells [1, 7]. Another example is the combination of immunotherapy with oncolytic virotherapy. As shown in Fig. 8.3, the viruses replicate inside the cancer cells and they burst to release virions, cytokines, TAA, and tumor cell debris. This will attract the attention of more circulating lymphocyte to the tumor micro-environment. In general, compared to monotherapy, combination therapy-based treatments demonstrate improved patient outcome in terms of delayed tumor relapse, reduced drug toxicity and drug resistance, and improved patient survival [2, 8].

Due to the encouraging outcomes of combination therapy, many novel combinations are currently under investigation to disseminate better treatment options for various types of cancers [9, 10]. This new trend, in turn, poses several open questions regarding the optimal combination of drug doses and treatment schedules. Along with the animal model-based experiments and clinical trials, mathematical model-based studies can be also used to conduct cost-effective and risk-free investigations to draw mechanistic insights in this regard. However, not all combination therapy approaches that are currently being practiced have corresponding mathematical models. Hence, in the first four sections of this chapter, some of the mathematical models of combination therapy that are available in the literature are discussed and then specific research gaps are pointed out in Sect. 9.5.

R. Padmanabhan et al., *Mathematical Models of Cancer and Different Therapies*, Series in BioEngineering, https://doi.org/10.1007/978-981-15-8640-8_9

Table 9.1 Notations used to model the drug dynamics term of various therapies discussed in this chapter

Var.	Description	Var.	Description
$U_{\mathrm{Ch}}(t)$	Concentration of chemotherapeutic drug	$U_{\mathrm{Im}}(t)$	Concentration of immunotherapeutic drug
$U_{\mathrm{An}}(t)$	Concentration of anti-angiogenic agent	$V(t)$	Number of viruses
$U_{\mathrm{Ab}}(t)$	Concentration of antibody (immune therapy, targeted therapy)		

In the case of combination therapy, there will be more than one control input. Hence, the drug effect function ($\mathscr{D}(\cdot)$) defined in the general model (1.1) and the drug dynamics model given by (1.2) can be rewritten as $\mathscr{D}_i\left(a, C_{\mathrm{p1}}(t), U_j(t)\right)$ and

$$\frac{\mathrm{d}U_j(t)}{\mathrm{d}t} = \mathscr{D}_{\mathrm{C_i}}\left(d_{\mathrm{U}_i}, U_j(t), u_i(t)\right), \quad U_j(0) = u_{j0}, \tag{9.1}$$

where i, $i = 1, 2, 3, \ldots$, denotes the number of therapies used and $j =$ Ch, Im, An, and Ab represent chemotherapy, immunotherapy, anti-angiogenic therapy, and targeted therapy (anti-body), respectively. Note that, in this book, the notation $U(t)$ is used to denote the concentration of drug or biochemicals and $u(t)$ denote drug input. In the case of oncolytic virotherapy, as the drug input is oncolytic virus, the notation $V(t)$ is used instead of $U(t)$ to depict the drug (virus) dynamics. Notations used to model the drug dynamics of various therapies that are discussed in this chapter are summarized in Table 9.1. Tables 9.2 and 9.3 summarize variable and parameter notations used in this chapter.

As mentioned earlier, even though many combinations of therapeutic strategies are currently used for cancer management, only a few mathematical models are reported

Table 9.2 Different types of cells and biochemicals in various therapies

Var.	Description	Var.	Description
$A(t)$	Number of cancer cells	$A_{\mathrm{U}}(t)$	Number of uninfected cancer cells
$A_{\mathrm{V}}(t)$	Number of viral infected cancer cells	$E(t)$	Number of active immune cells
$E_{\mathrm{NK}}(t)$	Number of natural killer cells	$E_{\mathrm{CL}}(t)$	Number of circulating lymphocytes
$U_{\mathrm{Ab}}(t)$	Amount of bound antibody	$U_{\mathrm{Af}}(t)$	Amount of free antibody
$U_{\mathrm{Pin}}(t)$	Amount of internalized paclitaxel	$U_{\mathrm{Pf}}(t)$	Amount of free paclitaxel
$V_{\mathrm{b}}(t)$	Variable carrying capacity in terms of vascular development	$U_{\mathrm{cp}}(t)$	Plasma concentration of drug
$N_{\mathrm{G}}(t)$	Number of normal glial cells	$N_{\mathrm{N}}(t)$	Number of normal neurons
$u(t)$	Control input	$U^{50}(t)$	Drug resistance dependent concentration for half-maximal response

Table 9.3 Parameter notations used in this chapter

Param.	Description	Param.	Description
r	Growth rate of cell population	g	Half-saturation constant related of cell population or cytokine
m	Mutation rate of a cell population	a	Drug induced cell-kill rate
b	Reciprocal carrying capacity of a cell population	k_c	Carrying capacity of a cell population
d	Rate of apoptosis or depletion of cell population	d_U	Depletion of drug
s	Influx rate or recruitment rate of immune cells	γ_P	Reduction in potential (cytotoxicity) of chemodrug
α_P	Rate of cellular uptake of chemodrug	α_T	Virus transfection rate
θ_{Ab}	Rate of antibody binding	θ_R	Average expression of receptors
σ	Synergy index	ξ_I	Angiogenic inhibition due to endothelial cell death
ξ_S	Angiogenic stimulatory effect of tumor	α	Drug absorption rate
β	Drug elimination rate	β_v	Virus production (burst) rate
$\bar{\psi}$	Loss influence related to neurons	ψ	Rate of inhibition of immune cells by a cell population
t_x	Drug toxicity of a drug	U_θ	Concentration threshold
δ_r	Capacity to resist drug		

in the literature. In this chapter, the mathematical models of following combination therapies are presented, namely:

- chemotherapy and immunotherapy,
- chemotherapy and virotherapy,
- chemotherapy and HER2 targeted therapy, and
- immunotherapy and anti-angiogenic therapy.

9.1 Chemotherapy and Immunotherapy

Recall that, in Chaps. 3 and 4, several different mathematical models that represent various aspects of cancer dynamics under chemotherapy and immunotherapy are discussed. The main difference between these two methods is that while the former involves the use of agents that directly kill cancer cells, the latter mainly invokes immune cells to kill cancer cells (Figs. 3.1 and 4.4).

As explained in Chap. 4, the immune system in the human body uses two ways to tackle external invaders. One is through nonspecific immunity (innate immunity), in which the lymphocytes such as NK cells take action against the external invaders irrespective of the type of invader. The second one is through specific immunity (adaptive immunity) which is facilitated by immune cells such as B cells, helper T cells, and cytotoxic T cells ($CD8^{+}T$) (Fig. 4.5). The overall immune response is facilitated by the orchestrated action of various cells by means of (1) identification of the type of antigen (a foreign body that initiates the immune response), (2) activation of immune cells, and (3) counteraction via appropriate antibodies (Fig. 4.1). Summarizing the discussion on immunotherapy strategy in Chap. 4, one can identify that immunotherapy can be facilitated mainly by (1) using monoclonal antibodies (mAbs), (2) small molecule inhibitors, or (3) via vaccines. Moreover, as shown in Fig. 4.4, immunotherapeutic agents mainly fall under two categories those which increase the response of the immune system and those which increase the immunogenicity of the tumor micro-environment.

Chemotherapeutic agents can be used to enhance the potency of immunotherapy. For instance, chemotherapeutic agents can be used to facilitate the release of tumor-associated antigens (TAA) in the tumor micro-environment or can cause depletion of T regulatory cells and other myeloid suppressive cells [11]. The main side effect associated with chemotherapy is the drug toxicity and related side effects due to the less target specificity of the agents used. On the other hand, one of the main advantages of immunotherapy is its target specificity that enables to selectively kill abnormal cells leaving host cells least effected. Moreover, immunotherapy often leaves antigen-experienced memory immune cells in the body which can restrict relapse of the disease by continuing immunosurveillance in the body even after the treatment period [12]. In addition to that, the abscopal effect (shrinkage of distant, undetected, and untreated tumor) mediated by the immune system also makes immunotherapy a common factor in many combination therapeutic strategies [12]. However, there is much more to be known regarding the right order and amount of drug administration required for a better outcome. In this section, two mathematical models that combine chemotherapy and immunotherapy are discussed, namely:

- chemotherapy, IL-2 injection, and vaccine therapy and
- chemo-immuno model that accounts for heterogeneous cell clones.

9.1.1 Chemotherapy, IL-2 Injection, and Vaccine Therapy

In [8], the effects of a chemotherapeutic drug and two immunotherapeutic agents on the tumor dynamics by using a mathematical model is presented which accounts for:

- the response of the tumor micro-environment for direct immunotherapy via IL-2 injection,
- a vaccine-based immunotherapy via activated tumor-infiltrating lymphocyte (TIL) injection, and
- the use of a chemotherapeutic drug.

Therapeutic cancer vaccines are prepared by deriving samples from the cancer cells in the patients (autologous). Such samples can be modified in an *in vitro* culture to

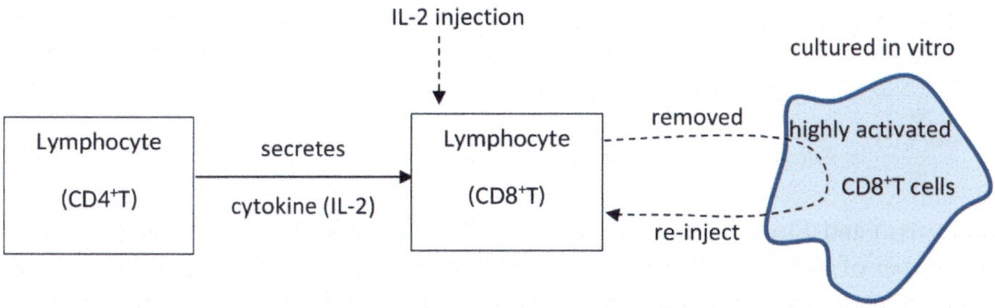

Fig. 9.1 Illustrative diagram showing the immunotherapy approach modeled in (9.2)–(9.7). The CD4$^+$T lymphocytes secrete IL-2 to activate CD8$^+$T lymphocytes. Additionally, an IL-2 injection (external input) is used to activate CD8$^+$T lymphocytes. Activated lymphocytes are removed from the patient's blood to culture in an *in vitro* set up and then injected back to the patient. IL-2 injection and TIL re-injection correspond to $u_1(t)$ and $u_2(t)$ in (9.2)–(9.7)

generate highly activated TIL which can be used to stimulate the immune system to act against the tumor cells. Figure 9.1 illustrates the use of IL-2 and TIL injections to boost immunity.

IL-2 is a cytokine secreted by the lymphocyte CD4$^+$T and has multiple immune functions and can mediate expansion, differentiation, and survival of CD8$^+$T cells. As illustrated in Fig. 9.1, the model accounts for two means of immunotherapy approaches such as (1) injecting IL-2 and (2) re-injection of TILs to boost the immune response. Apart from external IL-2 injection, some of the CD8$^+$T cells extracted from the patient's body are cultured *in vitro* and the highly activated T cells are injected back. Since cytotoxic T lymphocytes (CTL) will be directed towards the tumor micro-environment, such injections are called TIL injections. Figure 9.1 also shows the natural activation of CD8$^+$T cells mediated by the cytokine, IL-2, secreted by the CD8$^+$T cells. The model for combination therapy of chemotherapeutic drugs and immunotherapeutic agents is given by [8]:

$$\begin{aligned}\frac{\mathrm{d}A(t)}{\mathrm{d}t} =& r_1 A(t)(1-b_1 A(t)) - c_1 E_{\mathrm{NK}}(t)A(t) - \mathscr{D}\big(a_1, E(t), A(t)\big)A(t)\\ &- a_2\left(1-\mathrm{e}^{-U_{\mathrm{Ch}}(t)}\right)A(t),\end{aligned} \tag{9.2}$$

$$\begin{aligned}\frac{\mathrm{d}E_{\mathrm{NK}}(t)}{\mathrm{d}t} =& m_1 E_{\mathrm{CL}}(t) - d_1 E_{\mathrm{NK}}(t) + r_2\frac{A^2(t)}{g_2 + A^2(t)}E_{\mathrm{NK}}(t) - \psi_1 E_{\mathrm{NK}}(t)A(t)\\ &- a_3\left(1-\mathrm{e}^{-U_{\mathrm{Ch}}(t)}\right)E_{\mathrm{NK}}(t),\end{aligned} \tag{9.3}$$

$$\begin{aligned}\frac{\mathrm{d}E(t)}{\mathrm{d}t} =& r_3\frac{\left(\mathscr{D}(a_1, E(t), A(t))\right)^2 A^2(t)}{g_3 + \left(\mathscr{D}(a_1, E(t), A(t))\right)^2 A^2(t)}E(t) - d_2E(t) - \psi_2 E(t)A(t) - \psi_3 E_{\mathrm{NK}}(t)E^2(t)\\ &+ (r_4E_{\mathrm{NK}}(t) + r_5E_{\mathrm{CL}}(t))A(t) - a_4\left(1-\mathrm{e}^{-U_{\mathrm{Ch}}(t)}\right)E(t) + \frac{r_6E(t)U_{\mathrm{Im}}(t)}{g_4 + U_{\mathrm{Im}}(t)} + u_1(t),\end{aligned} \tag{9.4}$$

$$\frac{\mathrm{d}E_{\mathrm{CL}}(t)}{\mathrm{d}t} = s_1 - d_3 E_{\mathrm{CL}}(t) - a_5\left(1 - \mathrm{e}^{-U_{\mathrm{Ch}}(t)}\right) E_{\mathrm{CL}}(t), \tag{9.5}$$

$$\frac{\mathrm{d}U_{\mathrm{Im}}(t)}{\mathrm{d}t} = -d_{\mathrm{U}_1} U_{\mathrm{Im}}(t) + u_2(t), \tag{9.6}$$

$$\frac{\mathrm{d}U_{\mathrm{Ch}}(t)}{\mathrm{d}t} = -d_{\mathrm{U}_2} U_{\mathrm{Ch}}(t) + u_3(t), \tag{9.7}$$

where $A(t)$ and $E_{\mathrm{NK}}(t)$ are the number of cancer and NK cells, $E(t)$ and $E_{\mathrm{CL}}(t)$ are the number of CD8$^+$T cells and circulating lymphocytes, and $U_{\mathrm{Ch}}(t)$ and $U_{\mathrm{Im}}(t)$ are the concentration of chemotherapeutic and immunotherapeutic agents, respectively.

In (9.2), the first term models the growth of tumor cells in terms of the growth rate r_1 and the reciprocal carrying capacity b_1. The second term accounts for the reduction in the cancer cell number due to the invasion of NK cells. Compared to notations used in the general model given by (1.1)–(1.2), here the cell-kill rate is categorized as c_1 instead of a_1 as the term $c_1 E_{\mathrm{NK}}(t)A(t)$ accounts for the natural immune attack and competition for resource between NK cells and cancer cells, and not the drug-induced cell-kill. Specifically, the attack of NK cells on non-ligand transduced cancer cells is modeled in the term $c_1 E_{\mathrm{NK}}(t)A(t)$. The third term $\mathscr{D}\big(a_1, E(t), A(t)\big)A(t)$ accounts for the death of the cancer cells mediated by the CD8$^+$T cells. Note that the proliferation and activation of CD8$^+$T cells are enhanced by the immunotherapeutic agents. Hence, the recruitment term $\mathscr{D}\big(a_1, E(t), A(t)\big)$ is given by

$$\mathscr{D}\big(a_1, E(t), A(t)\big) = a_1 \frac{\big(E(t)/A(t)\big)^{\gamma_1}}{g_1 + \big(E(t)/A(t)\big)^{\gamma_1}}, \tag{9.8}$$

where a_1 denotes the drug-induced cell-kill rate related to immunotherapy, γ_1 is the steepness coefficient, and g_1 is the half-saturation constant associated with the recruitment of CD8$^+$T cells and the annihilation of cancer cells. Note that (9.8) is in the form of a modified Michaelis-Menten equation. The last term in (9.2), $a_2\left(1 - \mathrm{e}^{-U_{\mathrm{Ch}}(t)}\right)A(t)$, models the cell-kill mediated by the chemotherapeutic agent. This term accounts for the linear relationship between the cell-kill rate and drug concentration at a low concentration which gets saturated (plateau) at higher concentrations of the drug. Thus, the last two terms in (9.2) model the effect of immunotherapy and chemotherapy in annihilating cancer cells.

Signal transduction and cell-priming are two cellular mechanisms used by the immune system to facilitate the immune response. Signal transduction (also called cell-signaling) is the process of mediating cellular information via ligand-receptor binding between the exterior and interior of a cell and the recruitment of NK and CD8$^+$T cells are mediated by this process. Note that when the T cells come in contact with antigens present on the invader cells (also called cell priming), they start differentiating and proliferating. The increase in the number of NK and CD8$^+$T cells in response to the presence of tumor cells are supported by the clinical evidence given in [13]. The cell dynamics of NK cells and CD8$^+$T cells are modeled in (9.3) and (9.4), respectively.

In (9.3), the dynamics of the complex cascaded events that lead to the stimulation of NK cells is modeled based on some simplifying assumptions [8]. First of all, it is assumed that a proportion of circulating lymphocytes is converted into NK cells (Fig. 1.3 in Chap. 1). This is modeled by the term $m_1 E_{\mathrm{CL}}(t)$, where m_1 is the cell conversion rate. The second term models the death of NK cells in terms of the death rate d_1. The third term in (9.3), $r_2 \frac{A^2(t)}{g_2+A^2(t)} E_{\mathrm{NK}}(t)$, models the recruitment of NK cells due to the presence of tumor cells, where r_2 is the maximum growth rate of NK cells induced by the ligand-transduced cancer cells and g_2 is associated steepness coefficient. Note that the cell-priming by the ligand-transduced cancer cells has a key role in recruiting NK cells. The term $\psi_1 E_{\mathrm{NK}}(t) A(t)$ accounts for the reduction in the NK cell count due to the inhibitory effects of the cancer cells, where ψ_1 is the rate of inhibition. The last term in (9.3) accounts for the effect of the chemotherapeutic drug, where a_3 is the fractional cell-kill rate.

In (9.4), the first term accounts for the recruitment of the $\mathrm{CD8^+T}$ cells, where r_3 is the recruitment parameter that models the effect of tumor-specific antigen on the recruitment of $\mathrm{CD8^+T}$ cells and g_3 is the steepness coefficient of the recruitment curve. Note that, as shown in Fig. 9.1, the number of $\mathrm{CD8^+T}$ cells will increase in a nonlinear fashion due to the TIL re-injection as well. This effect is also captured by the first term in (9.4). The term $d_2 E(t)$ accounts for the death of $\mathrm{CD8^+T}$ cells at a rate d_2. The term $\psi_2 E(t) A(t)$ accounts for the inactivation or inhibition of $\mathrm{CD8^+T}$ cells by the cancer cells, where ψ_2 is the rate of inhibition. Similarly, $\psi_3 E_{\mathrm{NK}}(t) E^2(t)$ accounts for the inhibition of $\mathrm{CD8^+T}$ cells mediated by the NK cells. Many clinical data suggest that the proliferation, activation, and recruitment of $\mathrm{CD8^+T}$ cells are initiated by the presence of tumor cells and cell-debris due to tumor-immune cell (NK cells or $\mathrm{CD8^+T}$) encounter [8]. This is modeled using the growth parameters r_4 and r_5 in (9.4). Specifically, r_4 accounts for the increase in $\mathrm{CD8^+T}$ cell count due to the interaction of NK cells and cancer cells, whereas r_5 accounts for the increase in the $\mathrm{CD8^+T}$ cell count due to the interaction of circulating lymphocytes with the tumor cells. The term $a_4 \left(1 - \mathrm{e}^{-U_{\mathrm{Ch}}(t)}\right) E(t)$ accounts for the reduction in $\mathrm{CD8^+T}$ cell count due to the adverse effects of chemotherapeutic drug. As illustrated in Fig. 9.1, IL-2 secreted by the $\mathrm{CD4^+T}$ cells and the external IL-2 injection stimulates the growth of $\mathrm{CD8^+T}$ cells. The term $\frac{r_6 E(t) U_{\mathrm{Im}}(t)}{g_4+U_{\mathrm{Im}}(t)}$ models the increase in the number of $\mathrm{CD8^+T}$ cells due the stimulative effect of IL-2 injection, where r_6 is the growth rate and g_4 is the steepness coefficient. The last term $u_1(t)$ models TIL injection.

In (9.5), the parameters s_1 and d_3 model the rate of influx of circulating lymphocytes and death, respectively. The term $a_5 \left(1 - \mathrm{e}^{-U_{\mathrm{Ch}}(t)}\right) E_{\mathrm{CL}}(t)$ accounts for the reduction in the number of circulating lymphocytes as a side effect of chemotherapy. Finally, (9.6) and (9.7) account for the dynamics of immunotherapeutic and chemotherapeutic agents, where d_{U_1} and d_{U_2} are the respective drug decay rates and $u_2(t)$ and $u_3(t)$ are the drug infusion rates.

Table 9.4 summarizes the parameter values of the chemotherapy and vaccine therapy model (9.2)–(9.8) [8]. Three sets of initial conditions are given for the variables in model (9.2)–(9.8). To reflect an experimental case in which an initial tumor cell number of 10^6 is implanted in a mouse, $A(0) = 10^6$ (cells), $E_{\mathrm{NK}}(0) = 5 \times 10^4$ (cells), $E(0) = 100$ (cells), and $E_{\mathrm{CL}}(0) = 1.1 \times 10^7$ (cells) are used. To reflect

Table 9.4 Parameter values of the chemotherapy and vaccine therapy model (9.2)–(9.8) [8]

Parameter	Value (unit)	Parameter	Value (unit)
r_1	4.31×10^{-1} (days^{-1})	b_1	2.17×10^{-8} (cells^{-1})
c_1	7.13×10^{-10} (cells^{-1}days^{-1})	a_1	8.17 (days^{-1})
a_2	9×10^{-1} (days^{-1})	m_1	1.29×10^{-3} (days^{-1})
d_1	4.12×10^{-2} (days^{-1})	r_2	4.198×10^{-1} (days^{-1})
g_2	2.02×10^{7} (cells^{2})	ψ_1	1×10^{-7} (cells^{-1}days^{-1})
a_3, a_4, a_5	6×10^{-1} (days^{-1})	r_3	9.96×10^{-1} (days^{-1})
g_3	3.03×10^{5} (cells^{2})	d_2	2×10^{-2} (days^{-1})
ψ_2	3.42×10^{-10} (cells^{-1}days^{-1})	ψ_3	1.80×10^{-8} (cells^{-2}days^{-1})
r_4	1.1×10^{-7} (cell^{-1}days^{-1})	r_5	3×10^{-11} (cells^{-1}days^{-1})
r_6	1.25×10^{-1} (days^{-1})	g_4	2×10^{7} (cells^{2})
s_1	1.21×10^{5} (cells days^{-1})	d_3	1.2×10^{-2} (days^{-1})
g_1	6.18×10^{-1}	γ_1	6.57×10^{-1}
d_{U_1}	9×10^{-1} (days^{-1})	d_{U_2}	10 (days^{-1})

a weakened immune case, $A(0) = 10^6$ (cells), $E_{NK}(0) = 10^3$ (cells), $E(0) = 10$ (cells), and $E_{CL}(0) = 6 \times 10^8$ (cells) are used. To analyze the parameter value (c_1) of the model for which the system goes to high tumor state or zero tumor state, $A(0) = 6.89 \times 10^6$ (cells), $E_{NK}(0) = 3.97 \times 10^9$ (cells), $E(0) = 7.15 \times 10^3$ (cells), and $E_{CL}(0) = 1.65 \times 10^9$ (cells) are used.

9.1.2 Model of Chemotherapy and Immunotherapy that Accounts for Heterogeneous Cell Clones

Combination therapy is emerging as a mainstay treatment option to curtail drug resistance development and disease relapse. One of the reasons for the development of drug resistance is the presence of heterogeneous cell populations that respond differently to drugs. Hence, in this section, a model that accounts for the effect of chemotherapy and immunotherapy in two variants of cancer cells (clones) in the tumor micro-environment is discussed [14]. Immunotherapy is facilitated by a dendritic cell vaccine (DCV) mediated by adenovirus (Ad-p53), which will recruit cytotoxic T lymphocytes (CTL) to the tumor micro-environment. The model is given by [14]:

$$\begin{aligned}\frac{\mathrm{d}A_1(t)}{\mathrm{d}t} &= r_1 A_1(t)\big(1 - b_1 A_1(t)\big) - (c_1 A_2(t) + c_2 E(t)) b_1 A_1(t) \\ &\quad - U_{\mathrm{Ch1}}(t) A_1(t) - b_1 U_{\mathrm{Im}}(t) A_1(t) E(t),\end{aligned} \tag{9.9}$$

$$\frac{\mathrm{d}A_2(t)}{\mathrm{d}t} = r_2A_2(t)\big(1 - b_2A_2(t)\big) - (c_3A_1(t) + c_4E(t))b_2A_2(t)$$
$$- U_{\mathrm{Ch2}}(t)A_2(t) - b_2U_{\mathrm{Im}}(t)A_2(t)E(t), \tag{9.10}$$
$$\frac{\mathrm{d}E(t)}{\mathrm{d}t} = r_3E(t)\left(1 - \frac{E(t)}{\theta_1}\right) + s_1A_1(t)\left(\frac{E(t)}{\theta_1}\right) + s_2A_2(t)\left(\frac{E(t)}{\theta_1}\right), \tag{9.11}$$

where $A_i(t)$, $i = 1, 2$ denote the number of cancer cells in the cell clone 1 and 2, respectively, $E(t)$ represents the immune response, $U_{\mathrm{Ch}i}(t)$ $i = 1, 2$ are the concentration of chemotherapeutic agent in the cell clone 1 and 2, respectively, and $U_{\mathrm{Im}}(t)$ is the concentration of immunotherapeutic agent.

The first term in (9.9) models the growth of cell clone 1 in the absence of treatment and competition from the cell clone 2, where r_1 and b_1 denote the growth rate and reciprocal carrying capacity, respectively. The second term accounts for the limitation in growth due to the competition between two cell clones and the influence of immune cells, where c_1 and c_2 are respective competition rates. The last two terms account for the effect of chemotherapy and immunotherapy.

In (9.10), the first term models the growth of cell clone 2 in the absence of treatment and competition due to the presence of cell clone 1, where r_2 and b_2 denote the growth rate and reciprocal carrying capacity. The second term accounts for the limitation in growth due to competition between two cell clones and the influence of immune cells, where c_3 and c_4 are respective competition rates. The last two terms account for the effect of chemotherapy and immunotherapy.

In (9.11), the first term models the growth of various immune cells, where r_3 and θ_1 denote the growth rate and immune threshold parameter. The last two terms account for the influx or recruitment of immune cells triggered by the two cell clones, where s_1 and s_2 are the respective immune cell influx rates.

In [14], parameters pertaining to non-small cell lung cancer (NSCLC) are used to evaluate the right combination of chemotherapy and immunotherapy. Using the model-based simulation study, it is shown that, low doses of chemotherapy (erlotinib) with immunotherapy have similar results when compared to monotherapy using higher doses of erlotinib. Moreover, low-dose combination therapy has the advantage of fewer side effects from chemotherapy and slower drug resistance development. Compared to the earlier model (9.2)–(9.7), which used steepness coefficients denoted by g_i, $i = 1, \ldots, 4$, to account for the restrictions or regulatory actions on the nonlinear interaction curves, in (9.9)–(9.11) the reciprocal carrying capacity b_i, $i = 1, 2$, and immune threshold parameter θ_1 are used to model such restrictions. The model (9.9)–(9.11) incorporates the heterogeneity in the cell population, which is an important aspect that should be explored more to study the reasons and conditions that lead to tumor relapse after treatment. However, this model is a drastic simplification of the actual dynamics in the tumor micro-environment.

Table 9.5 summarizes the parameter values of the chemotherapy and immunotherapy model given by (9.9)–(9.11) [14]. The initial conditions for the variables in model (9.9)–(9.11) are $A_1(0) = 9 \times 10^4$ (cells), $A_2(0) = 4 \times 10^4$ (cells), and $E(0) = 5 \times 10^2$ (cells).

Table 9.5 Parameter values of the chemotherapy and immunotherapy model given by (9.9)–(9.11) [14]

Parameter	Value (unit)	Parameter	Value (unit)
r_1	0.15 (days^{-1})	b_1, b_2	0.2×10^{-7} (cells^{-1})
c_1, c_3	0.01–1 (days^{-1})	c_2, c_4	5.5 (days^{-1})
r_2	0.11 (days^{-1})	r_3	0.8 (days^{-1})
θ_1	3×10^5 (cells)	s_1, s_2	1.8×10^{-3} (days^{-1})

9.2 Chemotherapy and Oncolytic Virotherapy

The main advantage of combining chemotherapy with virotherapy is in the amalgamation of selective infectious power of viruses and the high cytotoxicity of chemotherapeutic agents. In the case of chemovirotherapy, the success rate depends on the efficacy of oncolytic viruses and chemotherapeutic drugs that are used in this context. Moreover, as discussed in Sect. 8.2 and illustrated in Fig. 8.3, oncolytic virotherapy triggers the immune response as well. In this section, the mathematical modeling of combined administration of chemotherapeutic agents and oncolytic viruses is discussed using the following two models;

- chemotherapy and oncolytic virotherapy with various drug inputs and
- chemotherapy and oncolytic virotherapy for glioma.

9.2.1 Chemotherapy and Oncolytic Virotherapy with Various Drug Inputs

The models discussed in this subsection is similar to the models (8.11)–(8.12) and (8.13)–(8.18) discussed in Sects. 8.2.1 and 8.2.2. Main difference is the additional effect of chemotherapy. The combined model for chemotherapy and oncolytic virotherapy presented in [15] is as follows:

$$\frac{\mathrm{d}A_{\mathrm{U}}(t)}{\mathrm{d}t} = r_1 A_{\mathrm{U}}(t)\Big(1 - b\big(A_{\mathrm{U}}(t) + A_{\mathrm{V}}(t)\big)\Big) - \alpha_{\mathrm{T}} A_{\mathrm{U}}(t)V(t) - a_1 A_{\mathrm{U}}(t)U_{\mathrm{Ch}}(t), \tag{9.12}$$

$$\frac{\mathrm{d}A_{\mathrm{V}}(t)}{\mathrm{d}t} = \alpha_{\mathrm{T}} A_{\mathrm{U}}(t)V(t) - a_2 A_{\mathrm{V}}(t) - a_3 A_{\mathrm{V}}(t)U_{\mathrm{Ch}}(t), \tag{9.13}$$

$$\frac{\mathrm{d}V(t)}{\mathrm{d}t} = \beta_{\mathrm{v}} a_2 A_{\mathrm{V}}(t) - \alpha_{\mathrm{T}} A_{\mathrm{U}}(t)V(t) - d_1 V(t), \tag{9.14}$$

$$\frac{\mathrm{d}U_{\mathrm{Ch}}(t)}{\mathrm{d}t} = -d_{\mathrm{U}} U_{\mathrm{Ch}}(t) + u(t), \tag{9.15}$$

Table 9.6 Parameter values of the chemotherapy and oncolytic virotherapy model (9.12)–(9.15) [15]

Parameter	Value	Parameter	Value	Parameter	Value
r_1	0.206	b	10^{-6}	α_T	0.001
a_1	0.005	a_2	0.5115	a_3	0.006
β_v	10	d_1	0.001	d_U	4.16

where $A_U(t)$ and $A_V(t)$ denote the amount of uninfected and infected cancer cells and $U_{Ch}(t)$ and $V(t)$ denote the amount of chemotherapeutic drug and viruses, respectively.

In (9.12), the first term models the growth of uninfected cancer cells and limitation due to the carrying capacity in terms of the growth rate r_1 and the carrying capacity b. The second term, $\alpha_T A_U(t)V(t)$, in (9.12) and (9.14) models the viral transfection dynamics, where α_T is the virus replication rate. The last term, $a_1 A_U(t)U_{Ch}(t)$, in (9.12) models the death of uninfected cancer cells due to chemotherapy, where a_1 is the cell-kill rate. In (9.13), the term $a_2 A_V(t)$ models the death of infected cells due to viral infection, where a_2 is the virus-induced cell-kill rate and the last term $a_3 A_V(t)U_{Ch}(t)$ models the reduction in infected cell population due to the effect of chemotherapeutic drug. Please refer to Fig. 8.3 for an illustrative diagram of oncolytic virus attacking cancer cells.

In (9.14), the term $\beta_v a_2 A_V(t)$ models the increase in the number of virus due to the rupture of infected cells due to viral burden, where β_v is the virus production (burst) rate and the last term in (9.14) models the death of virus. Finally, in (9.15), drug dynamics is modeled in terms of the drug decay rate d_U and rate of infusion $u(t)$, where $u(t) = u_1$, $u(t) = u_1 e^{-d_U t}$, and $u(t) = u_1 \sin^2(d_U t)$, can be used to account for constant, exponential, or periodical inputs.

As shown in Fig. 8.3, when the cancer cells burst to release virions, they also release cytokines, tumor-associated antigens (TAA), and tumor cell debris which often attract more immune cells to the tumor micro-environment. This enhanced virus-induced immune response is ignored in (9.12)–(9.15). Hence, it is imperative to extend the current model by incorporating relevant cell dynamics to better understand the dynamics pertaining to chemovirotherapy. Table 9.6 summarizes the parameter values of the chemotherapy and oncolytic virotherapy model (9.12)–(9.15) [15]. The initial conditions for the variables in model (9.12)–(9.15) are $A_U(0) = 1$, $A_V(0) = 0$, $V(0) = 0.1$, and $U_{Im}(0) = 0.1$. One unit of A_U corresponds to 10^6 cells and 1 unit of time is equivalent to 2 days.

9.2.2 *Chemotherapy and Oncolytic Virotherapy for Glioma*

In [16], a combination therapy model that uses chemotherapy and oncolytic virotherapy for managing glioma is discussed. Specifically, in [16], a mathematical model that depicts the dynamics of normal glial cells, cancerous glial cells (glioma), neurons, and chemotherapy given in [17] are extended to add the effects of oncolytic virotherapy. Gliomas are brain tumors that originate from glial cells. Glial cells are the star-shaped cells that are as abundant as the neurons whose main function is to provide nutritional and physical support to the neurons and clear debris in the brain. The model corresponding to chemotherapy and oncolytic virotherapy for glioma is given as [16]:

$$\frac{\mathrm{d}N_{\mathrm{G}}(t)}{\mathrm{d}t} = r_1 N_{\mathrm{G}}(t)\big(1 - bN_{\mathrm{G}}(t)\big) - c_1 N_{\mathrm{G}}(t) A_{\mathrm{U}}(t) - \frac{a_1 N_{\mathrm{G}}(t) U_{\mathrm{Ch}}(t)}{g_1 + N_{\mathrm{G}}(t)}, \tag{9.16}$$

$$\frac{\mathrm{d}N_{\mathrm{N}}(t)}{\mathrm{d}t} = \bar{\psi} \dot{N}_{\mathrm{G}}(t) F(-\dot{N}_{\mathrm{G}}(t)) N_{\mathrm{N}}(t) - \frac{a_2 N_{\mathrm{N}}(t) U_{\mathrm{Ch}}(t)}{g_2 + N_{\mathrm{N}}(t)}, \tag{9.17}$$

$$\begin{aligned}\frac{\mathrm{d}A_{\mathrm{U}}(t)}{\mathrm{d}t} &= r_2 A_{\mathrm{U}}(t)\Big(1 - b\big(A_{\mathrm{U}}(t) + A_{\mathrm{V}}(t)\big)\Big) - c_2 N_{\mathrm{G}}(t) A_{\mathrm{U}}(t) - \frac{a_3 A_{\mathrm{U}}(t) U_{\mathrm{Ch}}(t)}{g_3 + A_{\mathrm{U}}(t)} \\ &\quad - \alpha_{\mathrm{T}} A_{\mathrm{U}}(t) V(t),\end{aligned} \tag{9.18}$$

$$\frac{\mathrm{d}A_{\mathrm{V}}(t)}{\mathrm{d}t} = \alpha_{\mathrm{T}} A_{\mathrm{U}}(t) V(t) - a_4 A_{\mathrm{V}}(t), \tag{9.19}$$

$$\frac{\mathrm{d}V(t)}{\mathrm{d}t} = \beta_{\mathrm{v}} a_4 A_{\mathrm{V}}(t) - \alpha_{\mathrm{T}} A_{\mathrm{U}}(t) V(t) - d_{\mathrm{U}_1} V(t), \tag{9.20}$$

$$\frac{\mathrm{d}U_{\mathrm{Ch}}(t)}{\mathrm{d}t} = -d_{\mathrm{U}_2} U_{\mathrm{Ch}}(t) + u_1(t), \tag{9.21}$$

where $N_{\mathrm{G}}(t)$ and $N_{\mathrm{N}}(t)$ denote normal glial cells and neurons, $A_{\mathrm{U}}(t)$ and $A_{\mathrm{V}}(t)$ denote uninfected glioma cells and infected glioma cells, $V(t)$ and $U_{\mathrm{Ch}}(t)$ represent viruses and concentration of chemotherapeutic drug (temozolomide), respectively and $\dot{N}_{\mathrm{G}}(t) = \frac{\mathrm{d}N_{\mathrm{G}}(t)}{\mathrm{d}t}$.

The first and second terms in (9.16) model the growth of the normal glial cells and the growth limitation due to the carrying capacity and competition between normal and cancer cells, respectively, where r_1, b, and c_1 denote the growth rate, reciprocal carrying capacity, and competition rate, respectively. The last term in (9.16) accounts for the dose-dependent reduction in the normal glial cell count due to the influence of chemotherapy, where a_1 is the cell-kill rate and g_1 is the steepness coefficient.

Dynamics of neurons are modeled in (9.17), where the first term $\bar{\psi} \dot{N}_{\mathrm{G}}(t) F(\dot{N}_{\mathrm{G}}(t)) N_{\mathrm{N}}(t)$ models the reduction in the number of neurons due to glial cell death, $\bar{\psi}$ is the loss influence and F is the Heaviside function given by

$$F(x) = \begin{cases} 0 & x < 0 \\ \frac{1}{2} & x = 0 \\ 1 & x > 0 \end{cases} \tag{9.22}$$

The term $\frac{a_2 N_{\mathrm{N}}(t) U_{\mathrm{Ch}}(t)}{g_2 + N_{\mathrm{N}}(t)}$ in (9.17) accounts for the reduction in the number of neurons due to the effect of chemotherapy, where a_2 is the cell-kill rate and g_2 is the steepness coefficient.

In (9.18), the first and second terms model the growth of the uninfected cancer cells and the growth limitation due to the carrying capacity and competition between

Table 9.7 Parameter values of the chemotherapy and oncolytic virotherapy glioma model (9.16)–(9.21) [16]

Param.	Value (unit)	Param.	Value (unit)
r_1	0.0068 (days^{-1})	r_2	0.012 (days^{-1})
b	0.167×10^{-12} (cells^{-1})	c_2	3.0769×10^{-16} ($\text{cells}^{-1}\text{days}^{-1}$)
c_1	3.0769×10^{-15} (cells^{-1} days^{-1})	a_3	2.808×10^{8}($\text{m}^2\text{mg}^{-1}\text{days}^{-1}\text{cells}$)
a_1, a_2	2.808×10^{5} ($\text{m}^2\text{mg}^{-1}\text{days}^{-1}\text{cells}$)	α_T	1.2×10^{-10} (viruses $\text{cells}^{-1}\text{days}^{-1}$)
g_1, g_2, g_3	6×10^{12} (cells)	a_4	0.5 $\text{cells}^{-1}\text{days}^{-1}$
$\bar{\psi}$	3.418×10^{-13} (cells^{-1})	β_v	1000
d_{U_1}	24 ($\text{viruses}^{-1}\text{days}^{-1}$)	d_{U_2}	0.2 (days^{-1})

normal and cancer cells, where r_2, b, and c_2 denote the growth rate, carrying capacity, and competition rate, respectively. The term $\frac{a_3 A_\text{U}(t) U_\text{Ch}(t)}{g_3 + A_\text{U}(t)}$ accounts for the effect of chemotherapy, where a_3 is the cell-kill rate and g_3 is the steepness coefficient. The term $\alpha_\text{T} A_\text{U}(t) V(t)$ models the infection rate of uninfected glioma cells by the virus, where α_T is the infection rate.

In (9.19), the dynamics of glioma cells that are infected by viruses are modeled, where α_T is the infection rate of uninfected cells and a_4 is the death rate of virus infected cells. In (9.20), dynamics of virus population is modeled. The first term accounts for the increase in the number of viruses due to the bursting of infected cells, where β_v is the viral burst rate. The term $\alpha_\text{T} A_\text{U}(t) V(t)$ is used in this equation to account for the usage of viruses to infect a cell. The last term models the efficiency reduction of viruses at a rate of d_{U_1}.

Finally, in (9.21), the first term accounts for the drug infusion rate of chemotherapeutic drug (temozolomide) and the last term models the drug clearance at a rate of d_{U_2}. Note that the virus is genetically engineered to selectively attack cancer cells. Hence, virus induced infection ($\alpha_\text{T} A_\text{U}(t) V(t)$) and cell death ($a_4 A_\text{V}(t)$) are modeled in (9.18) and (9.19), whereas the effect of chemotherapy is reflected in normal and cancer cells. Table 9.7 summarizes the parameter values of the chemotherapy and oncolytic virotherapy glioma model (9.16)–(9.21) [16]. The initial conditions for the variables in model (9.16)–(9.21) are $N_\text{G}(0) = N_\text{N}(0) = 5.94 \times 10^{12}$ (cells), $A_\text{U}(0) = 6 \times 10^{10}$ (cells), and $A_\text{V}(0) = 0$ (cells). Chemotherapy input is $u_1(t) = 400$ mg m^{-2} day^{-1}.

9.3 Chemotherapy and HER2 Targeted Therapy

Targeted therapy, which works by targeting specific proteins, enzymes, or molecules are yet another important treatment modality that is discussed either separately or as part of the major methods such as immunotherapy, chemotherapy, anti-angiogenic therapy, and hormone therapy [18]. Examples of cancers that show poor response to general treatment strategies and thus require targeted therapy to annihilate cancer cells are those with HER2 (human epidermal growth factor receptor 2) or EGFR (epidermal growth factor receptor) mutations. Hence, anti-HER2 treatment for HER2$^+$ breast cancer, anti-EGFR treatment for prostate cancer, and lung cancer are used to manage such specific cancers [18–20]. Drugs that are designed to target specific mutations of genes namely BRAF and KRAS are also used to manage cancers with these particular mutations [19].

Similar to immunotherapy, targeted therapy is facilitated by antibodies and small molecule inhibitors [18]. The main difference between these two therapies is that immunotherapeutic drugs do not directly affect cancer cells, and they mainly boost immune cells to facilitate cancer lysis. However, targeted therapy-based drugs can directly modulate the cell-signaling process and result in an anti-proliferative effect and cell-cycle arrest. Some mAbs such as trastuzumab, which are used for targeted annihilation of HER2$^+$ breast cancer cells are capable of inducing antibody-dependent cellular toxicity (ADCC) as well. This means that, once the antibody binds to the targeted protein on the surface of the cancer cells, they will block growth signals and also attract immune cells which target antibody bound cancer cells.

As an example of combination therapy, in this subsection, a mathematical model pertaining to the use of paclitaxel (chemotherapy) and trastuzumab (mAb, anti-HER2) for the treatment of HER2$^+$ breast cancer patients is discussed [21]. Drug dynamics related to the binding properties of the antibody (trastuzumab) to the target site is also discussed in this model. The model is given by [21]:

$$\frac{\mathrm{d}A(t)}{\mathrm{d}t} = r\big(1 - \mathscr{D}_{\mathrm{Im}}(U_{\mathrm{Ab}}, t)\big)\left(1 - \frac{A(t)}{k_{\mathrm{c}} - \mathscr{D}_{\mathrm{Ch}}(U_{\mathrm{Pin}}, t)}\right)A(t), \tag{9.23}$$

$$\frac{\mathrm{d}U_{\mathrm{Ab}}(t)}{\mathrm{d}t} = \begin{cases} \theta_{\mathrm{Ab}}\Big(U_{\mathrm{Af}}(t) - U_{\mathrm{Ab}}(t)\Big)\Big(\theta_{\mathrm{R}}A(t) - U_{\mathrm{Ab}}(t)\Big), & U_{\mathrm{Af}}(t) > 0 \\ 0, & \text{otherwise} \end{cases}, \tag{9.24}$$

$$\frac{\mathrm{d}U_{\mathrm{Pin}}(t)}{\mathrm{d}t} = \begin{cases} \alpha_{\mathrm{P}}\Big(U_{\mathrm{Pf}}(t) - U_{\mathrm{Pin}}(t)\Big)A(t), & U_{\mathrm{Pf}}(t) > 0 \\ 0, & \text{otherwise} \end{cases} \tag{9.25}$$

where $A(t)$ is the amount of tumor cells, $\mathscr{D}_{\mathrm{Im}}(U_{\mathrm{Ab}}, t)$ and $\mathscr{D}_{\mathrm{Ch}}(U_{\mathrm{Pin}}, t)$ are functions that model the effect of immunotherapy and chemotherapy, respectively, given as:

$$\mathscr{D}_{\mathrm{Im}}(U_{\mathrm{Ab}}, t) = \begin{cases} a_1 U_{\mathrm{Ab}}(t), & t > t_{\mathrm{A}}^* \\ 0, & t \le t_{\mathrm{A}}^* \end{cases}, \tag{9.26}$$

$$\mathscr{D}_{\mathrm{Ch}}(U_{\mathrm{Pin}}, t) = a_2\left(e^{-\gamma_{\mathrm{P}}(t - t_{\mathrm{P}}^*)} + \sigma\right)U_{\mathrm{Pin}}(t), \tag{9.27}$$

$U_{\mathrm{Ab}}(t)$ and $U_{\mathrm{Af}}(t)$ are the amount of bound antibody and free antibody, respectively, and $U_{\mathrm{Pin}}(t)$ and $U_{\mathrm{Pf}}(t)$ are the amount of internalized and free chemotherapeutic agent (paclitaxel), respectively.

In (9.23), the effect of chemotherapy and HER2 targeted therapy on $HER2^+$ cancer is modeled, where r is the growth rate of cancer cells and k_c is the carrying capacity. In this model, the effect of chemotherapy is assumed to be reflected on the proliferation of cancer cells and that of HER2 targeted therapy on the carrying capacity of the tumor micro-environment. It can be seen that, when $\mathscr{D}_{Im}(U_{Ab}, t) = 0$ and $\mathscr{D}_{Ch}(U_{Pin}, t) = 0$, then (9.23) reduces to a logistic equation given by $\frac{dA(t)}{dt} = r\Big(1 - bA(t)\Big)A(t)$, where $b = \frac{1}{k_c}$ is the reciprocal carrying capacity. Specifically, chemotherapy and immunotherapy are assumed to reduce the proliferation of cancer cells and carrying capacity of the tumor micro-environment, respectively. These effects are modeled in (9.26) and (9.27), where a_1 represents the inhibition of proliferation due to the binding of the antibody with the respective receptor on the cancer cells, t_A^* denotes the delay between the drug administration and blocking of intracellular signal transduction resulting in an anti-proliferative drug effect of the antibody, a_2 represents the rate at which the carrying capacity is reduced due to the chemotherapeutic drug, γ_P accounts for the reduction in the cytotoxicity of the chemotherapeutic agent, and t_P^* denotes the time when the toxic effect of the chemotherapeutic drug falls below one and becomes zero as time passes. Thus, the term $e^{-\gamma_P(t-t_P^*)}$ models the immediate cytotoxicity caused by paclitaxel. The parameter σ in (9.26) accounts for the drug response due to the combined administration of two drugs. Specifically, $\sigma = 1$, when paclitaxel is administrated, and $\sigma > 1$ and $\sigma < 1$ correspond to synergistic and non-synergistic interactions of drugs, respectively.

In (9.24), the dynamics of the bounded antibody is modeled with respect to the amount of free antibody, where θ_{Ab} is the rate of antibody binding, and θ_R represents the average receptor expression on the cancer cells. Here, the binding of the antibody with the HER2 receptors on the cancer cells to block the growth signal is modeled. It is assumed that only one antibody binds to each HER2. In (9.24), $U_{Af}(t) > 0$ corresponds to the case when the free antibody is available in the blood or tumor micro-environment. Finally, in (9.25), the dynamics of the internalized paclitaxel is modeled in terms of the free paclitaxel, where α_P accounts for the rate of uptake of chemotherapeutic drug.

The main highlight of this model is the analysis of drug effects in terms of the antibody receptor binding and internalization of the drug. However, the model does not analyze the effect of immune cells on the cancer cells. Immune cell dynamics are important in this context as trastuzumab is known to cause ADCC which attracts more immune cells into the tumor micro-environment and enables cancer cell lysis [18]. Hence, apart from the anti-proliferative effect of trastuzumab, the immune enhancement effect should also be analyzed.

Table 9.8 summarizes the parameter values of the chemotherapy and HER2 targeted therapy model (9.23)–(9.27) [21]. The initial conditions for the variables in model (9.23)–(9.27) are $A(0) = 3.5 \times 10^4$ (cells), $U_{Ab}(0) = U_{Af}(0) = 0$ (molecules), and $U_{Pin}(0) = U_{Pf}(0) = 0$ (pmol).

Table 9.8 Parameter values of the chemotherapy and HER2 targeted therapy model (9.23)–(9.27) [21]

Parameter	Value (unit)	Parameter	Value (unit)
r	0.83 (time^{-1})	γ_P	6.35 (time^{-1})
a_1	2.51 (molecules^{-1})	θ_R	1.94×10^6 (receptors cell^{-1})
a_2	0.23×10^2(cells pmol^{-1})	θ_{Ab}	8.78 (receptors^{-1} time^{-1})
k_c	0.67 (cells)	σ	1
α_p	0.68 (cells^{-1} time^{-1})		

9.4 Immunotherapy Therapy and Anti-angiogenic Therapy

Angiogenesis is a milestone event that facilitates the quick progression of cancer [22, 23]. Hence, angiogenesis inhibitors are often used to treat cancers with poor prognosis such as NSCLC (non-small cell lung cancer) and liver cancer. Several clinical trials and animal model-based experiments suggest that the use of anti-angiogenic agents along with chemotherapy, radiotherapy, immunotherapy, and/or targeted therapy can improve the overall survival of patients with advanced cancers [24]. Notably, recent reviews call for more investigations to figure out the optimal combination of therapies [24]. Consequently, many anti-angiogenic agents such as bevacizumab, ramucirumab, and nintedanib which are FDA approved anti-angiogenic drugs for NSCLC are currently investigated for combination treatment with other agents.

In this section, a mathematical model of tumor dynamics under the combined use of anti-angiogenic therapy and immunotherapy is discussed. The association of angiogenesis and immunosuppression in the tumor micro-environment is a much-explored contemporary area of cancer research [25]. Many clinical trials shows improved efficacy when anti-angiogenesis and immunotherapy are practiced together [25, 26]. Evidence suggests that many key proteins associated with angiogenesis influence the immune system and result in immunosuppression. Such immunosuppressive pathways are even believed to create selective endothelium that restricts immune cells in favor of cancer cell survival [25].

These inter-dependencies between angiogenesis in tumor and the function of immune system components show that combined therapy strategies that can utilize anti-tumor pathways related to angiogenesis and immune action can significantly improve patient outcomes [25, 26]. Specifically, immunotherapy can be designed to bring about vascular remodeling in the tumors to favor immune action in the tumor micro-environment to accelerate the annihilation of tumor cells. The model discussed here is from [27], which is a combination of models in [28, 29] that is further extended to account for the dynamics of metastatic renal cell carcinoma. The model is given by [27]:

$$\frac{dA(t)}{dt} = -\upsilon_{11} A(t) \log\left(\frac{A(t)}{V_b(t)}\right) - a_1 A(t) E(t), \tag{9.28}$$

$$\frac{dV_b(t)}{dt} = -\upsilon_{12} V_b(t) + \xi_S A(t) - \xi_I V_b(t) A(t)^{\frac{2}{3}} - a_2 V_b(t) U_{An}(t), \tag{9.29}$$

$$\frac{dE(t)}{dt} = r_1 \left(A(t) - c_1 A^2(t)\right) E(t) - d_1 E(t) + s + a_3 E(t) U_{Im}(t), \tag{9.30}$$

where $A(t)$ is the tumor volume, $V_b(t)$ is the carrying capacity of the tumor in terms of the support via vascular network (endothelial volume), $E(t)$ represents the immune response, $U_{An}(t)$ is the concentration of the exogenous inhibitor administrated, and $U_{Im}(t)$ is the immunotherapy depend factor that boosts the effector cell count.

In (9.28), υ_{11} denotes a decreasing factor of the tumor volume with increase in the tumor size and a_1 denotes the rate of interaction between tumor cells and effector cells as well as the immunotherapy effect on tumor volume. In (9.29), υ_{12} denotes spontaneous loss of functional vasculature, ξ_S denotes the stimulatory effect of the tumor via secretion of growth factors such as VEGF, ξ_I denotes the inhibition effect of the tumor, and a_2 accounts for the anti-angiogenic drug dependent reduction in the volume of vasculature.

As a tumor progresses, it learns to suppress the immune response of our body [30–32]. The term $c_1 A^2(t)$, in (9.30) accounts for this reduction in immune action against tumor cells [33]. Note that $1/c_1$ represents the threshold value beyond which the immunological action is suppressed by the growing tumor. In (9.30), r_1 is the proliferation rate, c_1 is the inverse-threshold (interaction rate) for tumor suppression, d_1 is the death rate, and s is the influx rate of effector cells. Here, a_3 is a positive constant which quantifies the maximum dose of the immunotherapeutic agent to their effect (immune response).

In [27], the dynamics of the anti-angiogenic drug bevacizumab and immunotherapeutic drug atezolizumab using a two-compartmental model are discussed. The pharmacokinetics of these two drugs are represented as [27, 34]:

$$U_{cp_i}(t) = \frac{u_{Di}(\alpha - k_{21})}{V_c(\alpha - \beta)} e^{-\alpha t} + \frac{u_{Di}(k_{21} - \beta)}{V_c(\alpha - \beta)} e^{-\beta t}, \quad i = \text{An, Im}, \tag{9.31}$$

where $U_{cp_i}(t)$ is the concentration of ith drug in the central compartment (plasma concentration), u_D is the drug dose of the ith drug, α, β, k_{12}, and k_{21} are the distribution rate, elimination rate, distribution rate from compartment 1 to 2, and distribution rate from compartment 2 to 1, respectively. The pharmacodynamics of the drugs are modeled as

$$U_i(t) = \frac{(U_{cp_i}(t))^{\gamma_1}}{(U_i^{50}(t))^{\gamma_1} + (U_{cp_i}(t))^{\gamma_1}}, \quad i = \text{An, Im}, \tag{9.32}$$

where $U_i^{50}(t)$ is the half-saturation value of drug effect associated with each drug and γ_1 is the steepness coefficient. Note that, the concentration of the drug that causes 50% drug effect ($U_i^{50}(t)$) is modeled as a variable instead of a constant to account for the fact that cancer cells are capable of switching from drug-sensitive to drug-resistant variants according to the drug concentration in the plasma ($U_{\mathrm{cp}_i}(t)$, $i = \mathrm{An, Im}$) [35]. Thus, the drug resistance dependent half-saturation value is given by:

$$U_i^{50}(t) = f(t) U_{0i}^{50}, \tag{9.33}$$

$$f(t) = 1 + \delta_{\mathrm{r}} \int_0^t \max\left[0, U_\theta - U_{\mathrm{cp}_i}(\tau)\right] \mathrm{d}\tau, \tag{9.34}$$

where U_{0i}^{50} is the initial value of $U_i^{50}(t)$ before drug-resistant development, δ_{r} denotes the capacity of the cancer cells to resist the effect of the drug, and U_θ is the concentration threshold after which the pharmacodynamics of the drug varies considerably.

The next important effect of the drug is drug-induced toxicity. The grade of drug-induced toxicity may vary from mild to lethal. The drug toxicity, $T_{\mathrm{x}_i}, i = 1, 2$ for the anti-angiogenic and immunotherapeutic drug is used to find total drug toxicity as

$$T_{\mathrm{tot}} = \frac{T_{\mathrm{x}_1} + T_{\mathrm{x}_2}}{2}. \tag{9.35}$$

In general, the relationship between drug toxicity and drug concentration remains linear for low concentration. However, after a threshold concentration, the toxicity increases exponentially. In this model, it is assumed that drug toxicity does not affect drug kinetics and drug effect.

Compared to the other models discussed in this book, the main highlight of the model given by (9.28)–(9.35) is the addition of pharmacokinetics, pharmacodynamics, drug resistance, and drug toxicity of drugs along with the cancer dynamics. By bringing together the important after-effects of treatment such as drug resistance and toxicity, this model presents a very useful framework for analyzing prospective drug combinations and doses. However, as mentioned earlier, as there are several cascaded events and molecular pathways that are relevant in the context of angiogenesis, immunosuppression, and immunotherapy mediated vascular remodeling, it

Table 9.9 Parameter values of the model (9.28)–(9.30) [27–29]

Parameter	Value (unit)	Parameter	Value (unit)
r_1	3×10^{-5} (days^{-1})	d_1	0.37451
ν_{11}	0.025 (days^{-1})	ν_{12}	0.2 (days^{-1})
a_1	0.1 (days^{-1})	c_1	5×10^{-4}
a_2	1.35-11.25 (kg mg^{-1}days^{-1})	ξ_{S}	8.7 (days^{-1})
a_3	0.1-0.5 (kg mg^{-1})	ξ_{I}	8.73×10^{-3} (days^{-1}mm^{-2})
$T_{\mathrm{x}_1}, T_{\mathrm{x}_2}$	0–10	s	0.15

Table 9.10 Parameter values of the model (9.31)–(9.35) for anti-angiogenic drug (bevacizumab) and immunotherapy drug (atezolizumab) [27–29]

Parameter	Anti-angiogenesis	Immunotherapy
	Value (unit)	Value (unit)
u_D	0–15 mg kg^{-1}	0–20 mg kg^{-1}
α	0.4811 $days^{-1}$	0.5827 $days^{-1}$
V_c	2660 (mL)	3110 (mL)
β	0.0348 ($days^{-1}$)	0.0271 ($days^{-1}$)
k_{12}	0.223 ($days^{-1}$)	0.3 ($days^{-1}$)
k_{21}	0.215 ($days^{-1}$)	0.2455 ($days^{-1}$)
γ_1	1	1
U_{0i}^{50}	11.4274 (mg kg^{-1})	7.1903 (mg kg^{-1})

is imperative to extend this model by adding the dynamics of relevant cell populations and cytokines.

Tables 9.9 and 9.10 summarize the parameter values of the model (9.28)–(9.35) [27–29]. The initial conditions for the variables in model (9.28)–(9.35) are $A(0) = 300 - 10,000$ (mm^3), $V_b(0) = 625$ (mm^3), and $E(0) = 0.10$ (dimensionless). The range of values for $A(t)$ and $V_b(t)$ can go upto 18000 mm^3.

The unit of $U_{cp_i}(t)$ and u_D is mg kg^{-1}. Note that, to compare tumor growth with PK and PD dynamics, $U_{cp_i}(t)$ in mg kg^{-1} ml^{-1} is multiplied by V_c to get $U_{cp_i}(t)$ in mg kg^{-1}.

9.5 Summary

Cancer is a complicated disease that uses multiple cascaded pathways to combat many of the single agent-based therapeutic interventions and successfully reoccur after treatment. For stage IV breast and colorectal cancer, recurrence is reported for 31.1% and 55% of the patients, respectively [36]. As cancer cells can propagate cell signals via multi-molecular pathways, it is difficult to achieve complete annihilation by targeting a single pathway. Hence, current standard-of-care for majority of cancers involve a combination of several (neoadjuvant and adjuvant) therapies. In line with these developments, as discussed in Sects. 9.1–9.4 of this chapter, some mathematical models of combination therapies have also been developed mainly to investigate the optimal drug combinations and treatment schedules. Even though combination therapies that involve radiotherapy, hormone therapy, stem cell therapy, gene therapy, and oncolytic virotherapy are reported in clinical trials, corresponding mathematical models are yet to be devised. For instance, many of the hormone-derived cancers have a close correlation with altered gene regulation pathways. Hence, several adenovirus-mediated gene therapy approaches are investigated for prostate cancer after hormone therapy [37–40]. Similarly gene therapy combined with radiotherapy is presented in [41, 42]. However, a mathematical model of a combination of gene therapy with hormone therapy or radiotherapy is yet to report. Immunotherapeutic approaches based on immune checkpoint inhibitors are a relatively recent addition to the list of immune therapy drugs. Recently nivolumab, pembrolizumab, and atezolizumab are approved for NSCLC. However, a complete response is not reported with these monotherapies, and hence several combination therapies are undergoing clinical trials currently [23]. As immune checkpoint inhibitors are widely investigated with anti-angiogenic agents, developing related mathematical models can help to answer long-standing questions related to the complete response and disease-free-survival (DFS) of cancer patients.

Mathematical models for evaluating the dose-dependent mutation rate concerning the use of erlotinib for EGFR mutant NSCLC cancer are reported in [35]. This report suggests that mutation to a drug-resistant variant can have a different relationship to the concentration of drug dose used. For instance, the mutation rate can increase or decrease with drug concentration, or stay independent of the drug dose used. This means that, due to the development of drug resistance, the pharmacodynamics of patients varies with the use of various drug doses and drug combinations. In this context, developing mathematical models of various combination therapies that account for the varying pharmacodynamics as discussed in Sect. 9.4 of this chapter is an interesting future perspective.

References

1. N. Babaei, M.U. Salamci, Mixed therapy in cancer treatment for personalized drug administration using model reference adaptive control. Eur. J. Control **50**, 117–137 (2019)
2. C.J. Wheeler, A. Das, G. Liu, J.S. Yu, K.L. Black, Clinical responsiveness of glioblastoma multiforme to chemotherapy after vaccination. Clin. Cancer Res. **10**(16), 5316–5326 (2004)
3. J.H. Huang, S.N. Zhang, K.J. Choi, I.K. Choi, J.H. Kim, M. Lee, H. Kim, C.O. Yun, Therapeutic and tumor-specific immunity induced by combination of dendritic cells and oncolytic adenovirus expressing IL-12 and 4–1BBL. Mol. Ther. **18**(2), 264–274 (2010)
4. E. Piretto, M. Delitala, M. Ferraro, Combination therapies and intra-tumoral competition: insights from mathematical modeling. J. Theor. Biol. **446** (2018)
5. Z. Liu, C. Yang, A mathematical model of cancer treatment by radiotherapy followed by chemotherapy. Math. Comput. Simul. **124**, 1–15 (2016)
6. R. Serre, S. Benzekry, L. Padovani, C. Meille, N. André, J. Ciccolini, F. Barlesi, X. Muracciole, D. Barbolosi, Mathematical modeling of cancer immunotherapy and its synergy with radiotherapy. Cancer Res. **76**(17), 4931–4940 (2016)
7. D.E. Citrin, Recent developments in radiotherapy. New England J. Med. **377**(11), 1065–1075 (2017)
8. L.G. de Pillis, W. Gu, A.E. Radunskaya, Mixed immunotherapy and chemotherapy of tumors: modeling, applications and biological interpretations. J. Theor. Biol. **238**(4), 841–862 (2006)
9. M. Wang, Y. Liu, Y. Cheng, Y. Wei, X. Wei, Immune checkpoint blockade and its combination therapy with small-molecule inhibitors for cancer treatment. Biochim. Biophys. Acta (BBA)-Rev. Cancer **1871**(2), 199–224 (2019)

10. S. George, B.I. Rini, H.J. Hammers, Emerging role of combination immunotherapy in the first-line treatment of advanced renal cell carcinoma: a review. JAMA Oncol. **5**(3), 411–421 (2019)
11. S.E. Park, S.H. Lee, J.S. Ahn, M.J. Ahn, K. Park, J.M. Sun, Increased response rates to salvage chemotherapy administered after PD-1/PD-L1 inhibitors in patients with non-small cell lung cancer. J. Thor. Oncol. **13**(1), 106–111 (2018)
12. W. Ngwa, O.C. Irabor, J.D. Schoenfeld, J. Hesser, S. Demaria, S.C. Formenti, Using immunotherapy to boost the abscopal effect. Nat. Rev. Cancer **18**(5), 313–322 (2018)
13. T. Osada, H. Nagawa, Y. Shibata, Tumor-infiltrating effector cells of α-galactosylceramide-induced antitumor immunity in metastatic liver tumor. J. Immune Based Ther. Vaccines **2**, 7 (2004)
14. E. Piretto, M. Delitala, M. Ferraro, How combination therapies shape drug resistance in heterogeneous tumoral populations. Lett. Biomath. **5**(sup1), S160–S177 (2018)
15. J. Malinzi, Mathematical analysis of a mathematical model of chemovirotherapy: effect of drug infusion method. Comput. Math. Methods Med. **2019** (2019)
16. E. Urenda-Cázares, A. Gallegos, J. Macías-Díaz, A mathematical model that combines chemotherapy and oncolytic virotherapy as an alternative treatment against a glioma. J. Math. Chem. **58**(3), 544–554 (2020)
17. K.C. Iarosz, F.S. Borges, A.M. Batista, M.S. Baptista, R.A. Siqueira, R.L. Viana, S.R. Lopes, Mathematical model of brain tumour with glia-neuron interactions and chemotherapy treatment. J. Theor. Biol. **368**, 113–121 (2015)
18. R. Padmanabhan, H.S. Kheraldine, N. Meskin, S. Vranic, A.E. Al Moustafa, Crosstalk between HER2 and PD-1/PD-L1 in breast cancer: from clinical applications to mathematical models. Cancers **12**(3), 636 (2020)
19. C. Stangl, J.B. Post, M.J. van Roosmalen, N. Hami, I. Verlaan-Klink, H.R. Vos, R.M. van Es, M.J. Koudijs, E.E. Voest, H.J. Snippert et al., Diverse BRAF gene fusions confer resistance to EGFR-targeted therapy via differential modulation of BRAF activity. Mol. Cancer Res. (2020)
20. Y. Yuan, Z. Sheng, Z. Liu, X. Zhang, Y. Xiao, J. Xie, Y. Zhang, T. Xu, CMTM5-v1 inhibits cell proliferation and migration by downregulating oncogenic EGFR signaling in prostate cancer cells. J. Cancer **11**(13), 3762 (2020)
21. A.M. Jarrett, A. Shah, M.J. Bloom, M.T. McKenna, D.A. Hormuth, T.E. Yankeelov, A.G. Sorace, Experimentally-driven mathematical modeling to improve combination targeted and cytotoxic therapy for HER2+ breast cancer. Sci. Rep. **9**(1), 1–12 (2019)
22. S.E. Rebuzzi, F. Facchinetti, M. Tiseo, Anti-angiogenesis boosts chemo-immunotherapy in patients with EGFR mutations or baseline liver metastases: Insights from IMpower150 study. Transl. Cancer Res. (2019)
23. H. Liang, M. Wang, Prospect of immunotherapy combined with anti-angiogenic agents in patients with advanced non-small cell lung cancer. Cancer Manag. Res. **11**, 7707 (2019)
24. H. Qiang, Q. Chang, J. Xu, J. Qian, Y. Zhang, Y. Lei, B. Han, T. Chu, New advances in antiangiogenic combination therapeutic strategies for advanced non-small cell lung cancer. J. Cancer Res. Clin. Oncol. 1–15 (2020)
25. K. Khan, R. Kerbel, Improving immunotherapy outcomes with anti-angiogenic treatments and vice versa. Nat. Rev. Clin. Oncol. **15**, 310 (2018)
26. C. Stockmann, D. Schadendorf, R. Klose, I. Helfrich, The impact of the immune system on tumor: angiogenesis and vascular remodeling. Front. Oncol. **4**, 69 (2014)
27. F.F. Teles, J.M. Lemos, Cancer therapy optimization based on multiple model adaptive control. Biomed. Signal Process. Control **48**, 255–264 (2019)
28. P. Hahnfeldt, D. Panigrahy, J. Folkman, L. Hlatky, Tumor development under angiogenic signaling: a dynamical theory of tumor growth, treatment response, and postvascular dormancy. Cancer Res. **59**(19), 4770–4775 (1999)
29. U. Ledzewicz, M. Faraji, H. Schättler, Optimal controls for a mathematical model of tumor-immune interactions under targeted chemotherapy with immune boost. Discrete Contin. Dyn. Syst. Ser. B **4** (2013)

30. N. Stepnova, Course of the immune reaction during the development of a malignant tumor. Biophysics **24**(5), 917–923 (1980)
31. I. Hwang, N. Nguyen, Mechanisms of tumor-induced T cell immune suppression and therapeutics to counter those effects. Arch. Pharmacal Res. **38**, 1415–1433 (2015)
32. K. Shimizu, T. Iyoda, M. Okada, S. Yamasaki, S.I. Fujii, Immune suppression and reversal of the suppressive tumor microenvironment. Int. Immunol. **30** (2018)
33. U. Ledzewicz, M. Naghnaeian, H. Schättler, Optimal response to chemotherapy for a mathematical model of tumor-immune dynamics. J. Math. Biol. **64**, 557–577 (2012)
34. M.A. Hedaya, *Basic Pharmacokinetics* (CRC Press, Boca Raton, 2012)
35. L.L. Liu, F. Li, W. Pao, F. Michor, Dose-dependent mutation rates determine optimum erlotinib dosing strategies for EGFR mutant non-small cell lung cancer patients. PloS One **10**(11) (2015)
36. T.D. Thompson, L.A. Pollack, C.J. Johnson, X.C. Wu, J.R. Rees, M.C. Hsieh, R. Rycroft, M. Culp, R. Wilson, M. Wu et al., Breast and colorectal cancer recurrence and progression captured by five US population-based registries: findings from national program of cancer registries patient-centered outcome research. Cancer Epidemiol. **64**, 101653 (2020)
37. Y. Nasu, T. Saika, S. Ebara, N. Kusaka, H. Kaku, F. Abarzua, D. Manabe, T.C. Thompson, H. Kumon, Suicide gene therapy with adenoviral delivery of HSV-tK gene for patients with local recurrence of prostate cancer after hormonal therapy. Mol. Ther. **15**(4), 834–840 (2007)
38. R.E. Tamura, M.G. Lana, E. Costanzi-Strauss, B.E. Strauss, Combination of cabazitaxel and p53 gene therapy abolishes prostate carcinoma tumor growth. Gene Ther. **27**(1), 15–26 (2020)
39. C. Spitzweg, A.B. Dietz, M. O'connor, E. Bergert, D. Tindall, C. Young, J. Morris, In vivo sodium iodide symporter gene therapy of prostate cancer. Gene Ther. **8**(20), 1524–1531 (2001)
40. Y. Tao, Q. Guo, K. Aihara, A mathematical model of prostate tumor growth under hormone therapy with mutation inhibitor. J. Nonlinear Sci. **20**(2), 219–240 (2010)
41. S.O. Freytag, B. Movsas, I. Aref, H. Stricker, J. Peabody, J. Pegg, Y. Zhang, K.N. Barton, S.L. Brown, M. Lu et al., Phase I trial of replication-competent adenovirus-mediated suicide gene therapy combined with imrt for prostate cancer. Mol. Ther. **15**(5), 1016–1023 (2007)
42. S.O. Freytag, K.R. Rogulski, D.L. Paielli, J.D. Gilbert, J.H. Kim, A novel three-pronged approach to kill cancer cells selectively: concomitant viral, double suicide gene, and radiotherapy. Human Gene Therapy **9**(9), 1323–1333 (1998)

Chapter 10
Control Strategies for Cancer Therapy

Novel drugs and treatment methods are introduced for the management of cancer at a very fast pace. Given the complexity and heterogeneity of the disease, decision making regarding the right choice of the drug, dose, drug combination, and treatment schedule has become a perplexing task. Cancer scientists and oncologists worldwide are looking at using the available treatment options in a judicious and more effective manner so as to improve the overall treatment outcome and life quality of the patients. Towards this end, optimal drug dose, treatment schedules, and treatment combinations should be identified.

In the case of aggressive cancers, oncologists often choose intensive treatment strategies to reduce the mortality rate and cancer remission. On the other hand, for less aggressive cancers, sometimes the clinician makes a choice between an intense treatment and an alternative less intensive treatment to reduce tumor burden, drug toxicity, and drug resistance development. Due to the benefits of such patient-specific (personalized) treatment strategies, over the past years, many conventional treatment protocols have been revamped for providing less toxic and more disease-free survival time for patients [1–3]. Such enhancement in treatment protocols is done with respect to the results obtained from the experimental, theoretical, and clinical studies conducted in this area.

As mentioned earlier, one of the main goals of conducting empirical and theoretical studies in cancer research is to reduce the intensity of therapy while achieving equally good treatment outcomes. There are several advanced genomic testing methods and imaging techniques that enable assessing the status of a tumor before and after treatment so as to plan treatment escalation and de-escalation strategies [4, 5]. Accordingly, the oncologists come up with new treatment protocols. For instance, considering the fact that chemotherapy and radiotherapy when used for Hodgkin's lymphoma have caused fatal side effects such as heart disease and secondary cancer, several methods are used to assess treatment outcomes and then the oncologists reduce or skip further radiation or chemotherapy dose. Similarly, with respect to various clinical assessments oncologists decide that early-stage $HER2^+$ subtype of breast

R. Padmanabhan et al., *Mathematical Models of Cancer and Different Therapies*, Series in BioEngineering, https://doi.org/10.1007/978-981-15-8640-8_10

cancer can be treated without chemotherapy [6]. Mathematical model-based simulations and theoretical analysis are also used to gain mechanistic insight in this regard. For instance, in [7], it is pointed out that compared to traditional pulsed chemotherapy, optimal control of chemotherapy facilitates drifting of system dynamics to the desired basin of attraction which represents a tumor-free state where the treatment is no longer required (Sect. 2.5).

As discussed in Chaps. 3–9, in order to conduct theoretical analysis, along with the model that depicts the dynamics of the cell population in the tumor microenvironment, models that represent the drug distribution (pharmacokinetics (PK) and pharmacodynamics (PD)) should also be included to get an overall picture of the drug dynamics and its effect in the patient. Moreover, including mathematical models of drug toxicity and the development of drug resistance will be useful in simulating the realistic dynamics of a patient in response to therapy. It is important to use a reliable mathematical model with adequate descriptive power and predictability to conduct such theoretical analysis (Sect. 2.4). In many cases, some of the parameters used in the mathematical model are assumed and not validated against experimental data [8]. Note that most of the mathematical models that are used to simulate patient dynamics are developed either using in vitro experiments or in vivo experiments (in animal models). Hence, there will be discrepancies between the model dynamics and the actual dynamics of the patient under treatment. These discrepancies will introduce uncertainties in the model parameter values and model mismatch. Even if the clinical data from patients is used for obtaining the model, one patient is different from another (inter-patient variability) and hence there can be a mismatch when such models are used to derive control input (drug infusion) for another patient [9].

Given the complexity of the system (cancer dynamics in a patient), it is apparent that having a no mismatch model is practically not possible. Hence, if the controller is designed with respect to a model, then measures to tackle model parameter mismatch should also be incorporated, or at least the performance of the model-based controller in a range of possible parameter variation should be studied. As it can be seen in the following parts of this chapter, there exist controller design strategies that can derive a drug infusion profile with or without using a mathematical model. Data-driven controller design methods (not based on model) overcome the issues due to model mismatch but they are heuristic methods and involve iterative procedures that are computationally costly.

In this chapter, various control methods that have been used with each treatment methods discussed in Chaps. 3–9 are reviewed and summarized in Tables 10.1, 10.2, 10.3, 10.4, 10.5, 10.6 and 10.7. In each table, the control strategy used, year of publication, reference number, the objective of the control strategy, and model used for controller design and/or simulations are discussed. As shown in Tables 10.1, 10.2, 10.3, 10.4, 10.5, 10.6 and 10.7, controller design strategies such as optimal control, robust control, model predictive control (MPC), adaptive control, feedback linearization control, state-dependent Ricatti equation (SDRE) control, and sliding mode control (SMC) have been used to derive drug dose regimen for various cancer treatment methods. Apart from the model-based methods, heuristic methods such as artificial neural network-based control, fuzzy logic control (FLC), reinforcement learning (RL)-based control, and evolution algorithm (EA)-based controllers are also suggested for the management of cancer treatment.

Various drug dosing patterns such as the ones with low dose control for a long period or an initial high dose followed by a low dose control are followed during cancer therapy [10]. Optimal control methods are used to derive an optimal solution based on the system model and the objective function defined [11]. According to the requirement, several control objectives can be defined. A common one is to minimize the tumor cell population at the final time or over the course of time. Along with this primary objective, several constraints such as keeping the drug concentration below a maximum tolerable dose (MTD), and number of normal cells, immune cells, or level of tumor-suppressing cytokines above a threshold are considered. Note that, the requirement of a reliable model and design complexity involved in deriving a control solution for a nonlinear system with complex dynamics, and difficulty in handling disturbances and parameter uncertainties are important challenges here. Robust control (e.g. H_∞ control) is specifically good at handling disturbance and parameter uncertainties. State feedback controllers which are designed based on linearization around the operating point allows adaptation of linear control theory for the control of nonlinear systems. However, a limited operating range is a drawback.

MPC is a control technique that updates the control solution with respect to the system trajectory predicted by the model of the system towards achieving optimal control objectives. MPC can handle multi-variable optimal control with constraints and it offers enhanced transient and steady-state performance as well. SDRE is another important method that can be used for achieving near-optimal control of systems that exhibits nonlinear dynamics such as that in the case of cancer. This method is known for the flexibility that it offers in the controller design that can be used to tackle singularity and controllability issues associated with optimal control problems.

Adaptive controllers are useful in addressing the time-varying characteristics of the system. For instance, in the case of combination therapy that includes chemotherapy with immunotherapy and anti-angiogenic therapy, as treatment progresses, due to the use of angiogenic inhibitor the carrying capacity of the system changes, similarly the immune boost due to immune therapy also changes the system parameters [12]. Such changes in the system can be accounted for using an adaptive control framework.

Artificial intelligence (AI) based algorithms have also been adopted for supporting decision making in the area of cancer treatments. Evolutionary algorithms come under the superset of AI which mainly follow the learning pattern and dynamics of organisms which involve reproduction, mutation, recombination, and selection [13]. RL-, ANN-, FL-, and EA-based control strategies are data-driven techniques that use AI algorithms to derive optimal infusion profiles for cancer management.

RL-based controllers are a set of data-driven controllers that can learn optimal control solutions based on the interactions with the system. Similar to the other data-driven techniques, the main advantage of this method is that it does not rely on a system model and thus issues related to system uncertainties and model mismatch do not come into the picture. RL-based controllers learn optimal control solution by maximizing the reward achieved for good control moves. However, RL-based methods involve the computationally expensive learning phase.

ANN-based controllers use a generic approximation of input-output relationships to derive control solutions. Since this method relies on self-tuning and adaptability, they are particularly suitable for controlling highly nonlinear systems that are difficult to represent using mathematical models. Even though ANN-based controllers do not require mathematical models, controller design involves computationally expensive training phase and tuning of many parameters in different layers of the network. Moreover, this heuristic method needs a large data set to develop reliable controllers.

Fuzzy logic control framework uses intuitive and knowledge-based rules to control nonlinear and complex systems. When ANN controllers are based on the structural and functional basis (neurons) of the human brain, FL utilizes the human reasoning power. Rapid control action, simplicity of design, and implementation are advantages of this method. However, it involves parameter tuning and relies on a comprehensive and reliable set of rules which may not be available always.

The evolutionary pattern-based algorithm such as genetic algorithm (GA) is also used for optimizing the drug infusion and control of nonlinear cancer dynamics. GA is based on favorable mutations that have accumulated over the years and have led to better adaptation and survival of organisms (e.g. human beings). GA is yet another heuristic method that can be used to search for the best solution among the available set of solutions. As GA is based on heuristic simulations, controller design involves long run time to evaluate multiple objectives [14]. Even though AI-based algorithms demand more computational resources, different methods to override such requirements by sharing workload over the internet are proposed. Other difficulties involved in heuristic genetic algorithms are the selection of the initial population and fixing parameter values of the initial population [15]. In order to override the issue of premature convergence of the genetic algorithm, an iterative dynamic programming technique that involves local search is also added [14].

In a clinical setup, implementation of an open-loop drug infusion or closed-loop control for a short duration (hours) is done with the help of controllable drug infusion pumps and measuring systems that quantify patient response to treatment. However, to implement such controlled drug infusion for a very long duration (months or years) the patient needs to have an implantable or portable drug delivery set up. Many such implantable portable drug-delivering apparatus and even e-drug delivery system are reported in several literature [16–23]. The fact that the FDA has approved an implantable drug delivery apparatus for treating patients with heart disease in 2018 is a motivation for working towards the development of such closed-loop (automatic) drug delivery systems for cancer management.

10.1 Control of Chemotherapy

In Chap. 3, various mathematical models and related biological aspects of cancer dynamics under chemotherapy are presented. Most of the chemotherapeutic drugs have severe side effects and they reach the targeted tumor site via systemic circulation.

Hence, it is important to use drug dosing strategies that will ensure an optimal use of drugs to minimize side effects and maximize desired effects due to treatment. In this section, previous works on the control of chemotherapy as summarized in Table 10.1 are reviewed.

In the case of chemotherapy, along with minimizing tumor burden, it is important to minimize the drug-induced detrimental effects on the healthy host cells. Many works in the literature propose an optimal control of chemotherapy [7, 8, 10, 24–26]. In [7, 8, 10], the optimal solution is derived based on the mathematical model of tumor-immune interaction discussed in Sect. 3.1. In [25], the optimization results of cancer chemotherapy treatment are verified with respect to the mathematical models discussed in [8, 24] using four different data sets. Comparing different objective functions used for optimization, it is pointed out that the value of weighing parameters in objective functions has considerable influence in the derived optimal solutions [26].

SDRE-based controllers are used in [27, 28] to derive a state feedback controller to drive the system to a desired equilibrium (tumor-free equilibrium) using the model discussed in Sect. 3.1. In [28], a state feedback-based controller is designed by using a state estimator to predict the unavailable states from the system measurements.

Model predictive control has been used to control the drug infusion of the chemotherapeutic drug tamoxifen in [29–31]. In all the three works, the cell-cycle model with the pharmacokinetics of the drug tamoxifen is used for controller design. The growth of cells is modeled using the Gompertz model. The pharmacodynamics of tamoxifen is adapted from [32]. Since tamoxifen is a chemotherapeutic drug that can affect various phases of cell-cycle (S-phase, G-phase, and M-phase), the performance of the controller in various phases of cell-cycle is evaluated [29, 30]. Compared to [29], in [30] optimization is done by relatively weighing the tumor volume and amount of drug. Moreover, in [30], an additional moving horizon estimation (MHE) is used to estimate parameters and to account for model uncertainty. In [31], a linear matrix inequality-based controller design framework is used to design a robust MPC that accounts for the model uncertainty.

In [9], an adaptive nonlinear MPC (NMPC) is used to derive a drug infusion profile for treating leukemia patients using the drug 6TGN while accounting for system parameter uncertainties and measurement noises. A personalized drug dose regimen for 6TGN is derived using a model presented in Sect. 3.6 such that the desired value of mean corpuscular volume (MCV) is maintained. Apart from bringing together the advantages of the NMPC in deriving the optimal control solution, this method also allows the use of available clinical measurements for updating the parameters of the controller as well as the model. Similar adaptive controllers are discussed in [33, 34]. A combination of SDRE technique and model reference adaptive control (MRAC) is used in [33], and a nonlinear adaptive control with online parameter identification is used in [34] for realizing optimal and patient-specific control of chemotherapy.

RL-based control algorithms are used in [38, 40] to control chemotherapy. In [38], a simple model that accounts for tumor volume and patient wellness is used. However, in [40], the popular model of tumor-immune interaction (Sect. 3.1) with normal cells, tumor cells, and immune cells are used to represent the simulated patient which is used to derive data for training the RL-controller. Controller performance

Table 10.1 Control of chemotherapy

Control strategy, year [ref]	Objective	Model used	Remark
Optimal control, 2001 [8]	Derive optimal drug dose to minimize tumor burden. Compare the optimal control solution with pulsed chemotherapy	Model in Sect. 3.1	Even though larger oscillation in tumor cell count are seen with optimal control, over the time lesser tumor size is achieved compared to pulsed therapy
EA, 2002 [35]	Optimal drug scheduling for chemotherapy with control and state constraints	A first-order growth kinetics model in [36]	Computational overload issue of the evolutionary algorithm is tackled by sharing workload among multiple computers in a network (internet)
Optimal control, 2007 [10]	Minimize total drug administrated and tumor volume using objective functions (1) quadratic in control (2) linear in control. Minimize tumor with state constraint to keep healthy immune cell level	Modified model of Sect. 3.1	Compared three optimal control strategies. Graphically analyzed possible existence of singular control
GA, 2007 [14]	Optimal control solution for multi-drug scheduling problem using a new memetic algorithm. Iterative dynamic programming is combined with adaptive elitist GA to form new memetic algorithm	Model in Sect. 3.2	Analyzed the effect of chemotherapy on drug-sensitive and drug resistive cell populations
NMPC, 2008 [29]	Derive optimal dose of tamoxifen to track the set point (desired tumor volume). The tumor growth model and PK-PD model of tamoxifen are used	Cell-cycle model with the pharmacokinetics of drug tamoxifen is used for controller design. Growth of cells is modeled using Gompertz model [37]. PD of tamoxifen in [32]	Compared controller performance in tracking the desired tumor volume with respect to models that account for drug effect in various phases of cell-cycles (S-, G-, M-phase). Performance of the controller is dependent on the cell-cycle phase of drug effect

(continued)

Table 10.1 (continued)

Control strategy, year [ref]	Objective	Model used	Remark
RL-based controller, 2009 [38]	Estimate Q-function using support vector regression and extremely randomized tree	An ODE model with two states to represent tumor size and patient's wellness is proposed and used	Model-free controller design to derive optimal drug dose regimen for chemotherapy while accounting for drug toxicity
Adaptive nonlinear MPC, 2010 [9]	Personalized treatment for childhood leukemia. Determine sequence of 6TGN doses to maintain desired MCV	Model in Sect. 3.6	Nominal values are updated to patient specific values using an adaptive method to obtain optimal and patient specific drug dosing
SDRE controller, 2010 [27]	Derive state feedback controller to drive the system to a desired equilibrium (tumor-free equilibrium)	Model in Sect. 3.1	Lesser overall drug administration is achieved using SDRE controller compared to traditional pulsed chemotherapy
SDRE, 2013 [28]	State-feedback-based controller by using a state estimator (EKF) to predict the unavailable states from the system measurements	Model in Sect. 3.1	Accounted for the age and other concurrent illnesses of the patient with cancer
Optimal linear control and nonlinear robust control, 2013 [26]	Compare three control approaches such as optimal linear regulation, nonlinear H_∞ control, and nonlinear optimal control based on the variation of extremals are compared under parameter uncertainty	Gompertz tumor growth model with three different treatment effects such Skippers log-kill model, Norton-Simon model, and sigmoid model is used (Sect. 2.3.4)	H_∞ control is found to be more robust and it provided optimal drug dosage for faster tumor reduction

(continued)

Table 10.1 (continued)

Control strategy, year [ref]	Objective	Model used	Remark
GA, 2016 [39]	GA is used to deduce parameters of two measurement-based PID controllers to control the drug concentration and drug toxicity pertaining to chemotherapy	Finite set of measured data is used	Two PID controllers are used. One in the inner loop to regulate drug concentration desired level and one in the outer loop to maintain the level of drug toxicity within safe limits. No mathematical model is used. Robustness with respect to system parameter variation is shown
RL-based controller, 2017 [40]	Estimate Q-function using ϵ-greedy Q-learning algorithm	Model in Sect. 3.1 is used as an in silico patient in the closed-loop	Model-free controller design to derive optimal drug dose regimen for chemotherapy. Accounted for the age and other concurrent illnesses of the patient with cancer

in the case of an elderly patient, pregnant women, and patients with other concurrent illnesses is also investigated in [40].

Evolutionary computing-based algorithms such as EA or GA-based control of chemotherapy is demonstrated in many literature [14, 35, 39, 41]. In [35], a meta-heuristic optimization algorithm (Paladin-distributed evolutionary computing (DEC) software) is utilized which does not require gradient information or hybridization as in the case of usual/conventional methods. As mentioned in Table 10.1, computational overload can be reduced by sharing the workload among multiple computers in a network. Optimization problems that involve multiple drugs can also be solved using such algorithms [14]. In [39], GA is used to derive parameters of proportional-integral-derivative (PID) controllers based on a finite set of measured data to achieve the desired drug concentration while maintaining the level of drug toxicity within safe limits.

10.2 Control of Immunotherapy

As discussed in Chap. 4, recently the use of immunotherapy for cancer management is becoming more and more popular mainly because it is a biological strategy that can enhance specific anti-tumor functionalities of our immune system. Compared to chemotherapeutic agents, due to the biological compatibility of the immunotherapeutic agents, drug toxicity is not a major concern. However, some of the agents such as immune checkpoint inhibitors which are a recent addition to immunotherapy report many side effects [42]. In this section, previous works on the control of immunotherapy as summarized in Table 10.2 are reviewed.

A common objective pertaining to the control of immunotherapy is minimizing tumor cells by maximizing effector cells using optimal amount of drug [43–50]. In [45], the model discussed in Sect. 4.1 is used to derive an optimal control of adoptive cellular immunotherapy (ACI) to maximize effector cells and IL-2 cytokine while minimizing the tumor cells. Similarly, optimal control of dendritic cell vaccines (DCV) and bacillus Calmette-Guerin (BCG) vaccine are investigated in [51–53]. Relapse of the disease towards the end of treatment and cyclic dynamics of cancer cells are observed in [45, 46, 51], but later on in [54] the complete tumor eradication is achieved by penalizing the final stage [43, 44]. The cost function is further expanded in [49] to include additional constraints to reduce toxicity. As per the review on various optimal control strategies for immunotherapy reported in [44], the most effective treatment schedule is the one with a high initial dose followed by repeated small doses.

Feedback linearization-based controller designing method is used in [55] for the tracking control of two control inputs such as lymphokine-activated killer cells (LAK) and tumor-infiltrating leukocyte (TIL) injections. Closed-loop control is demonstrated using clinically measured (cellometer cell-counter) cell counts and programmable infusion pump (Harvard PHD 2000). Desired tracking and disturbance decoupling are achieved for the multi-input multi-output (MIMO) tumor-immune interaction system.

In [56], a data-driven nonlinear inversion controller is used to control immunotherapy to drive tumor cell numbers close to zero while keeping required levels of effector cells and IL-2. First, an open-loop treatment phase is conducted to reduce the tumor burden as well as to collect data for designing a closed-loop controller. Analysis using Monte Carlo simulation on randomly perturbed patient models show reliable results. An adaptive fuzzy back-stepping controller [58] is used to realize a robust closed-loop MIMO controller to reduce the tumor burden using LAK and TIL injections.

Table 10.2 Control of immunotherapy

Control strategy, year [ref]	Objective	Model used	Remark
Optimal control, 2004 [45]	Minimize tumor cells by maximizing effector cells. Model with activated T cell injection is used for the design. Effect of IL-2 also investigated	Model in Sect. 4.1.	There is a relapse of cancer towards end of treatment (after 300 d)
Optimal control, 2005 [46]	Minimize tumor cells by maximizing effector cells and cytokine IL-2	Model in Sect. 4.1	Noted that cancer cells show cyclic dynamics and are not completely eliminated. Treatment quality is varied with different objective functional that is minimised
Optimal control, 2006 [51]	Minimize final tumor volume as well as the integral of time during which tumor volume is above certain threshold volume	Model in Sect. 4.2	Different injection schemes for DCV with TAA are investigated. The scheme with uniformly allocated injection is the best one
Optimal control, 2010 [54]	Minimize tumor cells by maximizing effector cells and IL-2 even at the end of treatment. An objective function with a linear penalty for the final stage is used	Model in Sect. 4.1	Complete tumor eradication within lesser time frame (150–250 days) of treatment is achieved by penalizing the final stage
Feedback linearization 2010 [55]	Feedback linearization controller for the tracking control of two control inputs such as LAK and TIL injections with almost disturbance decoupling	Model in Sect. 4.1	Closed-loop control using clinically measured (cellometer cell-counter) cell counts and programmable infusion pump (Harvard PHD 2000). Desired tracking and almost disturbance decoupling are achieved for the MIMO tumor-immune interaction system

(continued)

Table 10.2 (continued)

Control strategy, year [ref]	Objective	Model used	Remark
Data-driven model inversion, 2016 [56]	Obtain control inputs (T-cell or IL-2 injection) required to drive tumor cell numbers close to zero while keeping the required levels of effector cells and IL-2. Data-driven nonlinear inversion controller is used	Model in Sect. 4.1	This method involves a phase of open-loop treatment to reduce tumor burden as well as to collect data for controller design followed by a closed-loop phase. Analysis using Monte Carlo simulation on randomly perturbed patient models show reliable results
Optimal, 2017 [53]	Minimize BCG dose with isoperimetric constraint on drug dose to not to exceed experimental dose. Along with minimal dose the overall cost of vaccination is also minimized	Bladder cancer dynamics given in [57]	Optimal BCG treatment via intravesical therapy for a simulated bladder cancer patient is derived
Optimal control, 2017 [52]	Determine injection schedules that minimize final tumor mass	Modified version of model given in [51] is used	Restrictions to reach the lymph node and other immunosuppression mechanisms faced by the DC injections are incorporated in the model. Compared to the therapist suggested doses, the optimal injection schedules are derived using the modified model resulted in lesser total drug usage and final tumor burden
Fuzzy back-stepping control, 2018 [58]	Deduce suitable treatment schedule for multiple drug administration to reduce tumor burden using adaptive fuzzy algorithm (MIMO). LAK and TIL injections are the input	Model in Sect. 4.1	The robust performance of the closed-loop MIMO system for a wide range of the parameter values and uncertainties is shown

10.3 Control of Anti-angiogenic Therapy

As discussed in Chap. 5, angiogenesis marks the transition of avascular tumors to the vascular ones which increases the possibility of tumor metastasis via newly developed abnormally formed blood vessels [59]. Due to the potential of angiogenesis to switch a benign tumor to a malignant one, anti-angiogenesis is an important target of investigation for developing methods for effective cancer treatment. Consequently, many control strategies have been developed to optimize the dosing of the anti-angiogenic agent [60–67]. In this section, previous works on the control of anti-angiogenic therapy as summarized in Table 10.3 are reviewed.

In general, the anti-angiogenic therapy aims to restrict the formation of new blood vessels and thus to facilitate the tumor shrinkage due to inadequate resource supply. Optimal control method is proposed in [68–70] for anti-angiogenic therapy. In [69], a linear quadratic regulator (LQR) controller is designed based on a linearized model of the system at a given operating point. In [70], a binary search method is used to derive the optimal solution and a pole placement based state feedback controller with a state estimator is used in [71]. Similarly, controller design with feedback linearization and path tracking is given in the flat control framework [72]. A feedback linearization based flat control is used to reduce the tumor volume while keeping the level of anti-angiogenic inhibitor below the desired level. Even though the linear control in [69, 71] leads to a lesser control input, the flat control yields more physiologically relevant control input (infusion rate of anti-angiogenic agent). In [63], two controllers (flat control and switching control) are derived for the linearized system which are capable to drive the tumor volume to 1% of the initial volume and to keep the level of anti-angiogenic inhibitor below the desired level. However, the switching control results in a lesser drug usage.

Robust tracking controllers are used in [64, 73] to control anti-angiogenic therapy. H_∞ controller is used in [64] for deriving patient-specific therapy schedules. When controller characteristics are compared at different operating points, controllers designed for lower operating points are more robust against system nonlinearities [64]. Notably, in [73], a closed-loop system with controlled anti-angiogenic infusion is demonstrated using a profusion-system for synthetic vasculature supported by a oxygenation coil. The smooth robust controller is tested against model uncertainties and shows robust tracking of the desired carrying capacity.

Adaptive controller to track the desired optimal trajectory is used in [74] and similarly, in [75], an adaptive fuzzy logic based controller is designed for the optimal and patient parameter specific infusion of an anti-angiogenic agent. Simulation results with parameter perturbation (25%) are used to show the efficacy of the controller in handling the parameter uncertainty. A modified MPC with robust fixed-point transformations (RFPT) is used in [76] to handle measurement error and model uncertainties. An RL-based model-free controller is used in [77] to derive optimal infusion of an anti-angiogenic agent. A switching controller such as SMC is tested in [78] for the control of angiogenesis. To overcome the chattering issue with the switching controller and to derive a smooth infusion profile, a PID surface SMC is used. In [77,

Table 10.3 Control of anti-angiogenic therapy

Control strategy, year [ref]	Objective	Model used	Remark
Optimal control, 2005 [68]	Optimal scheduling of anti-angiogenic drug infusion	Model in Sect. 5.1	Shows that the choice of free final time for optimizing therapy leads to an unrealistic control solution
Adaptive controller, 2010 [74]	Optimum desired trajectory is designed. Two controllers are demonstrated to track defined optimum trajectory, one which relies on complete system knowledge and a second one that accounts for parameter uncertainties	Model in Sect. 5.1	The adaptive controller is able to track the defined optimal trajectory without the knowledge of the system parameters
Optimal control, 2011 [69]	LQR controller based on linearized form of system at certain operating point	Model in Sect. 5.1	The LQR controller leads to a control input with an intense increase in input for an initial period that considerably reduced the tumor population, then a control input of lesser magnitude is maintained
Flat control 2012, [72]	Derive therapeutic protocols for the use of anti-angiogenic agent using feedback linearization and path tracking	Model in Sect. 5.1	Even though the linear control in [69, 71] leads to a lesser control input, the flat control yields more physiologically relevant control input (infusion rate of anti-angiogenic agent)
Flat control and switching control, 2013 [63]	Design a controller to drive the tumor volume to 1% of initial volume in minimum time while keeping the serum level of anti-angiogenic inhibitor below the desired level	Model in Sect. 5.1	Both the controllers are able to drive the tumor volume to 1% of the initial volume and keep the level of anti-angiogenic inhibitor below the desired level. Comparatively the switching control results in a lesser drug usage

(continued)

Table 10.3 (continued)

Control strategy, year [ref]	Objective	Model used	Remark
Nonlinear smooth robust control, 2013 [73]	Tracking control of time-varying carrying capacity by considering a periodic measurement of state variables	Modified version of the model in [60] is used	A closed-loop system with controlled anti-angiogenic infusion is demonstrated using an experimental setup. The smooth robust controller is tested against model uncertainties and shows robust tracking of desired carrying capacity
Linear H_∞ control, 2014 [64]	Derive linear robust controller to track desired tumor volume while accounting for model uncertainties and sensor noise	Model in Sect. 5.1	The linearized system at different operating points is used to design linear H_∞ controllers. When controller characteristics are compared at different operating points, controllers designed for lower operating points are more robust against system nonlinearities
Adaptive fuzzy technique, 2014 [75]	Use adaptive fuzzy controller to attain minimal tumor volume using anti-angiogenic agent	Model in Sect. 5.1	The adaptive fuzzy controller is able to adapt to perturbation (25% variations) in model parameter values
Optimal discrete time control, 2017 [70]	Obtain optimal drug infusion rate at different sampling time using a binary search algorithm	Model in Sect. 5.1	Better result is obtained with a smaller sampling time
Nonlinear MPC, 2018 [76]	Derive robust optimal control input (infusion of anti-angiogenic agent) for the set point tracking of desired tumor volume	Simplified version of model in [60] is used (Sect. 5.1)	Combination nonlinear MPC and Robust fixed point transformations (RFPT) is used to account for measurement errors and model uncertainties

(continued)

Table 10.3 (continued)

Control strategy, year [ref]	Objective	Model used	Remark
Reinforcement learning, 2019 [77]	Derive optimal control inputs for the infusion of an anti-angiogenic agent to reduce the tumor volume to the desired value	Model in Sect. 5.1	A closed-loop learning-based controller is presented. In silico trials conducted with parameter variations show that the controller is robust to tumor growth parameter changes
SMC, 2020 [78]	Derive a robust controller to achieve $<1\%$ of the initial tumor volume in a finite duration	Model in Sect. 5.1	A PID surface SMC is used to obtain smooth infusion profiles. Parameter sensitivity of the controller is extensively studied

78], the performance of the controller against parameter variations is investigated and is within the acceptable ranges.

10.4 Control of Radiotherapy

In Chap. 6, the common ODE models used to represent cancer dynamics under radiation therapy are discussed and it is observed that radiation has opposing effects on endothelial cells and thus the level of oxygenation in the tumor micro-environment. At the low dose, blood vessels become more permeable and consequently the oxygen supply in the tumor is increased. At high doses ($>$6Gy), vessel death happens which increases hypoxia. It should be noted that the therapeutic effect of ionizing radiation is highly dependent on the presence of oxygen in the tumor micro-environment. Moreover, hypoxia is linked to favor the development of radioresistance [79]. These opposing and interlaced effects of radiation dose and the effect of therapy necessitate the use of optimal drug dosing strategies in designing radiation doses for cancer management. In this section, previous works on the control of radiotherapy as summarized in Table 10.4 are reviewed.

In [80, 81], the tumor dynamics under radiotherapy using four different control techniques such as constant control, linear control, feedback control, and periodic control methods are investigated. The effect of radiation on cancer cells alone is studied in [80], while in [81] the effect of radiation on cancer cells and healthy cells are analyzed.

Table 10.4 Control of radiotherapy

Control strategy, year [ref]	Objective	Model used	Remark
Constant, linear, feedback, and periodic control, 2005, [80]	Control of radiotherapy using constant control, linear control, feedback control, and periodic control methods. The effect of radiation on cancer cells alone is studied	Model in Sect. 6.1	Equilibrium point analysis for a range of parameter values is used to evaluate the four types of control. In general, with each type of control, there exists a certain parameter range wherein cancer is completely removed with radiotherapy if detected early enough
Constant, linear, feedback, and periodic control, 2009, [81]	Investigate tumor dynamics under radiotherapy using four different control techniques such as constant control, linear control, feedback control, and periodic control methods. The effect of radiotherapy on cancer cells and healthy cells are studied	Model in Sect. 6.1	Perturbed case (with spillover to healthy cells) is considered for analysis. Existence of a solution in all four cases is shown
RL-based controller, 2017 [82]	Optimize radiotherapy dose for fixed schedule but variable fractional size over the period of treatment	An agent-based model is developed that simulates the vascular tumor growth and are used as an *in silico* patient	An agent based-model and Q-learning based controller is very useful in investigating various dosing scenarios of radiotherapy and derive optimal radiation dose
Optimal control, 2018 [83]	Optimize radiotherapy scheduling for low-grade gliomas	Model in [84] is used	Optimization problem is solved using interior-point (IP) algorithm and sequential quadratic programming (SQP) algorithm

An RL-based controller is used in [82] to optimize radiotherapy doses for a fixed schedule. An agent-based model that simulates the vascular tumor growth is developed and is used as an *in silico* patient. Using simulation results, the agent based-model and Q-learning based controller are able to control various dosing scenarios of radiotherapy and to derive the optimal radiation dose. In [83], an optimal control problem specifically for the control of low-grade gliomas is considered. Towards this end, a mathematical model for low-grade glioma in [84] is used. Interior-point (IP) algorithm and sequential quadratic programming (SQP) algorithm are used to deduce optimal control solutions for the control of low-grade glioma.

Apart from ODE-based models, as treatment effects of radiotherapy can be well quantified using imaging techniques, several image-based spatio-temporal feature analyzing techniques are also used to adjust treatment. For instance, in [85], optimization of radiotherapy is investigated using a murine data-based computer model in which the tumor heterogeneity and resistance to radiotherapy are assessed by using image processing techniques.

10.5 Control of Hormone Therapy

As detailed in Chap. 7, one of the important fact that should be considered while deciding drug dose and treatment schedule for hormone therapy is that an inappropriate drug dosing regimen can induce treatment-induced mutation of hormone-dependent cancer cells to hormone-independent cells leading to the relapse of the disease after treatment. Such castration-resistant (hormone-independent) tumor cells are much more difficult to treat. Hence, optimization of treatment in terms of minimal drug usage and timely scheduling is important. In this section, previous works on the control of hormone therapy as summarized in Table 10.5 are reviewed.

MPC is used in [86] to derive an optimal schedule for drug administration based on a piecewise affine model that represents tumor dynamics under hormone therapy. In this paper, it is shown that the optimal control solution derived is far less (by half) than the amount of drug used in the case of conventional intermittent androgen suppression (IAS) therapy. Similarly, an optimal control strategy is demonstrated in [88] for treating castration-resistant prostate cancer cells based on a Lodka-Volterra competition model. In [88], an optimal control strategy is used to treat metastatic prostate cancer for castration-resistant (androgen-independent) cells. Note that this is not androgen deprivation therapy as here androgen-independent cancer cells are treated. Using simulation results, it is shown that compared to other high dose treatments using the drug abiraterone which induce increased mutation and development of drug-resistant variants, the use of optimal drug dose allows a long term control of prostate cancer.

As shown in Table 10.5, the applicability of very few control methods is investigated for hormone therapy. Even though PK-PD of several drugs used for hormone therapy is available which can be used to derive individualized drug dosing, such drug-specific controller design are yet to be reported in the case of hormone ther-

Table 10.5 Control of hormone therapy

Control strategy, year [ref]	Objective	Model used	Remark
MPC, 2010, [86]	Derive optimal schedule for drug administration using MPC based on a piecewise affine model that represents tumor dynamics under hormone therapy	Model in [87] is used to derive a piecewise affine model	The optimal control solution is far less (by half) than the amount of drug used in case of usual intermittent androgen suppression therapy
Optimal control, 2018 [88]	Derive optimal drug dose for treating castration resistant prostate cancer cells	A Lodka-Voltera competition model is defined in [88]	Compared to other high dose treatment using abiraterone which induce increased mutation and development of drug resistant variants, the use of optimal drug dose allows a long term control of prostate cancer

apy. For instance, suramin is a drug used for hormone therapy [89] and a maximum a priori Bayesian estimator is used to estimate the plasma concentration profile of suramin in each patient. Such information along with mathematical models of cancer dynamics can be used to derive drug-specific control of hormone therapy.

10.6 Miscellaneous Therapy

In Chap. 8, many mathematical models are discussed that represent cancer dynamics under gene therapy, oncolytic virotherapy, nanocarrier-based therapy, and stem cell therapy under the heading of miscellaneous therapy. In this section, previous works on the control of such miscellaneous therapies as summarized in Table 10.6 are reviewed.

Recall that as shown in Figure 8.1, viral and non-viral vectors are used to facilitate gene therapy. Nanocarriers and genetically altered DC or T cells are also used for gene therapy. As immunogenicity of the tumor can be enhanced by gene therapy, some literature discuss such methods under the heading of immunotherapy. Out of the gene therapy methods, optimal control of gene therapy mediated by small interfering RNA (siRNA) is discussed in [90–92]. In [90], an optimal use of gene therapy to annihilate tumor cells by modulating the immune action mediated by TGF-β and IL-2 cytokine is demonstrated. In [92], a multi-objective optimization algorithm based

Table 10.6 Control of miscellaneous therapy

Control strategy, therapy, year [ref]	Objective	Model used	Remark
MPC and ANN, nanotherapy, 2009 [96]	Using an ANN-based drug release model of chemotherapeutic drug doxorubicin, the application of ultrasound is optimized to facilitate controlled drug release at the target site. MPC is used to optimize reference signal tracking	A neural-network equivalent of the dynamic model that represents the drug release process is used	The MPC controller is capable of fine-tuning the ultrasound intensity, frequency, and pulse width to sustain constant release of doxorubicin
Optimal control, gene therapy, 2012 [90]	Derive optimal control solution of siRNA mediated to achieve desired tumor size using AVK (A.V. Kamyad) method to solve nonlinear problems with uncertain parameters (NPUP)	Model in Sect. 8.1.2	Treatment with siRNA is considered to reduce the effect of TGF-β. Moreover, the effect of IL-2 is used to minimize the tumor cell
SDRE, nanotherapy, 2016 [97]	Optimal control of drug-loaded nanoparticles to facilitate anti-angiogenesis (endostatin), chemotherapy (doxorubicin), and radiotherapy (yttrium-90) as monotherapy options for liver cancer	Hahnfeldt's model is used to investigate anti-angiogensis (Sect. 5.1) and extended to incorporate chemotherapy [10]. The LQ model (Sect. 6.2) of radiotherapy is used to study the controlled delivery of radioisotope	Controlled locoregional magnetic-bolus administration of nanoparticles enabled reduced treatment time and optimal targeted drug usage
Optimal control, gene therapy, 2018 [92]	Optimal control of siRNA (non-viral) mediated gene therapy. A multi-objective optimization algorithm that minimizes total inhibitory effect and cytotoxicity is used	A simple two compartmental model that represents siRNA pharmacokinetics is used	Optimized undesirable gene expression as well as cytotoxicity are considered by accounting for time constraints related to the problem

(continued)

Table 10.6 (continued)

Control strategy, therapy, year [ref]	Objective	Model used	Remark
Successive SDRE, virotherapy, 2019 [93]	To derive optimal infusion rate for virotherapy by successively solving associated SDRE	Model in [98] is used	The effect of the immune system on the dynamics of viruses and tumor cells is considered as a disturbance. Using the robust and optimal control of virotherapy, the number of cancer cells reduced but not completely removed
MPC, stem cell therapy, 2019, [99]	Optimal control of notch-signaling pathway inhibitor to control melanoma. Intravenous dual anti-platelet therapy (DAPT) is used to reduce tumor growth	Gompertz model is used to represent tumor growth. A mathematical model that describes DAPT in melanoma patients is developed using experimental results on mice model	Using the model proposed, the influence of drug resistance on the treatment efficacy is also investigated. With optimal treatment planning, the tumor growth is minimized despite the development of drug resistance
MPC and ANN, nanotherapy, 2020 [100]	Design a drug release NN-MPC controller based on a neural network-based model of the system. External ultrasound trigger is used to initiate drug (attached to liposome) release into the tumor micro-environment	An in vitro drug release set up is used to mimic the ultrasound triggered drug release into to tumor site. An artificial neural network (ANN) model is used to represent the controlled patient. The ANN-based model is developed with respect to in vitro experimental details	The acoustically controlled feedback drug release set up is able to keep a safe and effective therapeutical level of drug in the tumor micro-environment

on a simple two-compartmental model of siRNA pharmacokinetics is discussed. Similarly, robust and optimal control of virotherapy is reported in [93–95]. In [93], the optimal infusion rate for virotherapy by successively solving associated SDRE is discussed. Using the SDRE-based robust and optimal control of virotherapy, the number of cancer cells reduced but not completely removed.

As mentioned in the case of immunotherapy, incomplete annihilation of cancer cells points to the need of combining gene therapy with other treatment strategies towards achieving improved treatment with less toxicity. MPC of stem cell therapy for melanoma patients is discussed in [99]. Stem cell therapy is facilitated using intravenous dual anti-platelet therapy (DAPT). In [99], a mathematical model of DAPT is developed that accounts for drug resistance in melanoma patients using experimental results on mice model. With an optimal treatment planning, the tumor growth is minimized despite the development of drug resistance. Similarly, SDRE-based optimal control of drug-loaded nanoparticles to facilitate anti-angiogenesis (endostatin), chemotherapy (doxorubicin), and radiotherapy (yttrium-90) as monotherapy options for liver cancer is discussed in [97].

Several recent literature discuss the optimization of nanocarrier-based drug delivery for cancer treatment [96, 97, 100, 101]. There are some common features in the control strategies presented in [96, 100], and both works use MPC and artificial neural network (ANN) for control of nanotherapy, and in both cases, drug release is facilitated by external application of ultrasound. Moreover, a neural network equivalent to the dynamic model is used that represents the drug release process. Here, the MPC is used for fine-tuning the ultrasound intensity, frequency, and pulse width to sustain the constant release of the chemotherapeutic drug (doxorubicin). Compared with [96], in [100] an in vitro drug release set up is demonstrated and an ANN-based model is developed with respect to in vitro experiment. Using the ANN-based MPC and ANN-based drug release model, acoustic controlled feedback drug release set up is able to keep a safe and effective therapeutical level of drug in the tumor micro-environment.

10.7 Control of Combination Therapy

Some treatment strategies such as immunotherapy, anti-angiogenic therapy, and virotherapy, when used as a monotherapy are inadequate for the complete annihilation of cancer cells. Hence, often such therapies are used in combination with other treatment methods. In Chap. 9, mathematical models that represent cancer dynamics under various combinations of treatment strategies are discussed. In this section, previous works on the control of combination therapies as summarized in Table 10.7 are reviewed.

It can be seen in this table that out of the 11 works listed, the most widely investigated one is the control of combination therapy that include immunotherapy [102–107]. Considering all types of combinations therapy, it can be seen that the efficacy of optimal control, GA, SDRE, adaptive algorithm, and fuzzy logic-based controllers have been investigated for the controlled infusion of drugs used to facilitate combination treatment.

Control of chemotherapy when used in combination with immunotherapy, anti-angiogenic therapy, radiotherapy, and virotherapy are listed in Table 10.7. Several studies show that the final tumor size and tumor relapse time can be decreased with combination therapy compared to the case when chemotherapy alone is used [103, 104, 106–109]. Similarly, clinical evidences show a possible improved efficacy in

Table 10.7 Combination therapy

Control strategy, year [ref]	Objective	Model used	Remark
Optimal control, radiotherapy with anti-angiogenic therapy, 2003, [113]	Maximize tumor cure probability (calculated using poison model) which is commonly used to assess success of radiotherapy	Models in [60, 114] (Sects. 6.2 and 5.1) are used	Out of the possible combination strategies, optimal control suggested dose intensifies the drug dosing protocol
Optimal control, chemotherapy with anti-angiogenesis, 2009 [24]	Optimize the amount of chemotherapeutic and anti-angiogenic drugs required to eradicate tumor	A modified model in [60] that additionally accommodate chemotherapy infusion is used (Sect. 5.1)	Optimal control solution derived contains some singular segments which are practically not realizable. However, the provided theoretical analysis presents insights to derive realistic control solutions
GA, chemotherapy with immunotherapy, 2013 [104]	Optimize the use of chemotherapeutic agent (doxorubicin) and immunotherapy (adoptive-cell-transfer) using genetic algorithm. Multi-objective optimization along with post-Pareto-optimality analysis is used	A combined model given in [36, 115] is used	Final tumor size and tumor relapse time have been decreased with combination therapy compared to the case when chemotherapy is used alone
Optimal control, chemotherapy with immunotherapy, 2013 [103]	Optimize the use of chemotherapeutic drug and immunotherapeutic agents to minimize the number of cancer cells at a final time	Model discussed in [116] is used	Both qualitative and quantitative analysis pertaining to the optimal control solution are provided. The relative importance of the side effects is discussed using numerical simulation
Optimal control, chemotherapy with immunotherapy, 2013 [105]	Minimize the use of drugs and thus reduce drug toxicity and maximize T helper cells that boost immune cells. An optimization algorithm is used to solve the two-point boundary value problem	Mixed chemotherapy and immunotherapy model in [117] is used	Iterative forward and backward stepping algorithm is used to solve the two-point boundary value problem numerically

(continued)

Table 10.7 (continued)

Control strategy, year [ref]	Objective	Model used	Remark
SDRE control, chemotherapy with immunotherapy, 2014 [106]	Derive an optimal finite duration control solution to achieve a healthy state. Vaccine therapy is used to alter system parameters and chemotherapy is used to drive the system states to desired healthy state	A modified version of mixed chemotherapy and immunotherapy model in [117, 118] is used.	Accounts for the changing dynamics (tumor-immune interaction) during treatment
Optimal control, virotherapy with targeted control, 2016 [119]	Minimize the tumor volume and the use of MEK inhibitor	A mathematical model is proposed which is a modified version of the model discussed in Sect. 9.2.1	The model does not have a cure-equilibrium. Hence, the tumor can be cured by oncolytic virotherapy
Optimal control, chemotherapy with virotherapy, 2018 [108]	Optimize the use of chemotherapy and virotherapy such that combined tumor (infected and non infected) population is minimized adequately	An extended version of the model discussed in Sect. 9.2.1 using parameter values in [120–122] is used	Results show that success of combinational therapy depends on the infection rate, virus burst size, and the amount of drugs and the optimal chemotherapeutic drug and virus combination is half of the respective maximum tolerated doses (MTD)
Adaptive control, chemotherapy with anti-angiogenic therapy, 2019 [109]	Objective is to design an adaptive controller to follow an optimal trajectory	Model in [123] is used	Parameter estimation is done by recursive algorithm and the closed-loop stability of the system is shown using Lyapunov theory
Multiple model adaptive control, immunotherapy with anti-angiogenic therapy, 2019, [102]	Design a decision support system to optimize drug usage and reduce tumor volume and drug-induced toxicity for metastatic RCC. Along with tumor dynamics, the pharmacodynamic model, and toxicity model are used to represent the system	Models in [60, 103] are used	Unsupervised learning and clustering methods are used to select models from multiple patient models. Drug resistance, drug toxicity, pharmacodynamics of drug, and parameter uncertainties are accounted for

(continued)

Table 10.7 (continued)

Control strategy, year [ref]	Objective	Model used	Remark
Fuzzy control, chemotherapy and immunotherapy, 2020 [107]	Objective is to drive the system from malignant region to benign region wherein immune system can effectively inhibit the tumor growth	Takagi-Sugeno model is derived and used	Optimization problem is solved using convex optimization approach

treatment when chemotherapy is combined with hormone therapy [110], nanocarrier mediated siRNA (genetherapy) [111], and stem cell therapy [112]. However, mathematical models and control strategies of such combination treatment are yet to be investigated.

Next to chemotherapy, the most investigated combination therapy is the one that includes immunotherapy with other methods [102–107, 124, 125]. The main advantage of combining immunotherapy with chemotherapy is the reduced use of the chemotherapeutic agent which will in turn significantly decrease the drug-induced toxicity and resistance development. A combination of immunotherapy with chemotherapy and anti-angiogenic therapy are listed in Table 10.7. The potential benefit of combining immunotherapy with radiotherapy [126] and hormone therapy [127] have initiated several clinical trials. However, mathematical models and control strategies of such combination treatment are yet to be investigated.

The optimal control and adaptive control of anti-angiogenic therapy in combination with radiotherapy, chemotherapy, and immunotherapy are discussed in [24, 102, 109, 113, 128]. Combining anti-angiogenic therapy with virotherapy [129] and hormone deprivation therapy [130] show positive impacts in certain type of cancers. However, mathematical models and control strategies of such combination treatment are yet to be investigated.

Optimal control of virotherapy with a type of targeted (MEK inhibitor) therapy and chemotherapy is reported in [108, 119]. Results show that the success of combinational therapy that involves virotherapy depends on the infection rate, virus burst size, and the amount of drugs used. Moreover, in the case of combination therapy, the optimal chemotherapeutic drug and virus combination is half of the respective maximum tolerated doses (MTD).

10.8 Summary

As it can be seen from Tables 10.1, 10.2, 10.3, 10.4, 10.5, 10.6 and 10.7, the optimal control strategy is the most widely investigated method as it can account for state and control constraints and allows stability analysis of the system under control for certain parameter ranges. However, model dependence and difficulties in handling parameter uncertainty, disturbance, and measurement noise have motivated researchers to investigate the efficacy of adaptive control strategies for the control of various therapies. Apart from the optimal and adaptive methods, several computationally intense heuristic methods such as ANN-, EA-, RL-, and FL-based methods are also used. Most of these control methods are tested for general treatment type (e.g. chemotherapy, immunotherapy), only very few methods have been investigated for cancer-specific treatments (e.g. chemotherapy for multiple myeloma) or drug-specific (e.g. control of tamoxifen or 6TGN). Given that the cancer dynamics vary with the type of cancer and mechanism (PK-PD) of action of drug used, conducting more disease-specific and drug-specific analysis of controllers can enhance the reliability of such methods for the use of cancer management. Moreover, validation of results using real patient data is also desirable [131].

As detailed in Chap. 9, combination therapy is preferred over monotherapy for the management of cancer due to the evidence of reduced drug toxicity, disease relapse, and the development of drug resistance [132]. Consequently, several mathematical models and controller design strategies that account for the combination of chemotherapy, immunotherapy, and anti-angiogenic therapy are studied. However, combination therapies that include hormone therapy, radiotherapy, virotherapy, and stem cell therapy are yet to be explored widely.

Evidences suggest that optimizing the treatment scheduling of immunotherapy improves the treatment efficacy of radiation therapy [133–135]. Similarly, short-term androgen deprivation and radiotherapy are suggested for prostate cancer [136, 137]. Studies show that there exist an immune modulation under hormone suppression and radiation therapy [138]. Based on this evidence, several studies point out the synergy that needs to be exploited in the area of treating hormone-dependent cancer cells with immunotherapy [139–142]. Hence, more research is required in this area towards the development of mathematical models and control strategies.

As an effective approach of targeting the drug to the tumor site while minimizing leakage to the systemic circulation, nanocarrier based therapy is a game-changer in cancer treatment. Several recent reviews report possible enhancement of immunotherapy using nanomedicines [97, 143, 144]. There exist many studies that investigate the enhanced treatment efficacy, when nanocarrier are used for drug-specific (e.g. docetaxel, doxorubicin) and cancer-specific (e.g. prostate cancer) treatment [145]. Similarly, nanocarrier is investigated in dendritic cell-based targeting of cancer stem cells (tumor re-initiating cells) in gynecological cancers [146].

One of the recent addition to immunotherapy such as immune checkpoint inhibitors has been showing positive results when combined with several conventionally used drugs. Immune checkpoint inhibitors are drugs that restrict the immune evasion by cancer cells. For instance, the use of immune checkpoint inhibitors has improved treatment outcomes of aggressive and difficult to treat cancers such as triple-negative and $HER2^+$ breast cancers [147]. Similarly, oncolytic viruses can enhance the infiltration of TILs into the tumor micro-environment and thus enhance the efficacy of immune checkpoint inhibitors (anti-PD-1) [148]. Immune evasion being one of the important hallmarks of cancer, it is imperative to develop mathematical models and controller design strategies that account for the action of immune checkpoint inhibitors in cancer treatment.

References

1. C.M. Craig, G.J. Schiller, Acute myeloid leukemia in the elderly: conventional and novel treatment approaches. Blood Rev. **22**(4), 221–234 (2008)
2. R. Ramakrishnan, D.I. Gabrilovich, Novel mechanism of synergistic effects of conventional chemotherapy and immune therapy of cancer. Cancer Immunol. Immunother. **62**(3), 405–410 (2013)
3. M. Gerwing, K. Herrmann, A. Helfen, C. Schliemann, W.E. Berdel, M. Eisenblätter, M. Wildgruber, The beginning of the end for conventional RECIST-novel therapies require novel imaging approaches. Nat. Rev. Clin. Oncol. **16**(7), 442–458 (2019)
4. M.J. Xu, Z. Kornberg, A.J. Gadzinski, D. Diao, J.E. Cowan, S.Y. Wu, L. Boreta, D.E. Spratt, S.C. Behr, H.G. Nguyen et al., Genomic risk predicts molecular imaging-detected metastatic nodal disease in prostate cancer. Eur. Urol. Oncol. **2**(6), 685–690 (2019)
5. G. Lee, S. H. Bak, H. Y. Lee, J. Y. Choi, H. Park, Radiomics and imaging genomics for evaluation of tumor response, in *Therapy Response Imaging in Oncology* (Springer, 2020), pp. 221–238
6. A. Llombart Cussac, J. Cortés, L. Paré, P. Galván, B. Bermejo, N. Martínez, M. Vidal, S. Pernas, R. López, M. Muñoz, et al., HER2-enriched subtype as a predictor of pathological complete response following trastuzumab and lapatinib without chemotherapy in early-stage HER2-positive breast cancer (PAMELA): An open-label, single-group, multicentre, Phase 2 trial. Lancet Oncol. **18**(4), 545–554 (2017)
7. L.D. Pillis, A. Radunskaya, The dynamics of an optimally controlled tumor model: A case study. Math. Comput. Model. **37**(11), 1221–1244 (2003)
8. L.G.D. Pillis, A. Radunskaya, A mathematical tumor model with immune resistance and drug therapy: an optimal control approach. Comput. Math. Methods Med. **3**(2), 79–100 (2001)
9. S.L. Noble, E. Sherer, R.E. Hannemann, D. Ramkrishna, T. Vik, A.E. Rundell, Using adaptive model predictive control to customize maintenance therapy chemotherapeutic dosing for childhood acute lymphoblastic leukemia. J. Theor. Biol. **264**(3), 990–1002 (2010)
10. L.G.D. Pillis, W. Gu, K.R. Fister, T.A. Head, K. Maples, A. Murugan, T. Neal, K. Yoshida, Chemotherapy for tumors: an analysis of the dynamics and a study of quadratic and linear optimal controls. Math. Biosci. **209**(1), 292–315 (2007)
11. H. Schättler, U. Ledzewicz, *Optimal Control for Mathematical Models of Cancer Therapies*, vol. 42 (Springer, 2015)
12. X. Han, Dynamical analysis of chemotherapy models with time-dependent infusion. Nonlinear Anal.: Real World Appl. **34**, 459–480 (2017)
13. R.J. Preen, L. Bull, A. Adamatzky, Towards an evolvable cancer treatment simulator. Biosystems **182**, 1–7 (2019)
14. S.M. Tse, Y. Liang, K.S. Leung, K.H. Lee, T.S.K. Mok, A memetic algorithm for multiple-drug cancer chemotherapy schedule optimization. IEEE Trans. Syst. Man Cybern. Part B (Cybern.) **37**(1), 84–91 (2007)
15. H. Sbeity, R. Younes, Review of optimization methods for cancer chemotherapy treatment planning. J. Comput. Sci. Syst. Biol. **8**, 074–095 (2015)
16. P.J. Blackshear, Implantable drug-delivery systems. Sci. Am. **241**(6), 66–73 (1979)
17. S.R. Baker, R.H. Wheeler, W.D. Ensminger, J.E. Niederhuber, Intraarterial infusion chemotherapy for head and neck cancer using a totally implantable infusion pump. Head Neck Surg. **4**(2), 118–124 (1981)
18. C. Zhao, H. Feng, L. Zhang, Z. Li, Y. Zou, P. Tan, H. Ouyang, D. Jiang, M. Yu, C. Wang et al., Highly efficient in vivo cancer therapy by an implantable magnet triboelectric nanogenerator. Adv. Funct. Mater. **29**(41), 1808640 (2019)

19. E.M. Tucker, Drug administration systems for infusion chemotherapy, in *Cancer Chemotherapy by Infusion* (Springer, 1987), pp. 41–58
20. A.G. Nanninga, E.G. de Vries, P.H. Willemse, B.E. Oosterhuis, D.T. Sleijfer, H.J. Hoekstra, N.H. Mulder, Continuous infusion of chemotherapy on an outpatient basis via a totally implanted venous access port. Eur. J. Cancer Clin Oncol. **27**(2), 147–149 (1991)
21. Y. Inoue, M. Kusunoki, Advances and directions in chemotherapy using implantable port systems for colorectal cancer: A historical review. Surg. Today **44**(8), 1406–1414 (2014)
22. H. Kaurav, D.N. Kapoor, Implantable systems for drug delivery to the brain. Therap. Del. **8**(12), 1097–1107 (2017)
23. K.S. Yadav, S. Kapse-Mistry, G. Peters, Y. Mayur, E-drug delivery: a futuristic approach. Drug Discovery Today (2019)
24. A. d'Onofrio, U. Ledzewicz, H. Maurer, H. Schättler, On optimal delivery of combination therapy for tumors. Math. Biosci. **222**(1), 13–26 (2009)
25. M. Engelhart, D. Lebiedz, S. Sager, Optimal control for selected cancer chemotherapy ODE models: a view on the potential of optimal schedules and choice of objective function. Math. Biosci. **229**(1), 123–134 (2011)
26. H. Moradi, G. Vossoughi, H. Salarieh, Optimal robust control of drug delivery in cancer chemotherapy: a comparison between three control approaches. Comput. Methods Programs Biomed. **112**(1), 69–83 (2013)
27. T. Çimen, Systematic and effective design of nonlinear feedback controllers via the state-dependent Riccati equation (SDRE) method. Ann. Rev. Control **34**(1), 32–51 (2010)
28. Y. Batmani, H. Khaloozadeh, Optimal chemotherapy in cancer treatment: state dependent Riccati equation control and extended Kalman filter. Opt. Control Appl. Methods **34**(5), 562–577 (2013)
29. J.A. Florian Jr., J.L. Eiseman, R.S. Parker, Nonlinear model predictive control for dosing daily anticancer agents using a novel saturating-rate cell-cycle model. Comput. Biol. Med. **38**(3), 339–347 (2008)
30. T. Chen, N.F. Kirkby, R. Jena, Optimal dosing of cancer chemotherapy using model predictive control and moving horizon state/parameter estimation. Comput. Methods Programs Biomed. **108**(3), 973–983 (2012)
31. P. Bumroongsri, S. Kheawhom, Optimal dosing of breast cancer chemotherapy using robust MPC based on linear matrix inequalities. Eng. J. **19**(1), 97–106 (2015)
32. S.P. Robinson, S.M. Langan Fahey, D.A. Johnson, V.C. Jordan, Metabolites, pharmacodynamics, and pharmacokinetics of tamoxifen in rats and mice compared to the breast cancer patient. Drug Metabol. Disposit. **19**(1), 36–43, (1991)
33. N. Babaei, M.U. Salamci, Personalized drug administration for cancer treatment using model reference adaptive control. J. Theor. Biol. **371**, 24–44 (2015)
34. M. Sharifi, H. Moradi, Nonlinear composite adaptive control of cancer chemotherapy with online identification of uncertain parameters. Biomed. Signal Process. Control **49**, 360–374 (2019)
35. K.C. Tan, E.F. Khor, J. Cai, C. Heng, T.H. Lee, Automating the drug scheduling of cancer chemotherapy via evolutionary computation. Artif. Intell. Med. **25**(2), 169–185 (2002)
36. R. Martin, Optimal control drug scheduling of cancer chemotherapy. Automatica **28**(6), 1113–1123 (1992)
37. J. Florian Jr, J. Eiseman, and R. Parker, Approximating cancer tumor growth dynamics using cell-cycle models in series, in *AIChE Annual Meeting*, p. 439ab (2003)
38. Y. Zhao, M.R. Kosorok, D. Zeng, Reinforcement learning design for cancer clinical trials. Stat. Med. **28**(26), 3294–3315 (2009)
39. S. Khadraoui, F. Harrou, H.N. Nounou, M.N. Nounou, A. Datta, S.P. Bhattacharyya, A measurement-based control design approach for efficient cancer chemotherapy. Inf. Sci. **333**, 108–125 (2016)
40. R. Padmanabhan, N. Meskin, W.M. Haddad, Reinforcement learning-based control of drug dosing for cancer chemotherapy treatment. Math. Biosci. **293**, 11–20 (2017)

41. K. Badakhshan, H. Khaloozadeh, Optimal control for cancer chemotherapy using genetic algorithm. WSEAS Trans. Biol. Biomed. **2**(1), 109–115 (2005)
42. F. Scotté, R. Ratta, P. Beuzeboc, Side effects of immunotherapy: a constant challenge for oncologists. Curr. Opin. Oncol. **31**(4), 280–285 (2019)
43. B. Piccoli, F. Castiglione, Optimal vaccine scheduling in cancer immunotherapy. Phys. A **370**(2), 672–680 (2006)
44. A. Konstorum, A.T. Vella, A.J. Adler, R.C. Laubenbacher, Addressing current challenges in cancer immunotherapy with mathematical and computational modelling. J. R. Soc. Interface **14**(131), 20170150 (2017)
45. T.N. Burden, J. Ernstberger, K.R. Fister, Optimal control applied to immunotherapy. Discret. Contin. Dyn. Syst. Ser. B **4**(1), 135–146 (2004)
46. K.R. Fister, J.H. Donnelly, Immunotherapy: an optimal control theory approach. Math. Biosci. Eng. **2**(3), 499 (2005)
47. A. Hamdache, S. Saadi, I. Elmouki, Nominal and neighboring-optimal control approaches to the adoptive immunotherapy for cancer. Int. J. Dyn. Control **4**(3), 346–361 (2016)
48. H. Basirzadeh, S. Nazari, T-lymphocyte cell injection cancer immunotherapy: an optimal control approach. Iran. J. Oper. Res. **3**(1), 46–60 (2012)
49. F. Castiglione, B. Piccoli, Cancer immunotherapy, mathematical modeling and optimal control. J. Theor. Biol. **247**(4), 723–732 (2007)
50. M. Alkama, A. Larrache, M. Rachik, I. Elmouki, Optimal duration and dosage of BCG intravesical immunotherapy: a free final time optimal control approach. Math. Methods Appl. Sci. **41**(5), 2209–2219 (2018)
51. F. Castiglione, B. Piccoli, Optimal control in a model of dendritic cell transfection cancer immunotherapy. Bull. Math. Biol. **68**(2), 255–274 (2006)
52. J. Rangel Reyes, J.C. Chimal Eguia, E. Castillo Montiel, Dendritic immunotherapy improvement for an optimal control murine model. *Comput. Math. Methods Med.* **2017** (2017)
53. I. Elmouki, S. Saadi, BCG immunotherapy optimization on an isoperimetric optimal control problem for the treatment of superficial bladder cancer. Int. J. Dyn. Control **4**(3), 339–345 (2016)
54. A. Ghaffari, N. Naserifar, Optimal therapeutic protocols in cancer immunotherapy. Comput. Biol. Med. **40**(3), 261–270 (2010)
55. T. Chien, C. Chen, C. Huang, Feedback linearization control and its application to MIMO cancer immunotherapy. IEEE Trans. Control Syst. Technol. **18**(4), 953–961 (2010)
56. C. Novara, M. Karimshoushtari, A data-driven model inversion approach to cancer immunotherapy control, in *2016 IEEE 55th Conference on Decision and Control (CDC)* (IEEE, 2016), pp. 5047–5052
57. S. Bunimovich Mendrazitsky, E. Shochat, L. Stone, Mathematical model of BCG immunotherapy in superficial bladder cancer, Bull. Math. Biol. **69**(6), pp. 1847–1870
58. H. Nasiri, A.A. Kalat, Adaptive fuzzy back-stepping control of drug dosage regimen in cancer treatment. Biomed. Signal Process. Control **42**, 267–276 (2018)
59. A. Anderson, M. Chaplain, Continuous and discrete mathematical models of tumor-induced angiogenesis. Bull. Math. Biol. **60**(5), 857–899 (1998)
60. P. Hahnfeldt, D. Panigrahy, J. Folkman, L. Hlatky, Tumor development under angiogenic signaling: a dynamical theory of tumor growth, treatment response, and postvascular dormancy. Cancer Res. **59**(19), 4770–4775 (1999)
61. U. Ledzewicz, H. Schättler, Antiangiogenic therapy in cancer treatment as an optimal control problem. SIAM J. Control Optim. **46**(3), 1052–1079 (2007)
62. U. Ledzewicz, H. Schattler, A. Berman, On the structure of optimal controls for a mathematical model of tumor anti-angiogenic therapy with linear pharmacokinetics, in *2009 IEEE Control Applications, (CCA) Intelligent Control, (ISIC)* (2009), pp. 71–76
63. A. Szeles, D.A. Drexler, J. Sápi, I. Harmati, L. Kovács, Model-based angiogenic inhibition of tumor growth using feedback linearization, in *52nd IEEE Conference on Decision and Control* (2013), pp. 2054–2059

64. L. Kovács, A. Szeles, J. Sápi, D.A. Drexler, I. Rudas, I. Harmati, Z. Sápi, Model-based angiogenic inhibition of tumor growth using modern robust control method. Comput. Methods Programs Biomed. **114**(3), e98–e110 (2014)
65. A. Swierniak, Control problems in anti-angiogenic therapy-comparison of six models. IFAC Proc. Vol. **41**(2), 10313–10318 (2008)
66. C. Tunceroglu, U. Hasirci, Controller and observer design for anti-angiogenic tumor treatment, in *2017 International Conference on Circuits, System and Simulation (ICCSS)* (IEEE, 2017), pp. 54–58
67. U. Ledzewicz, H. M. Schättler, *Optimal control for a system modelling tumor anti-angiogenesis* (2006). Citeseer
68. U. Ledzewicz, H. Schättler, A synthesis of optimal controls for a model of tumor growth under angiogenic inhibitors, in *Proceedings of the 44th IEEE Conference on Decision and Control* (2005), pp. 934–939
69. D.A. Drexler, L. Kovács, J. Sápi, I. Harmati, Z. Benyó, Model-based analysis and synthesis of tumor growth under angiogenic inhibition: a case study. IFAC Proc. Vol. **44**(1), 3753–3758 (2011)
70. D.A. Drexler, J. Sápi, L. Kovács, Optimal discrete time control of antiangiogenic tumor therapy. IFAC-PapersOnLine **50**(1), 13504–13509 (2017)
71. J. Sápi, D. A. Drexler, I. Harmati, Z. Sápi, L. Kovács, Linear state-feedback control synthesis of tumor growth control in antiangiogenic therapy, in *10th International Symposium on Applied Machine Intelligence and Informatics (SAMI)* (2012), pp. 143–148
72. D.A. Drexler, J. Sápi, A. Szeles, I. Harmati, A. Kovács, L. Kovács, Flat control of tumor growth with angiogenic inhibition, in *7th IEEE International Symposium on Applied Computational Intelligence and Informatics (SACI)* (2012), pp. 179–183
73. U. Hasirci, T.C. Burg, R.E. Groff, Closed-loop nonlinear smooth robust control of anti-angiogenic tumor therapy, in *2013 American Control Conference* (IEEE, 2013), pp. 2301–2306
74. N. Nath, T. Burg, D. M. Dawson, E. Iyasere, Optimizing antiangiogenic therapy for tumor minimization, in *Proceedings of the 2010 American Control Conference* (IEEE, 2010), pp. 1242–1247
75. A. Szeles, D. Drexler, J. Sápi, I. Harmati, L. Kovács, Model-based angiogenic inhibition of tumor growth using adaptive fuzzy techniques. Period. Polytech. Electr. Eng. **58**, 29 (2014)
76. B. Czakó, L. Kovács, Nonlinear model predictive control using robust fixed point transformation-based phenomena for controlling tumor growth. Machines **6**(4), 49 (2018)
77. P. Yazdjerdi, N. Meskin, M. Al Naemi, A.E. Al Moustafa, L. Kovács, Reinforcement learning-based control of tumor growth under anti-angiogenic therapy. Comput. Methods Prog. Biomed. **173**, 15–26 (2019)
78. R.Ö. Doruk, Angiogenic inhibition therapy, a sliding mode control adventure. Comput. Methods Programs Biomed. **190**, 105358 (2020)
79. J. Overgaard, M.R. Horsman, Modification of hypoxia-induced radioresistance in tumors by the use of oxygen and sensitizers. Semin. Radiat. Oncol. **6**(1), 10–21 (1996)
80. G. Belostotski, H.I. Freedman, A control theory model for cancer treatment by radiotherapy. Int. J. Pure Appl. Math. **25** (2005)
81. H.I. Freedman, G. Belostotski, Perturbed models for cancer treatment by radiotherapy. Differ. Equ. Dyn. Syst. **17**, 115–133 (2009). Apr
82. A. Jalalimanesh, H.S. Haghighi, A. Ahmadi, M. Soltani, Simulation-based optimization of radiotherapy: agent-based modeling and reinforcement learning. Math. Comput. Simul. **133**, 235–248 (2017)
83. E. Fernández Cara, J. Límaco, L. Prouvée, Optimal control of a two-equation model of radiotherapy. Math. Control Rel. Fields **8**(1), 117 (2018)
84. T. Galochkina, A. Bratus, V.M. Pérez García, Optimal radiation fractionation for low-grade gliomas: insights from a mathematical model. Math. Biosci. **267**, 1–9 (2015)
85. P. Paul Gilloteaux, V. Potiron, G. Delpon, S. Supiot, S. Chiavassa, F. Paris, S.V. Costes, Optimizing radiotherapy protocols using computer automata to model tumour cell death as a function of oxygen diffusion processes. Nat. Sci. Rep. **7**, 1–12 (2017)

86. T. Suzuki, N. Bruchovsky, K. Aihara, Piecewise affine systems modelling for optimizing hormone therapy of prostate cancer. Philos. Trans. R. Soc. A: Math. Phys. Eng. Sci. **368**(1930), 5045–5059 (2010)
87. T. Shimada, K. Aihara, A nonlinear model with competition between prostate tumor cells and its application to intermittent androgen suppression therapy of prostate cancer. Math. Biosci. **214**(1), 134–139 (2008)
88. J.J. Cunningham, J.S. Brown, R.A. Gatenby, K. Staňková, Optimal control to develop therapeutic strategies for metastatic castrate resistant prostate cancer. J. Theor. Biol. **459**, 67–78 (2018)
89. H.I. Scher, D.I. Jodrell, J.M. Iversen, T. Curley, W. Tong, M.J. Egorin, A. Forrest, Use of adaptive control with feedback to individualize suramin dosing. Cancer Res. **52**(1), 64–70 (1992)
90. E.K. Kiani, A.V. Kamyad, H. Shirzad, Optimal immunotherapy control of aggressive tumors growth. Intell. Control Autom. **3** (2012)
91. E. Jamili, V. Dua, Modelling and optimal control of non-viral siRNA delivery, in *26th European Symposium on Computer Aided Process Engineering. Computer Aided Chemical Engineering*, vol. 38 (Elsevier, 2016), pp. 673–678
92. E. Jamili, V. Dua, Optimal model-based control of non-viral siRNA delivery. Biotechnol. Bioeng. **115**(7), 1866–1877 (2018)
93. A.K. Arum, D. Handayani, R. Saragih, Robust control design for virotherapy model using successive method, in *Journal of Physics: Conference Series*, vol. 1245 (IOP Publishing, 2019), p. 012054
94. A.K. Arum, R. Saragih, D. Handayani, Bilinear robust control design for virotherapy model, in *2019 19th International Conference on Control, Automation and Systems (ICCAS)* (2019), pp. 82–86
95. D.P. Army, Optimal control of drug therapy and virotherapy via linear parameter varying (LPV) approach. Jurnal Matematika dan Sains **23**(1), 7–10 (2019)
96. G.A. Husseini, F.S. Mjalli, W.G. Pitt, N.M. Abdel Jabbar, Using artificial neural networks and model predictive control to optimize acoustically assisted doxorubicin release from polymeric micelles. Technol. Cancer Res. Treat. **8**(6), 479–488 (2009)
97. L. Mellal, D. Folio, K. Belharet, A. Ferreira, Modeling of optimal targeted therapies using drug-loaded magnetic nanoparticles for liver cancer. IEEE Trans. Nanobiosci. **15**(3), 265–274 (2016)
98. J.J. Crivelli, J. Földes, P.S. Kim, J.R. Wares, A mathematical model for cell cycle-specific cancer virotherapy. J. Biol. Dyn. **6**(sup1), 104–120 (2012)
99. A. Javadi, F. Keighobadi, V. Nekoukar, M. Ebrahimi, Finite-set model predictive control of melanoma cancer treatment using signaling pathway inhibitor of cancer stem cell. IEEE/ACM Trans. Comput. Biol. Bioinf. (2019)
100. H.G. Moussa, G.A. Husseini, S.E. Ahmad, N. Awad, The use of artificial neural networks to control the concentration of a model drug released acoustically. Emerg. Mater. 1–11 (2020)
101. H. G. Moussa, G. A. Husseini, N. Abel Jabbar, S.E. Ahmad, Use of model predictive control and artificial neural networks to optimize the ultrasonic release of a model drug from liposomes. IEEE Trans. NanoBiosci. **16**(3), 149–156 (2017)
102. F.F. Teles, J.M. Lemos, Cancer therapy optimization based on multiple model adaptive control. Biomed. Signal Process. Control **48**, 255–264 (2019)
103. U. Ledzewicz, M. Faraji, H. Schättler, Optimal controls for a mathematical model of tumor-immune interactions under targeted chemotherapy with immune boost. Discret. Contin. Dyn. Syst. Ser. B **4** (2013)
104. K.L. Kiran, S. Lakshminarayanan, Optimization of chemotherapy and immunotherapy: in silico analysis using pharmacokinetic-pharmacodynamic and tumor growth models. J. Process Control **23**(3), 396–403 (2013)
105. S. Zouhri, S. Saadi, I. Elmouki, A. Hamdache, M. Rachik, Mixed immunotherapy and chemotherapy of tumors: optimal control approach. Int. J. Comput. Sci. Issues **10**(4), 81 (2013)

106. A. Ghaffari, M. Nazari, F. Arab, Optimal finite cancer treatment duration by using mixed vaccine therapy and chemotherapy: State dependent Riccati equation control. J. Appl. Math. **2014** (2014)
107. E. Ahmadi, J. Zarei, R. Razavi Far, M. Saif, A dual approach for positive T-S fuzzy controller design and its application to cancer treatment under immunotherapy and chemotherapy. Biomed. Signal Process. Control **58**, 101822 (2020)
108. J. Malinzi, R. Ouifki, A. Eladdadi, D.F.M. Torres, K.A.J. White, Enhancement of chemotherapy using oncolytic virotherapy: mathematical and optimal control analysis. Math. Biosci. Eng. **15**, 1435 (2018)
109. P. Khalili, R. Vatankhah, Derivation of an optimal trajectory and nonlinear adaptive controller design for drug delivery in cancerous tumor chemotherapy. Comput. Biol. Med. **109**, 195–206 (2019)
110. G. Ceresoli, F. V. De, M. Sauta, M. Bonomi, P. Zucali, Role of chemotherapy in combination with hormonal therapy in first-line treatment of metastatic hormone-sensitive prostate cancer. Q. J. Nucl. Med. Mol. Imaging: Off. Publ. Italian Assoc. Nucl. Med. (AIMN)[and] the Int. Assoc. Radiopharmacol. (IAR),[and] Sect. Soc. of.. **59**(4), 374–380 (2015)
111. N.S. Gandhi, R.K. Tekade, M.B. Chougule, Nanocarrier mediated delivery of siRNA/miRNA in combination with chemotherapeutic agents for cancer therapy: Current progress and advances. J. Control. Release **194**, 238–256 (2014)
112. G.A. Yanik, J.E. Levine, K.K. Matthay, J.C. Sisson, B.L. Shulkin, B. Shapiro, D. Hubers, S. Spalding, T. Braun, J.L. Ferrara et al., Pilot study of iodine-131-metaiodobenzylguanidine in combination with myeloablative chemotherapy and autologous stem-cell support for the treatment of neuroblastoma. J. Clin. Oncol. **20**(8), 2142–2149 (2002)
113. A. Ergun, K. Camphausen, L.M. Wein, Optimal scheduling of radiotherapy and angiogenic inhibitors. Bull. Math. Biol. **65**(3), 407–424 (2003)
114. J.F. Fowler, The linear-quadratic formula and progress in fractionated radiotherapy. Br. J. Radiol. **62**(740), 679–694 (1989)
115. V.A. Kuznetsov, I.A. Makalkin, M.A. Taylor, A.S. Perelson, Nonlinear dynamics of immunogenic tumors: parameter estimation and global bifurcation analysis. Bull. Math. Biol. **56**(2), 295–321 (1994)
116. U. Ledzewicz, M. Naghnaeian, H. Schättler, Optimal response to chemotherapy for a mathematical model of tumor-immune dynamics. J. Math. Biol. **64**, 557–577 (2012). Feb
117. L.G. de Pillis, W. Gu, A.E. Radunskaya, Mixed immunotherapy and chemotherapy of tumors: modeling, applications and biological interpretations. J. Theor. Biol. **238**(4), 841–862 (2006)
118. H. Freedman, S. Pinho, Stability criteria for the cure state in a cancer model with radiation treatment. Nonlinear Anal.: Real World Appl. **10**(5), 2709–2715 (2009)
119. Y. Su, C. Jia, Y. Chen, Optimal control model of tumor treatment with oncolytic virus and MEK inhibitor. BioMed. Res. Int. **2016** (2016)
120. S.T.R. Pinho, D.S. Rodrigues, P.F.A. Mancera, A mathematical model of chemotherapy response to tumour growth. Canad. Appl. Math. Q. **19**, 369–384 (2011)
121. Ž. Bajzer, T. Carr, K. Josić, S.J. Russell, D. Dingli, Modeling of cancer virotherapy with recombinant measles viruses. J. Theor. Biol. **252**(1), 109–122 (2008)
122. D. Le, J.D. Miller, V.V. Ganusov, Mathematical modeling provides kinetic details of the human immune response to vaccination. Front. Cell. Infect. Microbiol. **4**, 177 (2015)
123. S. Pinho, F. Bacelar, R. Andrade, H. Freedman, A mathematical model for the effect of anti-angiogenic therapy in the treatment of cancer tumours by chemotherapy. Nonlinear Anal.: Real World Appl. **14**(1), 815–828 (2013)
124. S. Sharma, G. Samanta, Analysis of the dynamics of a tumor-immune system with chemotherapy and immunotherapy and quadratic optimal control. Differ. Equ. Dyn. Syst. **24**(2), 149–171 (2016)
125. F.A. Rihan, S. Lakshmanan, H. Maurer, Optimal control of tumour-immune model with time-delay and immuno-chemotherapy. Appl. Math. Comput. **353**, 147–165 (2019)
126. J. Kang, S. Demaria, S. Formenti, Current clinical trials testing the combination of immunotherapy with radiotherapy. J. Immunother. Cancer **4**(1), 51 (2016)

127. A. Nicolini, A. Carpi, P. Ferrari, P. Mario Biava, G. Rossi, Immunotherapy and hormone-therapy in metastatic breast cancer: a review and an update. Cur. Drug Targets **17**(10), 1127–1139 (2016)
128. U. Ledzewicz, H. Schättler, Multi-input optimal control problems for combined tumor anti-angiogenic and radiotherapy treatments. J. Optim. Theory Appl. **153**(1), 195–224 (2012)
129. M. Bazan Peregrino, R. Sainson, R. Carlisle, C. Thoma, R. Waters, C. Arvanitis, A. Harris, R. Hernandez-Alcoceba, L. Seymour, Combining virotherapy and angiotherapy for the treatment of breast cancer. Cancer Gene Ther. **20**(8), 461–468 (2013)
130. Z. Melegh, S. Oltean, Targeting angiogenesis in prostate cancer. Int. J. Mol. Sci. **20**(11), 2676 (2019)
131. K.H. Shain, D. Hart, A. Siqueira Silva, R. Alugubelli, G. De Avila, P.R. Sudalagunta, A. Tungesvik, A. Kulkarni, C. Blancuicett, H. Dai, et al., Reinforcement learning to optimize the treatment of multiple myeloma. Blood **134** (2019)
132. E. Piretto, M. Delitala, M. Ferraro, How combination therapies shape drug resistance in heterogeneous tumoral populations. Lett. Biomath. **5**(sup1), S160–S177 (2018)
133. K.H. Young, J.R. Baird, T. Savage, B. Cottam, D. Friedman, S. Bambina, D.J. Messenheimer, B. Fox, P. Newell, K.S. Bahjat et al., Optimizing timing of immunotherapy improves control of tumors by hypofractionated radiation therapy. PLoS ONE **11**(6), e0157164 (2016)
134. S.C. Formenti, S. Demaria, Combining radiotherapy and cancer immunotherapy: a paradigm shift. J. Natl Cancer Inst. **105**(4), 256–265 (2013)
135. S. Demaria, E.B. Golden, S.C. Formenti, Role of local radiation therapy in cancer immunotherapy. JAMA Oncol. **1**(9), 1325–1332 (2015)
136. C.U. Jones, D. Hunt, D.G. McGowan, M.B. Amin, M.P. Chetner, D.W. Bruner, M.H. Leibenhaut, S.M. Husain, M. Rotman, L. Souhami et al., Radiotherapy and short-term androgen deprivation for localized prostate cancer. N. Engl. J. Med. **365**(2), 107–118 (2011)
137. J.M. Crook, C.J. O'Callaghan, G. Duncan, D.P. Dearnaley, C.S. Higano, E.M. Horwitz, E. Frymire, S. Malone, J. Chin, A. Nabid et al., Intermittent androgen suppression for rising PSA level after radiotherapy. N. Engl. J. Med. **367**(10), 895–903 (2012)
138. J.L. Kalina, D.S. Neilson, A.P. Comber, J.M. Rauw, A.S. Alexander, J. Vergidis, J.J. Lum, Immune modulation by androgen deprivation and radiation therapy: implications for prostate cancer immunotherapy. Cancers **9**(2), 13 (2017)
139. E.M. Rutter, Y. Kuang, Global dynamics of a model of joint hormone treatment with dendritic cell vaccine for prostate cancer. Discret. Contin. Dyn. Syst.-B **22**(3), 1001 (2017)
140. J.B. Aragon Ching, K.M. Williams, J.L. Gulley, et al., Impact of androgen-deprivation therapy on the immune system: implications for combination therapy of prostate cancer. Front. Biosci. **12**(4957), 71 (2007)
141. X. Lu, J.W. Horner, E. Paul, X. Shang, P. Troncoso, P. Deng, S. Jiang, Q. Chang, D.J. Spring, P. Sharma et al., Effective combinatorial immunotherapy for castration-resistant prostate cancer. Nature **543**(7647), 728–732 (2017)
142. M. Burotto, N. Singh, C.R. Heery, J.L. Gulley, R.A. Madan, Exploiting synergy: immune-based combinations in the treatment of prostate cancer. Front. Oncol. **4**, 351 (2014)
143. J. Nam, S. Son, K.S. Park, W. Zou, L.D. Shea, J.J. Moon, Cancer nanomedicine for combination cancer immunotherapy. Nat. Rev. Mater. **4**(6), 398–414 (2019)
144. N.L. Syn, L. Wang, E.K.H. Chow, C.T. Lim, B.C. Goh, Exosomes in cancer nanomedicine and immunotherapy: prospects and challenges. Trends Biotechnol. **35**(7), 665–676 (2017)
145. K. Li, W. Zhan, Y. Chen, R.K. Jha, X. Chen, Docetaxel, doxorubicin codelivery by nanocarriers for synergistic treatment of prostate cancer. Front. Pharmacol. **10** (2019)
146. A. Bhargava, D.K. Mishra, S.K. Jain, R.K. Srivastava, N.K. Lohiya, P.K. Mishra, Comparative assessment of lipid based nano-carrier systems for dendritic cell based targeting of tumor re-initiating cells in gynecological cancers. Mol. Immunol. **79**, 98–112 (2016)

147. R. Padmanabhan, H.S. Kheraldine, N. Meskin, S. Vranic, A.E. Al Moustafa, Crosstalk between HER2 and PD-1/PD-L1 in breast cancer: from clinical applications to mathematical models. Cancers **12**(3), 636 (2020)
148. A. Ribas, R. Dummer, I. Puzanov, A. VanderWalde, R.H. Andtbacka, O. Michielin, A.J. Olszanski, J. Malvehy, J. Cebon, E. Fernandez et al., Oncolytic virotherapy promotes intratumoral T cell infiltration and improves anti-PD-1 immunotherapy. Cell **170**(6), 1109–1119 (2017)

Chapter 11
Conclusions

Our understanding of cancer has improved remarkably over the last few decades. In parallel, the emergence of many therapeutic measures against cancer has led to an impressive improvement in the disease-free and overall survival of patients. For instance, the advent of immuno-modulatory drugs including checkpoint inhibitors has opened up novel treatment strategies to manage rare breast cancer subtype such as TNBC with very poor prognosis. Similarly, stage IV melanoma, another cancer which has been considered as a terminal disease, is now a much more manageable disease [1, 2]. All these hopeful results emphasize the capabilities of the empirical and theoretical studies conducted in the area of cancer dynamics in making a difference in the management of this disease.

However, millions of new cases of cancer are reported every year [3, 4]. Even though reduced, still a significantly high percentage of mortality and functional impairments are reported in cancer patients [2, 5–8]. Moreover, our understanding of the biological and theoretical aspects of the initiation and progression of this highly complex disease is quite incomplete which hinders the development of appropriate treatment strategies. Even though many novel remedies are put forward, reports on side effects are also mounting with the ongoing use of many of these novel and promising treatment strategies [9]. The rising cost of treatment is another important concern associated with the management of cancer that is intimidating the existence of mankind [10, 11]. Consequently, more investigations are imperative to improve the overall therapeutic efficacy and patient outcome along with reducing the treatment costs. Following are some of the ways identified to mitigate the cost and improve patient outcome [2, 9–13]:

- Optimizing treatment schedules and drug usage as an optimal usage of drugs not only reduces the treatment cost and associated side effects, but it also reduces the chance of drug resistance development.
- Identifying patient-specific and cancer-type-specific treatment protocols so as to reduce unsuccessful treatment episodes and related side effects.
- Streamlining the high-cost associated with clinical trials and pharmaceutical research.

R. Padmanabhan et al., *Mathematical Models of Cancer and Different Therapies*, Series in BioEngineering, https://doi.org/10.1007/978-981-15-8640-8_11

- Reducing the overall time and resource utilization involved in the process of taking a novel drug from bench to bedside so as to curtail the overall treatment cost involved.

Mathematical model-based analysis has been contributing heavily to optimize the cost and time associated with drug screening, drug usage, and treatment scheduling [12]. Utilizing technical advancements including mathematical and computational tools to analyze clinical situations are more desirable due to the cost and safety advantages [12–14]. The overall therapeutic efficacy and the patient outcome can be improved significantly by using a judicious combination of empirical and theoretical approaches [10, 12, 13].

More collaborative efforts are required to translate the in-depth understanding and experience of cancer biologists and oncologists into reliable mathematical models. Such models can be used to further decipher the complex multi-path interactions in the tumor micro-environment that is favoring the survival of cancers in humans. This book is an attempt to provide a unified framework for the mathematical modeling of cancer therapies so as to meet the future expectations of the clinical community from the area of integrative mathematical oncology. In this book, a general overview of the cancer dynamics, types of therapies used for the cancer management, mathematical models pertaining to each therapy modes, and a survey on various control strategies in literature are discussed. Clinically observed phenomena pertaining to each therapeutic approach that are yet to be explained through mathematical models are also highlighted at the end of each chapter. Some of the general research gaps in the area of mathematical modeling of cancer dynamics are discussed henceforth.

Many recent reviews in this area point out the need to improve the mathematical models to answer critical questions regarding tumor relapse, development of drug resistance, and drug toxicity [15–17]. The capability of cancer cells to proliferate and survive in large numbers even in the presence of many disturbance and adverse effects are sometimes called *cancer robustness* [14, 18]. The cell heterogeneity of the tumor population is considered as one of the factors that contribute to the robustness of cancer biology. Heterogeneity in the cell population is the reason why the tumor can maintain a stable function despite various perturbations that they encounter in the form of immune attack, therapy, etc. It is well known that there can be several genetically different (heterogeneous) sub-populations in a tumor micro-environment. These sub-populations exhibit different growth rates, de-differentiation, immunogenicity, metastatic potential, and biochemistry [16, 19]. Investigating more about heterogeneity in tumor cells is considered a promising approach to explain many clinical observed phenomena such as cancer recurrence, tumor dormancy, and drug resistance. For instance, due to the presence of different types of cancer cells in a single neoplasm, it is more likely that when one cell type is annihilated by a certain chemotherapeutic drug, the other type of cancer cells which are insensitive to that drug will make use of the excess resource availability due to less competition and tend to proliferate more [17, 20]. Therefore, it may not be just the change of cells to a resistant type that causes tumor relapse and instead, the relapse of the disease may be also due to the survival of the fittest among the heterogeneous clones [21]. More investigation is required in this regard.

It is known that cancer cells use several mechanisms including metabolic reprogramming and switching of cellular signaling pathways that mediate cell growth and division to retain the characteristics of the disease and escape from the adversities caused by the anti-cancer agents [13, 22]. Even though enormous empirical and theoretical works have been done in this area, most models discuss cell transition dynamics (drug-sensitive to drug resistance variant) and ignore the influence of the immune system and vascular supply [17, 20]. Mathematical models that depict drug resistance can be used to evaluate the long-term efficacy of novel therapeutic agents, their combinations, or a new hypothetical treatment strategy [12]. In [23], the need to develop mechanistic models that depict drug penetrability and resistance and incorporate the propagation of drug resistance to predict treatment efficacy is pointed out. Such models can be used in treatment scheduling to figure out maximum allowable treatment free period between end of the current treatment and prior to the recurrence [23].

As mentioned in Chaps. 1 and 2, the survival rate of the patients heavily depends on the type and stage of cancer when diagnosed, the age of the patient, and on the type of the treatment strategies adopted [24]. For many types of cancers, there is ample time between the tumor initiation to lethal period. This points out to the scope for improvement of treatment outcome by using better diagnostics tools for cancer. But unfortunately, very less is known about the initiation of a tumor which restricts the diagnosis and treatment at an early stage [25, 26]. Mathematical models can be used to analyze the likelihood of tumor initiation within a clinically observable time. One such example is presented in [26] where a simplified mathematical model that accounts for the involvement of oncogenes and tumor suppressor genes and related mutations in initiating cancer is discussed. Similarly, the association of inherent population shrinkage at low densities (Allee effect) and feedback regulations in cancer stem cells should be investigated more to answer critical questions regarding tumor initiation, tumor persistence, spontaneous tumor remission, tumor invasion and metastasis, phenotypic plasticity, and feedback regulation in stem cells. In general, a model is used to investigate, what fraction of undamaged cancer cells left after a particular treatment can likely cause cancer relapse [27–29]. Even though several cell-signaling pathways and molecular networks that can be potential therapeutic targets for cancer cure are identified recently, mathematical modeling of such cell-signaling pathways and molecular networks deserves further exploration [30, 31].

Combination therapy is emerging as a promising mainstay treatment option to curtail drug resistance development and disease relapse. Several clinical trials and animal model-based experiments suggest that the use of anti-angiogenic agents along with chemotherapy, radiotherapy, immunotherapy, and/or targeted therapy can improve the overall survival of patients with advanced cancers [32]. Similarly, immunotherapy tends to be a common factor in many combination therapeutic approaches. This is mainly due to its advantages in invoking immunogenicity, enhancing the immune response, improving target specificity, and mediating abscopal effect [33–36]. Moreover, immunotherapy can modulate the adaptive immune system to leave memory

T cells for long-term immune effects. However, most of the combination therapy models rely on drastic simplification assumptions. Hence, existing mathematical models that analyze combination therapies should be extended to incorporate relevant dynamics. For instance, the model (9.2)–(9.7) discussed in Chap. 9, Sect. 9.1 accounts for the effect of immunotherapy (IL-2 injection and TIL vaccine) and chemotherapy. This model can be improved by adding important dynamics related to immunotherapy such as the dynamics of cytokines IL-2 and TGF-β which have a key role in the overall immune response [37]. Recall that a model ((4.13)–(4.21)) that discusses the dynamics of IL-2 cytokine, T helper cells, and T regulator cells under immunotherapy alone is discussed in Chap. 4.

In the case of combination treatments, the order of treatments can have a significant effect on the efficacy of overall treatment. For instance, in [38], based on an experimental study, it is shown that using anti-angiogenic agents for vascular normalization prior to the use of cytotoxic chemotherapeutic drugs can improve the survival rate of NSCLC patients. The anti-VEGF agent (e.g. bevacizumab) induces vascular normalization and thus heals the leaky tumor vasculature and improves drug delivery [39]. Hence, an optimal time gap should be provided between the use of anti-angiogenic and chemotherapeutic agents. A mathematical model is used in [40] to find an optimal delay between the use of an anti-angiogenic agent and cytotoxic agent for efficient treatment [40, 41]. Conducting a similar analysis in case of scheduling various combination therapies is desirable. Even though combination therapies that involve radiotherapy, hormone therapy, stem cell therapy, gene therapy, and oncolytic virotherapy are reported in clinical trials, corresponding mathematical models are yet to be devised.

In the case of radiotherapy, most of the models discussed mainly account for the radiation-induced DNA damage and dose-dependent cell-kill at the tumor site. Evidence suggests that the efficacy of radiotherapy is positively correlated with the supply of oxygen and negatively correlated with the immune deficiency [42, 43]. Hence, while combining radiotherapy, with anti-angiogenic therapy and/or immunotherapy, an optimal treatment scheduling is essential to reap maximum benefits.

Similarly, more investigations are required to assess an optimal treatment scheduling of stem cell transplantation along with immunotherapeutic agents that include immuno-modulatory drugs, proteasome inhibitors, and mAbs [44]. In [44], the importance of induction treatment (chemotherapy) to reduce the tumor burden so as to increase the probability of achieving successful stem cell transplantation is highlighted. A mathematical model can be used to assess the optimal chemotherapeutic drug dose and the optimal time to wait until the tumor burden reduces below a threshold value so as to start the stem cell transplantation. Such an analysis facilitates successful engraftment with minimum toxicity on healthy hematopoietic cells [44]. Similarly, several drugs are used for the mobilization of blood cells from the BM to the PB [45–47]. The combinations of drugs (e.g. daratumumab, carfilzomib, lenalidomide, dexamethasone) that are promising for the treatment can also be assessed by using mathematical models that depict pharmacokinetics and pharmacodynamics specifically for multiple myeloma.

The rate of recruitment of hematopoietic cells to the PB considerably influences the number of harvested cell numbers for transplantation. In [45], a model of blood cell collection for transplantation using a continuous flow cell-separator based on the mobility of the cells from BM into PB is presented. A two-compartment PK-PD model for the mobilization of CD34+ cells by using the immunostimulant AMD3100 (plerixafor) based on 29 human subjects is presented in [46]. Such models can be combined with the stem cell dynamics model such as that discussed Sects. 8.4.3 and 8.4.2 in Chap. 8 to assess whether minimum threshold level of mobilization required for successful transplantation is achieved or not [44]. Such analysis using mathematical models can help to reduce repeated apheresis sessions [48, 49]. Stem cell models for specific allogeneic and autologous transplantation can be also used to predict treatment success, cell rejection probability, etc.

Targeted treatment strategies which include gene, nanocarrier, and mAb-based therapy can particularly annihilate cancer cells and cause comparatively less systemic toxicity. As mentioned in Chap. 8, there is no complete ODE-based mathematical model that represents the overall cancer dynamics under nanocarrier based therapy. Being an emerging area in cancer therapy, there is much more to be known regarding the drug and carrier-specific pharmacokinetics, pharmacodynamics, and cell dynamics under nanotherapy [50]. Gene therapy, nanocarrier mediated therapy, and stem cell-based therapy are novel areas of cancer research that need elaborate theoretical and experimental support to expand to their full potential [51–54]. In general, mathematical models that represent the overall dynamics under a therapy (or a combination) can provide significant insight regarding the possible therapeutic effects and post-treatment toxicities. Hence, more cancer-specific and therapy-specific mathematical models should be devised [55].

Finally, based on the general framework presented in Chap. 1, any new therapeutic strategy can be translated to a mathematical model by using the following steps: (1) list down the cell populations that are most relevant to the therapy under consideration, (2) identify the important biological mechanisms that affect the progression and regression of each cell population involved, (3) choose appropriate growth or decay pattern based on the intuitive idea of the biological mechanisms involved, (4) link the pharmacokinetics and pharmacodynamics of the drug(s) to the cell population dynamics, (5) model the dynamics related to drug sensitivity, toxicity, and resistance if any, (6) estimate parameters of the model using experimental results conducted or that are already in the literature, and (7) validate the model as and when more clinical and experimental data is available.

References

1. M. Smith, H. Smith, K. Joshi, M. Gore, D. Strauss, A. Hayes, J. Larkin, The impact of effective systemic therapies on surgery for stage IV melanoma. Eur. J. Cancer **103**, 24–31 (2018)
2. Y. Tokumaru, D. Joyce, K. Takabe, Current status and limitations of immunotherapy for breast cancer. Surgery **167**(3), 628–630 (2020)
3. Worldwide cancer statistics, Technical report, Cancer research, UK, https://www.cancerresearchuk.org/health-professional/cancer-statistics/worldwide-cancer
4. Cancer survival rate statistics by type of cancer. www.cancer.gov/statistics. Statistics from the period between 2003 and 2009, Accessed: 2019-08-31
5. Cancer statistics, Technical report, National Cancer Institute, https://www.cancer.gov/about-cancer/understanding/statistics
6. K.D. Miller, R.L. Siegel, C.C. Lin, A.B. Mariotto, J.L. Kramer, J.H. Rowland, K.D. Stein, R. Alteri, A. Jemal, Cancer treatment and survivorship statistics, 2016, CA: Cancer J. Clin. **66**(4), 271–289, (2016)
7. F.H. Wen, J.S. Chen, W.-C. Chou, W.C. Chang, W.C. Shen, C.H. Hsieh, S.T. Tang, Family caregivers' subjective caregiving burden, quality of life, and depressive symptoms are associated with terminally ill cancer patients' distinct patterns of conjoint symptom distress and functional impairment in their last six months of life. J. Pain Symp. Manage. **57**(1), 64–72 (2019)
8. W. Nadruz, E. West, M. Sengeløv, G.L. Grove, M. Santos, J.D. Groarke, D.E. Forman, B. Claggett, H. Skali, A. Nohria et al., Cardiovascular phenotype and prognosis of patients with heart failure induced by cancer therapy. Heart **105**(1), 34–41 (2019)
9. L. Wang, Q. Ma, R. Yao, J. Liu, Current status and development of anti-PD-1-PD-L1 immunotherapy for lung cancer. Int. Immunopharmacol. **79**, 106088 (2020)
10. A.E. Glode, M.B. May, Rising cost of cancer pharmaceuticals: Cost issues and interventions to control costs. Pharmacother.: J. Hum. Pharmacol. Drug Ther. **37**(1) (2017), pp. 85–93
11. K. Jackson, M.C. Nahata, Rising cost of anticancer medications in the United States. Ann. Pharmacother. **51**(8), 706–710 (2017)
12. R. Padmanabhan, H.S. Kheraldine, N. Meskin, S. Vranic, A.E. Al Moustafa, Crosstalk between HER2 and PD-1/PD-L1 in breast cancer: from clinical applications to mathematical models. Cancers **12**(3), 636 (2020)
13. A.R. Anderson, V. Quaranta, Integrative mathematical oncology. Nat. Rev. Cancer **8**(3), 227–234 (2008)
14. R.J. Preen, L. Bull, A. Adamatzky, Towards an evolvable cancer treatment simulator. Biosystems **182**, 1–7 (2019)
15. A. Yin, D.J.A. Moes, J.G. van Hasselt, J.J. Swen, H.-J. Guchelaar, A review of mathematical models for tumor dynamics and treatment resistance evolution of solid tumors. CPT: Pharmacomet. Syst. Pharmacol. **8**(10), 720–737 (2019)
16. G.P. Karev, A.S. Novozhilov, E.V. Koonin, Mathematical modeling of tumor therapy with oncolytic viruses: effects of parametric heterogeneity on cell dynamics. Biol. Direct **1**, 30 (2006)
17. J.M. Greene, J.L. Gevertz, E.D. Sontag, Mathematical approach to differentiate spontaneous and induced evolution to drug resistance during cancer treatment. JCO Clin. Cancer Inf. **3**, 1–20 (2019)
18. T. Tian, S. Olson, J.M. Whitacre, A. Harding, The origins of cancer robustness and evolvability. Integr. Biol. **3**(1), 17–30 (2011)
19. I. González García, R.V. Solé, J. Costa, Metapopulation dynamics and spatial heterogeneity in cancer. Proc. Natl. Acad. Sci. **99**(20), 13085–13089 (2002)
20. J.M. Greene, C. Sanchez-Tapia, E.D. Sontag, Mathematical details on a cancer resistance model. *BioRxiv*, p. 475533 (2018)
21. E. Piretto, M. Delitala, M. Ferraro, How combination therapies shape drug resistance in heterogeneous tumoral populations. Lett. Biomath. **5**(sup1), S160–S177 (2018)

22. M.A. Alaoui Jamali, J. Paterson, A.E. Al Moustafa, L. Yen, The role of ErbB-2 tyrosine kinase receptor in cellular intrinsic chemoresistance: mechanisms and implications. Biochem. Cell Biol. **75**(4), 315–325 (1997)
23. D.A. Botesteanu, S. Lipkowitz, J.M. Lee, D. Levy, Mathematical models of breast and ovarian cancers. Wiley Interdiscip. Rev.: Syst. Biol. Med. **8**(4), 337–362 (2016)
24. J. Rosenberg, Y.L. Chia, S. Plevritis, The effect of age, race, tumor size, tumor grade, and disease stage on invasive ductal breast cancer survival in the US SEER database. Breast Cancer Res. Treat. **89**(1), 47–54 (2005)
25. Z. Neufeld, W. von Witt, D. Lakatos, J. Wang, B. Hegedus, A. Czirok, The role of Allee effect in modelling post resection recurrence of glioblastoma. PLoS Comput. Biol. **13**(11), e1005818 (2017)
26. H. Enderling, M.A. Chaplain, A.R. Anderson, J.S. Vaidya, A mathematical model of breast cancer development, local treatment and recurrence. J. Theor. Biol. **246**(2), 245–259 (2007)
27. D. Kirschner, J.C. Panetta, Modeling immunotherapy of the tumor-immune interaction. J. Math. Biol. **37**(3), 235–252 (1998)
28. V.A. Kuznetsov, I.A. Makalkin, M.A. Taylor, A.S. Perelson, Nonlinear dynamics of immunogenic tumors: parameter estimation and global bifurcation analysis. Bull. Math. Biol. **56**(2), 295–321 (1994)
29. R. De Boer, P. Hogeweg, H. Dullens, R.A. De Weger, W. Den Otter, Macrophage T lymphocyte interactions in the anti-tumor immune response: a mathematical model. J. Immunol. **134**(4), 2748–2758 (1985)
30. B. Ji, J. Chen, C. Zhen, Q. Yang, N. Yu, Mathematical modelling of the role of Endo180 network in the development of metastatic bone disease in prostate cancer. Comput. Biol. Med. **117**, 103619 (2020)
31. A. Konstorum, A.T. Vella, A.J. Adler, R.C. Laubenbacher, A mathematical model of combined CD8 T cell costimulation by 4–1BB (CD137) and OX40 (CD134) receptors. Sci. Rep. **9**(1), 1–12 (2019)
32. H. Qiang, Q. Chang, J. Xu, J. Qian, Y. Zhang, Y. Lei, B. Han, T. Chu, New advances in antiangiogenic combination therapeutic strategies for advanced non-small cell lung cancer J. Cancer Res. Clin. Oncol. 1–15 (2020)
33. V. Velcheti, K. Schalper, Basic overview of current immunotherapy approaches in cancer. Am. Soc. Clin. Oncol. Edu. Book **36**, 298–308 (2016)
34. J. Kang, S. Demaria, S. Formenti, Current clinical trials testing the combination of immunotherapy with radiotherapy. J. Immunother. Cancer **4**(1), 51 (2016)
35. A. Nicolini, A. Carpi, P. Ferrari, P. Mario Biava, G. Rossi, Immunotherapy and hormone-therapy in metastatic breast cancer: a review and an update. Curr. Drug Targets **17**(10), 1127–1139 (2016)
36. N. Suek, L.F. Campesato, T. Merghoub, D.N. Khalil, Targeted APC activation in cancer immunotherapy to enhance the abscopal effect. Front. Immunol. **10**, 604 (2019)
37. M. Qomlaqi, F. Bahrami, M. Ajami, J. Hajati, An extended mathematical model of tumor growth and its interaction with the immune system, to be used for developing an optimized immunotherapy treatment protocol. Math. Biosci. **292**, 1–9 (2017)
38. R.S. Heist, D.G. Duda, D.V. Sahani, M. Ancukiewicz, P. Fidias, L.V. Sequist, J.S. Temel, A.T. Shaw, N.A. Pennell, J.W. Neal et al., Improved tumor vascularization after anti-VEGF therapy with carboplatin and nab-paclitaxel associates with survival in lung cancer. Proc. Natl. Acad. Sci. **112**(5), 1547–1552 (2015)
39. R.K. Jain, Normalizing tumor vasculature with anti-angiogenic therapy: a new paradigm for combination therapy. Nat. Med. **7**(9), 987–989 (2001)
40. S. Mollard, J. Ciccolini, D.-C. Imbs, R. El Cheikh, D. Barbolosi, S. Benzekry, Model driven optimization of antiangiogenics + cytotoxics combination: application to breast cancer mice treated with bevacizumab + paclitaxel doublet leads to reduced tumor growth and fewer metastasis. Oncotarget **8**(14), 23087 (2017)
41. S. Benzekry, C. Lamont, A. Beheshti, A. Tracz, J. Ebos, L. Hlatky, P. Hahnfeldt, Classical mathematical models for description and prediction of experimental tumor growth. PLoS Comput. Biol. **10**(8), e1003800 (2014)

42. C. Grassberger, S.G. Ellsworth, M.Q. Wilks, F.K. Keane, J.S. Loeffler, Assessing the interactions between radiotherapy and antitumour immunity. Nat. Rev. Clin. Oncol. 1–17 (2019)
43. R.S.A. Goedegebuure, L.K. de Klerk, A.J. Bass, S. Derks, V.L.J.L. Thijssen, Combining radiotherapy with anti-angiogenic therapy and immunotherapy: a therapeutic triad for cancer? Front. Immunol. **9**, 3107 (2019)
44. R. Al Hamed, A.H. Bazarbachi, F. Malard, J.L. Harousseau, M. Mohty, Current status of autologous stem cell transplantation for multiple myeloma. Blood Cancer J. **9**(4), 1–10 (2019)
45. J. Mayer, Z. Pospíšil, Z. Kořístek, Mathematical model of peripheral blood stem cell harvest kinetics. Bone Marrow Transp. **32**(8), 749–757 (2003)
46. N. Lack, B. Green, D. Dale, G. Calandra, H. Lee, R. MacFarland, K. Badel, W. Liles, G. Bridger, A pharmacokinetic-pharmacodynamic model for the mobilization of CD34+ hematopoietic progenitor cells by AMD3100. Clini. Pharmacol. Therapeutics **77**(5), 427–436 (2005)
47. F. Jost, J. Zierk, T.T. Le, T. Raupach, M. Rauh, M. Suttorp, M. Stanulla, M. Metzler, S. Sager, Model-based simulation of maintenance therapy of childhood acute lymphoblastic leukemia. Front. Physiol. **11**, 217 (2020)
48. A. Verlinden, A. Van de Velde, G.A. Verpooten, K. Janssen van Doorn, Determining factors predictive of CD34+ cell collection efficiency in an effort to avoid extended and repeated apheresis sessions. J. Clin. Apheresis **28**(6), 404–410 (2013)
49. J. Chen, C. Goss, S.T. Avecilla, H. Hong, E. Walsh, D. Wuest, P. Maslak, M.S. Pessin, Evaluation of peripheral blood mononuclear cell collection by leukapheresis. Transfusion **59**(5), 1765–1772 (2019)
50. S. Rawal, M.M. Patel, Threatening cancer with nanoparticle aided combination oncotherapy. J. Control. Release **301**, 76–109 (2019)
51. J. Arciero, T. Jackson, D. Kirschner, A mathematical model of tumor-immune evasion and siRNA treatment. Discret. Contin. Dyn. Syst. - B **4**, 39 (2004)
52. H.M. Horton, D. Anderson, P. Hernandez, K.M. Barnhart, J.A. Norman, S.E. Parker, A gene therapy for cancer using intramuscular injection of plasmid DNA encoding interferon α. Proc. Natl. Acad. Sci. **96**(4), 1553–1558 (1999)
53. H. Yoshizawa, Y. Morishita, M. Watanabe, K. Ishibashi, S. Muto, E. Kusano, D. Nagata, TGF-β 1-siRNA delivery with nanoparticles inhibits peritoneal fibrosis. Gene Ther. **22**(4), 333–340 (2015)
54. F.O. Aval, S.A. Amiri, A. Azadmehr, M. Oladnabi, P. Saadat, H. Ebrahimi, B. Baradaran, B. Mansoori, F. Pourabdolhossein, P. Torabian et al., Gene silencing of TGFβRII can inhibit glioblastoma cell growth. Asian Pac. J. Cancer Prev. **19**(9), 2681 (2018)
55. J.G. da Silva, R.M. de Morais, I.C.R. da Silva, P.F. Arruda Mancera, Mathematical models applied to thyroid cancer. Biophys. Rev. **11**, 183–189 (2019)

The manufacturer's authorised representative in the EU is Springer Nature Customer Service Centre GmbH, Europaplatz 3, 69115 Heidelberg, Germany. If you have any concerns regarding our products, please contact ProductSafety@springernature.com

Printed and bound by CPI Group (UK) Ltd, Croydon, CR0 4YY
24/07/2026
02175960-0001